LONGEVITY NOW

Paradise

Other books by David Wolfe

The Sunfood Diet Success System
Superfoods: The Food and Medicine of the Future
Eating for Beauty
Naked Chocolate
Amazing Grace
Chaga: King of the Medicinal Mushrooms

LONGEVITY NOW

A Comprehensive Approach to Healthy Hormones, Detoxification, Super Immunity, Reversing Calcification, and Total Rejuvenation

Written and created by
David "Avocado" Wolfe

Compiled and edited by David "Avocado" Wolfe and R. A. Gauthier

North Atlantic Books
Berkeley, California

Published by North Atlantic Books
P.O. Box 12327
Berkeley, California 94712

Cover photos: main image © Triff/Shutterstock.com, Inset of author © Michael Roud
Cover and book design by Brad Greene

Printed in the United States of America

MEDICAL DISCLAIMER: The following information is intended for general information purposes only. Individuals should always see their health care provider before administering any suggestions made in this book. Any application of the material set forth in the following pages is at the reader's discretion and is his or her sole responsibility.

Longevity Now: A Comprehensive Approach to Healthy Hormones, Detoxification, Super Immunity, Reversing Calcification, and Total Rejuvenation is sponsored by the Society for the Study of Native Arts and Sciences, a nonprofit educational corporation whose goals are to develop an educational and cross-cultural perspective linking various scientific, social, and artistic fields; to nurture a holistic view of arts, sciences, humanities, and healing; and to publish and distribute literature on the relationship of mind, body, and nature.

North Atlantic Books' publications are available through most bookstores. For further information, visit our website at www.northatlanticbooks.com or call 800-733-3000.

Library of Congress Cataloging-in-Publication Data

Wolfe, David.
    Longevity now : a comprehensive approach to healthy hormones, detoxification, super immunity, reversing calcification, and total rejuvenation / written and created by David Wolfe ; compiled and edited by David Wolfe and R. A. Gauthier.
        pages cm
    Summary: "Lose weight, boost your immunity, cleanse your blood and organs, and live longer and happier with this comprehensive five-part approach created by leading nutrition and raw food authority David Wolfe. In *Longevity Now,* Wolfe exposes the number-one cause of all degenerative illness and aging: calcification. Caused by an excess of calcium and the presence of nanobacteria, calcification can be found in some degree in virtually every adult and even some children. It leads to a plethora of illnesses and manifests as achy joints, hardened arteries, cellulite, cysts, kidney stones, gallstones, dental plaque, cataracts, and bone spurs, among many other health problems. By breaking down calcification and removing parasites, heavy metals, and other 'unwanted guests' from your system, you can reverse the aging process and eliminate the prospect of degenerative disease from your future" —Provided by publisher.
    ISBN 978-1-58394-614-5 (hardback)
    1. Longevity. 2. Health behavior. 3. Self-care, Health. 4. Calcium in the body—Health aspects. I. Gauthier, R. A. II. Title.
    RA776.75.W65 2013
    613.2—dc23
                                                                        2013014381

1 2 3 4 5 6 7 8 9 SHERIDAN 18 17 16 15 14 13
Printed on recycled paper

ACKNOWLEDGMENTS

Special thanks to:

Mike Adams	Richard Grossinger
Steve Adler	Angela Hartman
Cem Akin	Tania Leilani
Dr. Stewart Blaikie	Andrea McGinnis
Truth Calkins	Krystyna Robin Chaga
Dr. Gabriel Cousens	McMillan
Groovinda Dasi	Douglas Mulhall
Wendy Dherin	Doug Reil
Len Foley	Michele Rogalin
Juliana Garske	Paul Stamets
L. J. Gauthier	Ron Teeguarden
M. A. Gauthier	Kevin Trudeau
R. A. Gauthier	Candice and Robert
Kathy Glass	Weismandel
Nick Good	Robert Williams

. . . and so many others, for their contribution to this project and research, as well as for being a catalyst for the best health ever for everyone.

Photo credits:

Juliana Garske
Michael Roud
Sacred Chocolate (www.sacredchocolate.com)
Shazzie (www.shazzie.com)
Christopher Wodtke (www.kirlian.com)
David Wolfe (www.davidwolfe.com)

DISCLAIMER

Longevity Now is for informational purposes only and is in no way intended as medical advice, as a substitute for medical counseling, or as a treatment or cure for any disease or health condition, nor should it be construed as such. The contents of this book are protected under freedom of speech and freedom of religion. Neither David Wolfe, Rebecca Gauthier, North Atlantic Books, nor any of their editors, partners, affiliates, or subsidiaries will be held accountable in any way for the use or misuse of the information presented herein. The authors and publishers of this work are not medical doctors, nor is this document to be considered in any way medical advice. Because there is always some risk when making any health changes, none of the abovementioned persons and entities involved with the development and distribution of this information are responsible for any adverse effects or consequences of any kind resulting from the use or misuse of any suggestions or procedures described within this book. Always work with a qualified health professional before making any changes to your diet, your prescription drug use, your lifestyle, or your exercise activities. This information is provided prima facie and the reader assumes all risks from the use, nonuse, or misuse of this information.

SAFETY INFORMATION AND GUIDELINES

By choosing to follow the recommendations outlined in *Longevity Now,* you are making decisions about your own health. The information in this book is *not* to be used as the basis for treating a disease or a particular symptom, nor does it replace any current treatment you may be undergoing. All the recommended guidelines in this book, as well as any individual formulations contained within the book, are for educational purposes and for building health.

Although every supplement and superherb contained in *Longevity Now* is safe to use, if you have any of the health conditions listed below, we recommend that you seek immediate professional attention instead of acting on the suggestions within this book. Please always make sure to consult a qualified health professional before embarking upon any program or changing anything about your diet and supplementation.

Do not adopt the Longevity Now approach if:

- you have an acute, active, life-threatening infection anywhere in your body
- you are recovering from a medical surgery, procedure, or therapy
- you experience extreme weakness and/or hypersensitivity, or have extreme nutrient and mineral deficiencies
- you are undergoing active treatment or taking prescription medicine regularly including: anticoagulant drugs, antiplatelet drugs, antihypertensives, antidepressants, chemotherapy, corticosteroids, diuretic drugs, heart medication, high blood pressure drugs, insulin, or radiation.

Also, do not use the Longevity Now approach if you are nursing, pregnant, or are trying to get pregnant.

IMPORTANT: This document (nor any portion of it) may not be reproduced or distributed without the express written consent of the author David Wolfe or his legally delegated representative.

Environmental Certificate

Printed on 70# Appleton 2: Xtra Green recycled stock.

Compared to standard 70# coated white stock, Appleton 2: Xtra Green saves:

Trees: 59   Water: 25,080 gallons

Energy: 41.82 million BTUs   Solid Waste: 2,775 pounds

Greenhouse Gases: 5,464 pounds CO_2 equivalent

CONTENTS

Longevity Now Shopping List . . . 345

Resources . . . 347

Notes . . . 351

Bibliography . . . 357

SIDEBARS

PREFACE

The information contained in *Longevity Now* is unique, revolutionary, evolutionary, and potentially an important contribution to the physical sciences of longevity. It is arriving just in time.

In the Age of Information, all knowledge becomes available. Ours is a time of crisis and, simultaneously, opportunity. Our time is truly the most extraordinary time ever to be alive in the history of the world. As the heirs to all the ages, we are endowed and gifted with the wisdom and knowledge of our ancestors and contemporaries. We are able to access this information more readily and easily now than ever before. I am convinced that the answer to any question we have ever had has been found. All we require now is the passion and willpower to decode the answers and put them into immediate action.

Longevity Now arrives as an answer to the questions I have been habitually asking myself for twenty years:

- "How do we experience the best health ever?"
- "How do we easily and enjoyably heal ourselves of 'chronic' physical conditions?"
- "What is the fundamental and primary cause of aging?"
- "How do we reverse aging immediately and achieve longevity right now?"
- "How do we achieve a state where we are never again sick or ill for any reason?"

Contemplate the concepts contained within this book. Put these ideas into action immediately and align them with your habits so they work for you in both the short term and the long term.

Longevity Now cuts to the point. I have done my best to avoid "fluffy" language. This book is designed to create an understanding of innovative strategies that are the core seed concepts and methods around which any longevity program may be designed.

Longevity Now is and shall remain a work in progress. It continues to evolve and develop. Ultimately, this work is a seed planted into the consciousness of humanity. The information revealed in this work along with discoveries to come will assist humanity with activating the noble dreams of our true human potential. What you have before you is the summation of my life's work (up to this moment) in the fields of nutrition, longevity, rejuvenation, increasing core vitality, and radiant health.

For maximum benefit from the contents of *Longevity Now,* the recommended mental state while reading and studying these pages is one of conscious inner calm that facilitates hyperlearning, as well as a spiritual attitude of lovingness and acceptance toward all that occurs in life, so that one can move forward with healing and the activation of superhero qualities.

This book focuses on more physical and energetic aspects of healing and longevity and less on the spiritual, relationship, and emotional aspects. I feel that these spiritual, relationship, and emotional aspects are extraordinarily important, yet are simply not the focus of this work. I recommend that you continue to pursue an education in what creates spiritual, relationship, and emotional well-being.

Longevity Now delivers natural, simple healing strategies to real underlying physical causes/symptoms of aging and degeneration— which, based on my twenty years of research, include challenges such as hormone imbalances, poor nutrition, environmental toxicity, and calcification.

Present-day science, conventional medicine, and the mindset of "better living through chemistry" have delivered their results, and they are less than excellent. Essentially, due to poor results, these methods no longer reign supreme. An opening has occurred; the opportunities are before us. A streaming beam of fractal laser light is currently illuminating new health, healing, and longevity options for an enormous portion of humanity.

The best news ever is here NOW.

— David "Avocado" Wolfe
Hawaii, January 2013

Introduction

Why We Get Old, and What We Can Do about It

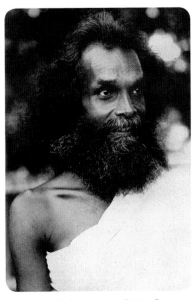

The Shivapuri Baba

How do we achieve extreme longevity like that of the great Taoist masters and Vedic yogis who lived to 130 and even 252 years of age, such as the Shivapuri Baba, who lived 137 years?

A big part of my work has been about focusing on the answer to that question. Obviously, they understood the mental, emotional, and spiritual aspects of longevity, yet it also appears they understood the nature of parasites, hormones, and the dangerous repercussions of calcification on our tissues. Armed with this knowledge, these great masters developed dietary approaches, herbal purges, physical tissue-cleansing strategies, and alchemical techniques; they sought out and bathed and drank from sacred high-mountain springs and glacial meltwater sources.

All these strategies are similar to what is outlined in this book. *Longevity Now* contains numerous concepts and strategies that I have learned from twenty years on the road in the health field. I believe that by understanding and utilizing the ideas in this book and by taking action you will be empowered to unlock your body's potential to become younger.

Chapter-by-Chapter Breakdown

Chapters 1 through 4 of this book are about excellent nutrition and elimination. From excellent organic, biodynamic, homegrown, and/or wild food nutrition, and a clean, healthy digestive tract, we begin the transformative process that creates a fertile bed for more advanced longevity strategies to develop and evolve within.

Chapter 5 of this book contains six specific strategies designed to level the hormonal playing field, in order to increase the effectiveness of your diet, immune system, youthening, and fitness regimes. The chapter on hormones focuses on amplifying what I call the "androgen"* hormones in your metabolism, negating hormonal triggers to disease, and removing bad estrogens and cortisol from your system.

After hormones, Chapter 6 details five specific strategies that are designed to break down and cleanse bad calcium from the body; to modulate the immune system; to ward off calcium-forming organisms and other parasites from multiplying in our bodies; and to create an overall superior level of health and well-being so that disease symptoms, illness, bacteria, viruses, and/or fungi cannot proliferate. These five specific strategies are more effective once nutrition and hormone suggestions have been heeded, so that the important health hormones are up and bad estrogen hormones and cortisol are down.

The more components of *Longevity Now* you incorporate over time, the more extraordinary levels of health and well-being you will experience in your life. The purpose of this approach is to gain the edge that will provide abundant health and longevity. The more comprehensive your engagement with your health, the deeper and more complete the transformation.

*My definition differs from the common scientific definition of the word "androgen." My definition of androgen hormones includes but is not limited to: progesterone, testosterone, DHEA, vitamin D3, thyroid hormone, androstenedione, and other hormones that preserve health, youth, and immunity, and oppose bad estrogens and cortisol.

The Real Causes of Aging

Longevity Now presents cutting-edge breakthroughs in nutrition, cellular cleansing, detoxification, weight loss, life extension, and immune system transformation by focusing on two key elements: creating hormone health and strategies to defeat calcification. These elements are the two intertwining trees of *Longevity Now.* The fertile soil these trees grow in is good—in fact, exceptional—nutrition. So if you are not getting the nutrition you need, you cannot start to grow these trees. *Longevity Now* gives you the best information on how to maximize your hormonal health and get rid of calcification, using nutrition—as well as some additional excellent strategies!

> **TIP** The best way to make use of the information in this book is to stack the odds in your favor by taking action on those concepts that make sense to you immediately. Everything else in this book may be considered as seeds to plant for the future.

Hormonal Imbalance

Unbalanced and low levels of hormones have been associated with numerous chronic health problems and age-related conditions. Along with many other actions, hormones are chemical messengers; they signal the cells to become younger or older, to slow or increase multiplication, to be immunologically responsive or lazy. As it turns out, the sex hormones are the health hormones, and (as adults) we require the sex hormones to be within a certain range individually and to maintain a certain ratio with one another; otherwise we could end up with potentially harmful conditions such as estrogen dominance and cortisol dominance.

Low levels of hormones and unbalanced hormones leading to estrogen dominance, cortisol dominance, or even thyroid disorders disable the immune system, interfere with energy production in the cells, and can signal the body to age.

Hormone irregularities are major contributing factors to joint disorders (such as arthritis), chronic inflammatory conditions, autoimmune conditions, etc. Essentially, hormone irregularities eventually erode our potential to experience optimal health and vibrancy. They inevitably affect every area of our life, including our natural state of well-being, ability to exercise, and sex life.

Calcification

Calcification is the hardening of body tissues by calcium salts or deposits. Although calcification itself is not considered a disease, it has been shown to be a significant contributing factor in nearly every known illness and aging condition, including heart disease, kidney stones, gallstones, chronic inflammation, arthritis, cancers, cataracts, eczema, psoriasis, and even wrinkles. If our androgen hormones (progesterone, testosterone, et al.) are chronically low and/or out of balance, this contributes to calcification. The higher our level of calcification, the more difficult it is to keep our skin, bones, joints, nervous system, and immune system running at a peak and youthful state.

Calcification is one of the most pervasive yet least understood health conditions on the planet. Historically, calcification has been identified as an effect and not a cause. Because calcification is so often overlooked in the process of diagnosis and treatment, it is not dealt with in the way it needs to be: as a major threat to our health and well-being. *Longevity Now* addresses calcification directly by outlining decalcification strategies to drive the "bad calcium" out of the body before it starts causing problems.

Calcification causes acute and chronic pain that disrupts our lifestyle and forces us to become increasingly dependent on drug treatments that mask pain and reduce suffering. These treatments only address the symptoms and not the underlying causes. *Longevity Now* helps us identify the sources of the pain and to intelligently address each cause, step by step.

It appears that the great undertakers found in Nature are parasites of different sorts and descriptions. These thieving organisms range from tapeworms, flukes, harmful bacteria, and viruses, to what appear to be calcium-forming microorganisms similar to microscopic coral. These parasites break down and often calcify even the most noble mammals, birds, reptiles, and amphibians. Where does this calcification come from? The answers to this question supplies the keys to medical and longevity research.

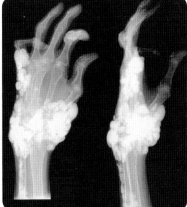

An X-ray of an arthritic hand. Notice the similarity to coral formation in the ocean.

Where Does Calcification Come from?

Hormone research indicates that once hormones begin to drop with age, calcification ensues. That is one piece in the puzzle.

Rudolf Steiner believed that calcification was caused by **telluric forces** (which originate in the Earth and exist within organisms) being overcome by energies of the atmosphere, heavens, planets, and cosmos. In other words, calcification is the result of being oxidized by the atmosphere (the free-radical theory), fried by radiation, overcome by a deficiency of electrons, losing the levitational qualities that emanate from the Earth, or however we can phrase the corrosive effects the atmosphere and cosmic radiation have on us over our lifetime.

Another theory is that the source of this calcification is water naturally contaminated by calcium-rich strata found in the Earth's crust. This **calcium-rich water** is thought to contain bad calcium (calcium harmful to us because of its insolubility and lack of electrons) and even spores of calcium-forming organisms (bacteria, archaea, and other extremophile microorganisms that are theorized to form shells like snails or coral). According to this theory, any calcium-rich (hard) waters, especially well and municipal-piped waters, must be avoided whenever possible. Continuing with this idea, we know that boiling the water does not extract calcium, nor does it appear to kill all calcium-forming microorganisms, as they are suspected of being extremophiles that can survive the heat.

According to a related **parasite** theory, all kinds of living creatures drink contaminated water of some type or another, and as a result these contaminants (including parasites) begin working their way into the food chain. Carnivores seek young prey not just because they're easier to catch, but also because they have a lower level of parasites as well as "juicier" tissue due to their lack of calcification. Many parasites and possibly calcium-forming microorganisms can be passed orally (mouth-to-mouth), by touch, or sexually.

The main problem of calcification is that insoluble, electron-deficient calcium acts like sand in our biological gears and eventually turns into clogging plaques. This causes inflammation (friction) and interferes with our implosion (double-spiral) blood and fluid flow, oxygenation, and the movement of white blood cells. As a result, calcification conditions can lead to dangerous infections and create the perfect staging ground for a myriad of chronic viral, bacterial, and fungal infections.

We know that animals in Nature are, for the most part, eating an original, raw, wild-food diet rich in minerals and vitamins. Based on the evidence, this is very likely the way we were intended to eat. Despite the fact that animals eat the best foods they can access, those animals do have a life span, and at some point they will die. What is it that takes out a wild animal? What is it that will cause, for example, a turtle or an eagle to die? It is clear that arthritic calcification causes the range of motion of even the most noble, long-lived animals to decrease and, ultimately, brings their life to an end.

Even if we eat the best diet ever (and I highly recommend that we do), we still may not achieve the longevity that is possible. Theoretically, we must maintain youthful, balanced hormone levels, avoid calcified, iron-rich, hard water, keep inflammation at an absolute minimum, dodge parasites, block the intake of dead calcium supplements, and escape the grip of calcification conditions, including arthritis, cancer, heart disease, stroke.

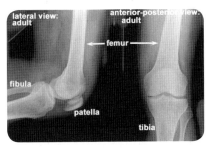

Healthy bones and joints

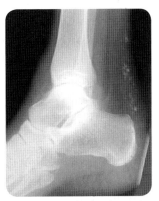

Achilles tendon showing the beginnings of calcification

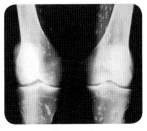

Calcification showing in the leg muscles

🌿 Toxins and a Poor Diet

As we will see in the nutrition portions of this book, nutrition is a critical factor in experiencing the best health ever. Not only does it affect how we feel on a daily basis, it also determines the future of our health. If we eat foods loaded with chemicals and toxins today, then tomorrow we will create deficiencies that will be counterproductive to experiencing the best health ever.

If we are serious about transforming our health, then we need to begin to create new eating habits and behaviors that help our body heal, rejuvenate, build energy, and increase immune intelligence. In order to do this, we should avoid eating things that are harmful. Toxic foods that are laden with chemicals, preservatives, artificial coloring, artificial flavoring, and addictive qualities keep us stuck in an unhealthy state—a state we often don't even realize we're in until we experience a substantial transformation in our food quality and fitness level.

If one is eating a chemicalized, cooked, animal-food-based diet, then the body is dealing with massive exposure to fertilizers, toxic metals, pesticides (even if one is washing conventionally raised foods), and antibiotics and hormones that have been injected into animals that are raised to be slaughtered for human consumption. According to some estimates, more than three thousand chemicals are added to our food supply and more than ten thousand chemicals are involved in food processing, storage, and preservation. The chances of being contaminated by this toxicity is high, and it has a cumulative effect that results in irregularities and disorders in the body and could eventually lead to hormone irregularities and calcification conditions.

If you eat conventional, mass-produced, industrial foods and beverages (tap water, soda, etc.) on a regular basis, it is highly likely that the toxic load generated by this exposure will impair your immune system and load your body with carcinogens. If you have been vaccinated, the contaminants in vaccines, including mercury and SV-40 virus, may still be continuing to impair your immune system. This inevitably creates opportunities for parasites of various sorts to penetrate into regions of energy stagnation along the body's complex nervous, circulatory, organ, and skeletal systems. A number of challenges may develop later in life, ranging from microscopic coral-like plaques in the blood flow, joints, and nerves, to oxidation and scarring damage within the body's various tissues.

It is very likely that the rise in debilitating chronic conditions is closely linked to the toxic load generated by the following substances and types of contamination:

- Toxins: Phthalates and bisphenol A used in plastics, furans, toluene, and xylene petrochemicals; polychlorinated biphenyls, perfluorooctanoic acids used to make stain-resistant, nonstick products; and polybrominated-diphenyl-ethers used in mattresses, couches, and carpets.
- Pesticides and fertilizers: anilazine, azinphos-methyl, benomyl, BHC, bifenthrin, captan, carbaryl, carbofuran, DDE, diazinon, dicofol, dieldrin, dimethoate, diphenyl 2-ethylhexyl phosphate, endosulfan I-II, endosulfan sulfate, folpet, iprodione, iprodione metabolite isomer, malathion, methamidophos, methiocarb, methomyl, mevinphos, omethoate, parathion-methyl, propargite, styrene, toxaphene, vinclozolin, etc. These are all pesticides that are commonly used and found on grocery store shelves. Only organic foods are free from these common dangerous pesticides.
- Hormonally altered substances: for example, rBGH milk.
- Genetically modified substances: soy, corn, potato, wheat, etc.
- Grain-fed factory-farmed meat: now known to be heavily contaminated with pesticides, larvicides, fungicides, and antibiotics. In addition, these animals are also fed artificial, genetically modified grain.

This is merely a short list of primary considerations of what to avoid when ingesting anything. To simplify, that means avoiding factory-farmed meat (i.e., normal meat bought in a grocery store), genetically modified (GMO) food of any kind (e.g., corn, wheat, soy, potato), hormonally altered milk substances, and all chemical-sprayed and fertilized foods. Essentially, only consume organic, homegrown, and/or wild-grown food. A more extensive list of foods to avoid is included later in this book. It is essential that you choose organic food, or even better-quality organic food as much as possible, just as a baseline health premise.

It is also important that we do our best to avoid some of the very severe toxic substances found in carpets, new mattresses, nonorganic couches, and other furniture. Although I recognize that it may not be immediately possible to remove these products from your everyday life,

I encourage you to seek ecofriendly alternatives as best you can and from this point forward to purchase only ecofriendly, non-outgassing furniture, fixtures, and carpets in order to reduce the burden on your immune system. As the research indicates, an immune system burdened with carcinogens will fail to control the growth of cancer.

Preparing for Transformation

Stepping into extreme longevity requires strategy, knowledge, spiritual research, emotional release work, inspired dedication, and determination. *Longevity Now* presents a number of insights that help us in our efforts to crack the code to extreme longevity, peak performance, and optimal physical health. By incorporating the Longevity Now approach into our lifestyle, we can optimize our hormone levels, get our immune system functioning intelligently, push calcification into a small corner, and really start living!

The transformative process that begins by focusing on the Longevity Now approach allows you to rebuild yourself at a deep level—in essence, to reshape yourself into a younger, more perfect work of art. It endows you with a newfound ability to resculpt your character, physique, and future—your potential. It inspires you to fully invest your time in the process of re-creating yourself as a masterpiece.

The tissue-terrain-transforming, hormone-enhancing, and decalcification strategies that make up the Longevity Now approach require us to add into our lifestyle as many nutritious foods, antioxidant-rich superfoods, adaptogenic superherbs, super-supplements, mineral compounds, longevity technologies, healthful habits, and positive emotions and thoughts as we can, in order to keep stacking the odds in our favor to push back aging. Stacking the odds in your favor is a powerful strategy to maximize optimal cleansing, detoxification, and longevity.

Let us all take as many preventative steps as possible to reduce damaging our bodies in the first place, along with the specific youthening actions outlined in this book as part of our longevity-enhancing one–two combination.

Results You Can Expect

The following results have been reported from incorporating the Longevity Now approach:

- enhanced mental clarity and focus
- improved immune function
- radical improvement of candida symptoms
- elimination of free radicals and free-radical cell damage
- increased energy and vitality
- reduced stress levels
- improved physical endurance and strength-building capabilities
- improved mineralization of bones, teeth, skin, nails, and hair
- balancing of metabolism and thyroid function
- healthy weight loss and long-term weight maintenance
- total-body alkalization and balancing of pH for optimal cell function
- relief from nasal congestion and environmentally caused allergies
- better balance of hormone levels and improvements in the endo-crine system
- reduction of painful PMS and menopausal symptoms
- improved ability to regenerate damaged tissues and recover from injury
- reversal of aging symptoms and restoration of our natural ability for longevity
- improvement in heart-rate variability
- improvement and normalization in cortisol levels
- regeneration of healthy cells
- improvements and eventual elimination of aches and pains
- less stiffness and more flexibility
- higher levels of energy
- incremental improvements in memory
- bone-density improvements
- increasing levels of hope and heartfelt joy
- improvement of calcification conditions

Continues

Continued

- improvement in androgenic hormones and lowering of bad estrogens
- increases in the range of motion of major joints and muscles
- continued increase in the will to live
- cleanse mucus, congestion, fermentation, and inflammation in the digestive tract
- purification of the blood

Read these benefits again and again, and feel how powerful they are. Actually feel the power of these benefits in your heart. Picture yourself feeling these benefits every day.

Making a Commitment

I designed Longevity Now as an approach that can be easily adapted and incorporated into your lifestyle, no matter what level of health you are at. Longevity Now cannot be compared with a cleanse or a diet. It is a long-term approach, a lifestyle that you can explore, experiment, evolve, and expand with throughout the years. The insights gained here will grow with you.

The whole idea of this book is relatively simple. If you have the discipline to brush your teeth every day, you can take on the Longevity Now approach!

NOW is the time for Action. NOW is the Best Time Ever. Without taking action on the ideas, strategies, and overall content of *Longevity Now*, we will continue the painful path of slow (or rapid) decay that comes with advancing age, just as our parents and grandparents experienced. Taking positive action now allows us to live longer—adding quality, pain-free life to our years—so we can be happier, healthier, more radiant versions of ourselves! By taking action on the ideas, strategies, and overall content of *Longevity Now,* we discover that an entirely new destiny is possible for ourselves.

Realize how fortunate you are to have access to information that increases hope and nourishes life.

Imagine yourself right now taking action daily on the ideas and concepts in *Longevity Now.* Visualize yourself ten years from now feeling and looking younger than you do today. This vision is possible and, in fact, probable. I have seen it happen for thousands of people. Nothing is as powerful as action. Action immediately destroys procrastination, doubt, and fear. Go for it, because NOW is the best time ever!

Conquering Doubt

Believe you can and you will. All behavior is belief-driven. Consider the following negative belief systems:

- "I don't have the discipline."
- "Life's not worth living anyway."
- "I'm not worth it."
- "I'm not smart enough."
- "I don't know."
- "I'm not capable."
- "I don't have good genes."
- "It's too complicated and confusing."

These belief systems are thoughts and ideas we have entirely made up and purchased. But we can return them at any time for a full refund. In each and every case, we can find numerous examples of individuals who could have bought into these belief systems, yet changed their mind and thus changed their lives.

Now consider the actual truth behind these beliefs:

- "I don't have the discipline."

    Yes, you do. You brush your teeth every day. If you have the discipline to do that twice a day, every day since you were a child, you can do anything. Not much discipline is required. Longevity Now is about taking as much action as you desire with ease and grace so that every part of the approach becomes second nature for you.

- "Life's not worth living anyway."

  This idea results from being in a low energy state. As you raise your energy with the recommendations in this approach, you will naturally increase your desire to live.

- "I'm not worth it."

  Yes, you are. Anybody who has made it this far and is reading these words right now is extraordinary for taking action on an approach like this.

- "I'm not smart enough."

  You can read and write. You were clever enough to get this book in front of you. Like other smart people, you are actually interested in the subjects of health and longevity.

- "I don't know."

  Yes, you do. Take your power back. You know many things. Say to yourself "I do know" or "I choose to know."

- "I'm not capable."

  You are capable of amazing feats. Recall a time in your life when you were capable and pulled off something amazing! Yes. You are capable.

- "I don't have good genes."

  This belief is always about removing responsibility. Instead, take responsibility. Know that you can change your genes with mineral-rich, nutrient-rich foods and herbs as well as exercise and pure water. Consider examples of short professional basketball players who could have quit as teenagers because they didn't have tall genes. Yet they made it all the way to the top.

- "It's too complicated and confusing."

  Longevity Now is as simple as you want to make it. It is designed so that any single piece of this approach is powerful by itself—let alone several or all the pieces working together. Taking action on one thing in this approach may be the most appropriate place to start.

> **TIP** More and more of us are becoming aware of the importance of having partners, mentors, and coaches in our life to help drive us toward our goals. Partners help keep us on track, maintain motivation, discern progress, and make participation more fun. Sharing your breakthroughs and discoveries with another is exciting!
>
> Find a Longevity Now partner. It is easier to get younger together than to get older together. That's why we can (if we choose) select a partner for our journey into and beyond Longevity Now. Taking action is easier with the help of others!

The Power of Adding

Multiply your results by adding. In order for any program, diet, or cleanse to work in the long term, one must align with one's own human nature. Human nature is such that we don't like being denied things. We don't like having things taken away permanently. As soon as we tell a child "No" s/he is immediately finding a way to "Yes." They'll do what they want if they can get away with it. This habit or quirk of human nature never changes—adults do the same thing. The key idea is that we have to get into complete psychological alignment with our own nature. What does that mean?

In the context of Longevity Now, that means we avoid taking away from ourselves too much of any flavor or joy. Instead, we *add* wonderful, clean, organic foods, raw superfoods, super supplements, adaptogenic superherbs, fitness concepts, tissue cleansing strategies, etc. Is it possible that the "good stuff" will make us feel so good that we'll naturally move away from the "bad stuff"? In my experience, the answer is *yes*.

Additionally, all the transformation in lifestyle is done without trying. Everything happens gracefully. That is the key idea. We are going for the essence of longevity—more years of life and more life in our years, with lots of joy and pleasure sprinkled all around. We focus on all the great-tasting, super-healthy supplements, superfoods, and super-herbs that we discover by simply adding them to our diet and lifestyle.

Any of the strategies recommended in *Longevity Now* can be *added* into one's existing lifestyle. Simply discover the ones you like and go for it. Find a partner, friend, or family member to join you in activating genius, increasing vital health, revving up healthy hormones, and breaking down inner calcification. Get out a blender and make entirely new types of lemonades, shakes, smoothies, elixirs, and beverages from super-supplements and superfoods. Design superfood trail mixes. Take your favorite adaptogen superherbs and make teas out of them.

The overall approach is to add the most powerful longevity strategies, allowing them to help you naturally diminish or drop all the other things you have been doing, because the old ways have become irrelevant. You will naturally and suddenly shed old habits through experiencing empowering results, positive momentum, and wonderful transformations in health, as well as greater flexibility, deeper nutrition, greater flavor, and joy.

> **TIP** The goal of Longevity Now is to add more life to your years, not just years to your life. Remember to have fun and to become inspired by your own personal transformation of health and well-being. We will come to recognize that each of us is ultimately the one who knows our own body best. Although it is perfectly normal to go through some detoxification effects during the course of Longevity Now, please proceed at a pace that is appropriate for your physical capacity.

CHAPTER 1

Eating Well

Major minerals like silicon, carbon, sulfur, phosphorus, zinc, sodium, potassium, calcium, magnesium, and iodine that construct our tissues are typically all derived from our food. If the foods we are eating lack these minerals and nutrients, then we will be missing crucial elements in our physical makeup. With the proliferation of super-drug sugars (high-fructose corn syrup) and artificial protein powders, as well as every kind of nutrition marketing scam, we must be keenly concerned with quality. We must be able to distinguish what is sugar-filled chemical garbage and what is valuable. To do this, I recommend that you reflect on the ancient wisdom of diet that has been time-tested over thousands of years: a wisdom that directs us to add certain foods, superfoods, and superherbs into our diet that will help us to automatically develop healthy and longevity-inducing eating habits.

You are going to discover that in one fell swoop it may be possible for you to go from zero to superhero. This means you will be able to go from food that's worthless all the way to superhero food because it's simple, easy, and enjoyable! Anybody can eat a goji berry, and it tastes awesome. The goji berry is perhaps the number-one-ranking superfood in the world.

Let's say you've been surviving on junk food; in one day you could go from zero to superhero. That day is now. This a powerful technology. We need this technology in our current situation—a situation that is, essentially, a dietary holocaust.

But in that dietary holocaust, massive opportunities for transformation and health and healing become available because nothing's out of balance in the universe. Everything is in a sort of balance—a dynamic disequilibrium that favors health and growth. And yes, there might be

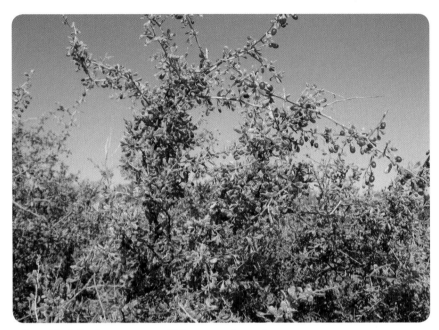

A wild Arizona goji berry bush

chaos, destruction, genetically modified GMO stuff, and fast food on one end of the spectrum; but on the other end of the spectrum guess what becomes available? *The best food ever.*

For me, "the best food ever" means the highest-quality, mineral-rich, organic, homegrown, or wild foods, superfoods, and superherbs. I have found that following this principle is not only the simplest way to choose what I eat, it is also the best way to bring about good health and spiritual transformation. Because of this, I have made my life's work a study of how to help as many people as possible succeed and prosper with super-healthy foods, superfoods, and superherbs.

I encourage anyone who wishes to experience the bounties of Nature to delve into eating what Nature provides us. That is: raw plant foods, superfoods, and superherbs. I encourage people to learn about what plants are most edible, to learn a new way of living, to experience the incredible health that Nature will give to you by accepting the foods she provides, and to live a life in harmony with the plants and animals. By doing so, you may experience and reclaim your own little bit of paradise!

You Are What You Eat

"You are what you eat" is the zip file that we received when we were emailed to the planet by God. "You are what you eat" is a quantum phenomenon. Quantum physics indicates that we are a mineral matrix consisting mostly of empty space (vast spaces between minerals or atoms). And that empty space is defined by an energy field that we call our body. According to the blossoming field of epigenetics, our energy field or body is dramatically affected by our environment—especially our internal environment. The substances we are putting inside our energy field day after day shape our internal environment; these include, most notably, our food, air, and water.

Eating poorly is similar to building a house or office complex with inferior materials that wear out in twenty years instead of two hundred years. This is the power of "you are what you eat." This maxim implies that you have control over your physical and mental destiny so that you can manifest your true phenotype and genotype. Specifically, eating healthfully allows your phenotype to fully express your genotype. This means you become capable of achieving a full expression of your genetics.

"You are what you eat" means that if we are eating junk food, we create a junk body. If we're eating fast food, then our body is going to burn up fast and we're not going to be around very long. If your "you are what you eat" bank account is bankrupt because the food you consume is full of empty calories, then you will consequentially lack the capability to manifest your real resources. Those resources can be tapped through the diet of foods, superfoods, superherbs, super-supplements, and technologies that I recommend in these pages.

By incorporating the information found in this book, we will, step by step, manifest our true abilities to control what we're eating. Eventually impulsive behaviors (such as going through half a bag of potato chips before we realize what's happening) start to lessen their grip upon us. It is important that we are very gentle with ourselves because it takes some time to change for the better.

Some of us can make a commitment to health and stick with it more easily than others can. But a lot of us are not there. We need to take simple, easy steps and gradually add foods that work for our body, foods that we enjoy—foods that have tremendous nutritional value. And then slowly we start letting go of all the foods and substances that we know are not good for us—foods that are actually working against us.

We do know what's good for us and what's not. Everybody knows that junk food is junk. Everybody knows that food you buy in a normal store is nutrient-deficient and mineral-deficient. Everybody knows that you can have better-quality food if you grow it in your own backyard. If you grow a garden, you know that your own tomatoes taste better based on personal experience!

One of the most important distinctions found within these pages is the fact that all foods are not created equal. Some foods are deficient in minerals and key nutrients, while other foods are packed with a powerhouse of valuable nutrients that can change your life, your health, and your body in a truly incredible way. Selecting those foods that also deliver the flavor, taste, and enjoyment that we are seeking will cause us to develop new, healthy eating habits that simultaneously satiate all our cravings. You can have salads that taste extraordinary! You can eat amazing foods like avocados and literally become hooked on them as your favorite snack food.

As a gastronaut, I have explored "you are what you eat" for more than twenty-five years. I've made a couple of appropriate observations about this famous phrase:

1. Eating superfoods and/or superherbs that are the products of long-lived plants helps you to live long. For example: green tea shrubs-trees are exceedingly long-lived (they can live over one thousand years) and impart that quality upon us; olive trees can live thousands of years (it is no wonder that olive oil has such strong research supporting its longevity-enhancing properties);

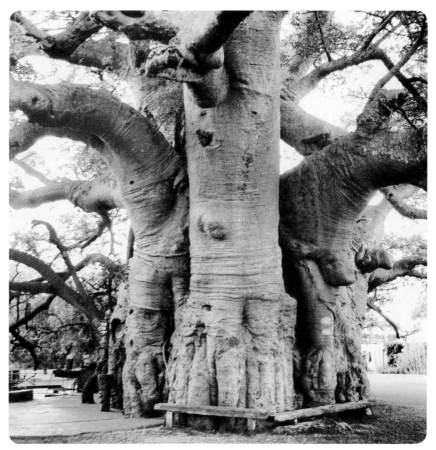

The Sunland baobab (Limpopo, South Africa), estimated to be anywhere from 1,700 to 6,000 years old. Theoretically, baobab fruit confers these longevity properties.

baobab trees can live thousands of years, with their longevity properties being potentially conferred in their baobab fruit; goji berry bushes and ginseng can live hundreds of years; etc.

2. Powerful pioneer plants that grow where the Earth has been disturbed, deforested, eroded, etc. often are good medicines for us. These include: chaga mushroom and its pioneering, medicinal host birch tree; astragalus and its power as a nitrogen-fixing

(soil-replenishing) superherb; noni and its ability to grow even on barren lava fields; grapes and their tendency to survive damaged ecosystems; mucuna and its antistimulant, nourishing qualities; Andean "grain" quinoa and its character of being able to survive even sterile soils; etc.

What we eat deeply and radically affects the way we think, feel, and behave. We are what we eat, and we eat what we are. Food affects every aspect of our being.

Every person is a work of art in progress. One can become progressively more beautiful, or one can follow the fate that aspects of our civilization have set out for us: decay, illness, and an untimely death. Each action taken determines which of these two destinies will be achieved. What we eat helps to guide our path. Eating determines what level of health our body will experience. Every bite of food put into the body should add to our strength, spirituality, and beauty. Each meal becomes part of who we are at the deepest level.

"You are what you eat" will have the final say.

The Benefits of Organic Food

Eating organic is critical, because it provides us with the most basic form of food to build a happy, healthy body. Organic food is the oldest form of agriculture known. It is completely natural. Organic foods are not sprayed, not genetically modified, and not grown with pesticides, herbicides, or fungicides—all chemicals specifically designed to kill living organisms. These chemicals should not be put into the Earth, sprayed on our foods, or fed to our children.

Spraying all kinds of growth hormones on plants to accelerate their production, and adding artificial fertilizers to the soil that are contaminated with petroleum and the slag from burning metals is not natural. This is harmful to our bodies and our children's bodies. This is a big mistake and a dangerous practice, and we need to stop it, reverse it, and go back to growing food naturally, with no artificial processes whatsoever.

Perhaps we have thought in the past that organic food was too expensive. My position is: if you have to spend $1 more, $5 more, or $20 more for organic produce, spend the extra money, because you are worth it. That investment in your health will come back to you a hundredfold. You can either pay a little more now for nutrient-filled, natural food, or you can pay later with sickness while in the hospital, racking up bills that your health insurance will not cover. The choice is yours. By eating organic, you will be investing in your health as well as supporting organic farmers and food distributors who are doing the right thing for a sustainable future.

Benefit #1: Organic foods are richer in minerals.

This is because all agriculture, and all nutrition, begins with mineral-rich soil. When more minerals are available to the plant, the plant's vitamin, polysaccharide, and enzyme content, as well as overall immune system, are improved. When we eat mineral-rich foods we directly absorb the nutrients that made the plant healthy. We also enjoy more conscious choices and freedom as the cells throughout our body become healthier and more vital. Entire books have been written on how rich soils helped build enormous civilizations; and how the subsequent mismanagement of crops and soil led to the loss of mineral-rich soil and a subsequent collapse of those civilizations.

The famous twelve-year Schuphan study tested the nutritional superiority of organically grown foods. Among other things, Schuphan found the following.[1]

- Organic foods have far higher mineral and trace mineral contents, with the exception of sodium. For example, organic produce contains far more iron, potassium, magnesium, and calcium than conventional crops. (Most studies of this type demonstrate that organic foods have two to ten times the mineral content of conventional foods—you really do get more value for the money.)
- Organic spinach contained 64 to 78 percent more vitamin C.

Love in the garden.
Love in the cabbage.

🌿 Organic savoy cabbage contained 76 to 91 percent more vitamin C.

🌿 Organic crops had a dry weight (after dehydration) of 69 to 96 percent more than conventional crops, demonstrating a higher food-value content.

In 1993 Bob Smith, a trace minerals laboratory analyst, began a small experiment. For two years he visited stores in Chicago and purchased four to fifteen samples of both organic and commercial produce. He brought these samples back to his laboratory and tested them for trace elements. His conclusions were as follows:[2]

🌿 Organically grown wheat had twice the calcium, four times the magnesium, five times the manganese, and thirteen times more selenium than commercial wheat.

🌿 Organically grown corn had twenty times more calcium and manganese, and two to five times more copper, magnesium, molybdenum, selenium, and zinc.

🌿 Organically grown potatoes had two or more times the boron, selenium, silicon, strontium, and sulfur, and 60 percent more zinc.

🌿 Organically grown pears had two to nearly three times more chromium, iodine, manganese, molybdenum, silicon, and zinc.

🌿 Overall, for twenty of the twenty-two beneficial trace minerals, the quantities found in organically grown food significantly exceeded that of the commercially grown crops. Organic foods also had lower quantities of toxic trace elements such as aluminum, lead, and mercury.

🌿 Benefit #2: Organic agriculture is sustainable.

Organic food production has existed for thousands of years (since the beginning of agriculture) and it will continue as long as humans live on the planet. Organic agriculture is nontoxic: it leaves no permanent toxicity. The pesticide and artificial fertilizer industries are toxic and nonsustainable. These industries have covered the entire planet with dangerous chemicals.

The story of DDT is known to nearly all of us. DDT went into commercial distribution in 1948. Because of its unsustainable toxicity, DDT was banned in the United States in 1972 and soon afterward was banned worldwide. DDT is a known neurotoxin, xenoestrogen, and carcinogen. Who was brought to justice after the facts of DDT were revealed? How many people, children, and animals have been injured by this chemical? How much longer will we continue to spray the Earth with poisons? These are critical questions that we have to ask ourselves. We now know that DDT has been found in the sweat of polar bears. It is in the tissues of animals, including the milk of human mothers. It is all over the planet. That is just one chemical. There are at least 77,000 different artificial chemicals that we have released into the biosphere, geosphere, and atmosphere.

We know that kids are being born today with hundreds of different chemicals in the blood of their umbilical cord. In one study, researchers from two major laboratories looked for the presence of toxic chemicals in the umbilical-cord blood of ten newborns born in U.S. hospitals in August and September 2004. Of the more than 400 chemicals tested for, 287 were detected in umbilical cord blood. Of these, 180 cause cancer in humans or animals, 217 are toxic to the brain or nervous system, and 208 cause birth defects or abnormal development in animals.[3] These are synthetic chemicals created by humankind that have gotten into the food supply and are brought into the baby by the mother. We used to believe that the baby was protected by the mother, that toxins were filtered by the umbilical cord and placenta. The truth is that the chemicals are not entirely filtered out. In my estimation, this is a key reason we have an explosion of autism. Now, 1 in 150 babies is born with autism. Estimates indicate that this number could become 1 in 50 babies born autistic in the future.[4]

These chemicals are also one of the reasons we have a massive explosion of cancer, especially cancer in children. It is one of the reasons kids have chronic asthma and allergies from birth. It is one of the reasons kids are suffering from skin diseases. It is from spraying chemicals in the air, in water, on food, and on everything. "Better living through chemistry" has been an experiment in suffering and genocide.

We must stop eating chemical-grown food and return to organic food to be healthy and maintain a sense of certainty, quality control, and safety. There is no other choice. What we choose to buy and eat is like voting. When we buy conventionally grown, we are voting for conventional farming. We are saying that we want more pesticides and chemicals. Anyone reading this right now knows that this is not what we want.

TIP Just a few thousand years ago, 100 percent of the human population was eating 100 percent wild food! Agriculture did not exist.

Wild food contains even *more* minerals than organically farmed food. Picking wild berries, fruits, vegetables (such as dandelion), and medicinal mushrooms (reishi, chaga, maitake, shiitake, poria, etc.) makes for a wonderful hobby. It reconnects us with Nature in a simple and enjoyable way. For an excellent field guide to discovering and harvesting wild food—in urban, suburban, and rural areas—read Sergei Boutenko's *Wild Edibles*.

If you cannot pick wild fruits and vegetables for at least 25 percent of your diet, it is recommended to include a raw organic green superfood powder in the diet, as well as fresh vegetable juices, to supply a full spectrum of alkaline minerals and nutrients.

Benefit #3: Organic food is safer for our endocrine system, which produces hormones.

When our endocrine system is disrupted, our hormones are thrown out of balance and/or hormone production stops altogether. We know that our reproductive system, thyroid system, thymus, immune system, and adrenals are all hormonally operated. We also know that estrogen-mimicking pesticides interfere with the function of the human hormone system.

Some better-known examples of highly toxic, endocrine-disrupting pesticides are:

- DDT and its metabolite DDE, which are both now known to exhibit their toxicity through antiandrogenic demasculinizing properties
- thinclosalin, a heavily used fungicide that is antiandrogenic
- endosulfan, a DDT relative with estrogenic properties that is found more often in food than any other pesticide
- atrazine, a weed killer with broad hormonal activity, contaminates the drinking water of about twenty million people in the United States

In addition, plastics are known to contain xenoestrogens, such as BPA, that interfere with hormones. Plastics need to sit for at least a year before coming into contact with liquids due to the volatility of plasticizers such as BPA. Typically, plastic bottles are blown and less than sixty seconds later filled with liquids such as drinking water. Plastic bottled water should be avoided.

Benefit #4: Eating organic foods, superfoods, and superherbs is safe, easy, and fun.

You can grow organic foods anywhere with seeds, nice soil, sunshine, sufficient moisture, smiles, and lots of love. Gardening skills are attractive and sexy and make for a safe, healthy hobby. Organic foods have been proven over thousands of years to be safe to eat. Conventional chemical-sprayed foods have been proven over fifty years to be unsafe to eat.

Make the determination to eat organic. It is the best thing you can do for yourself and your family. The only foods that have any value are organic foods or, even better, high-quality homegrown and/or wild foods.

If You Don't Have Access to Organic Foods

- Request organic food at your local store.
- Shop on the Internet and order organic foods to be delivered to your home.
- Start your own organic farm.
- If you do not have a yard, ask a friend if you can grow a garden in his or her yard and then share the delicious food you grow with them!
- Write an email to your local politicians, online magazines, and other media outlets, telling them how you feel about the difficulties of finding nonsprayed, natural foods in your area.
- Learn to forage and eat wild foods.
- Plant fruiting plants and trees wherever you legally can and enjoy the harvest each year.
- Consider moving to a location where higher-quality foods are available.
- Contact gardening advocacy groups and solicit their assistance.

The Benefits of Living Food

Let's start this section by addressing an incorrect assumption about food. It is so basic that it literally has slipped by us all for thousands of years. It's an assumption that was never really scientifically questioned until the twentieth century. And that is the assumption that cooked food is a normal and natural part of a daily balanced diet.

Cooking is something that was *invented.* It is not indigenous to the Planet Earth. Fire is indigenous, but cooking food is not. It is something we do that is different from every other creature on Earth. We humans and our domesticated animals are the only creatures on this planet who eat cooked foods. All animals living in the wild eat their food raw and, almost always, fresh. Cooked and processed foods are artificial. The cooking and processing of foods has become so common that most of us do not even question it.

The basis of human nourishment is obvious: it is raw plant foods. And Nature presents this to us in abundance. Raw plant foods are simple, easy to find, fun to eat, enjoyable, contain thousands of discovered

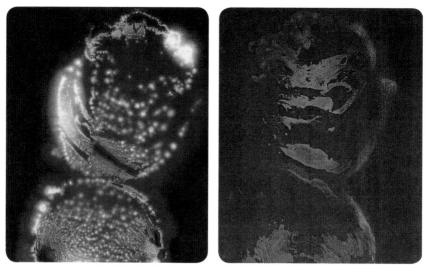

Kirlian imagery: raw cabbage on the left; cooked cabbage on the right

and yet-to-be-discovered health-giving nutrients, and conform to the biological design of the human digestive system. The Sun is the beating heart of all life, and raw plant foods represent the purest form of transformed sun energy.

> **TIP** If you eat cooked foods, try to eat a salad with your meal. This increases the amount of enzymes present in your diet. I also recommend that you add cultured vegetables, seaweeds, and superfoods because of their high enzyme content.

Eating a balanced mix of raw plants (and especially their juices) restores the body on a molecular level, builds strong cells, neutralizes oxidation damage (aging), raises alkalinity, and grounds the person in the natural world. Of course, the body resists shocking changes, so everyone should ease into the raw-food approach at an appropriate pace. Also, everyone should self-educate on this subject by visiting www.thebestdayever.com and other online sources, reading raw-food books, attending lectures, and talking to others so that the common mistakes are avoided.

I strongly recommend that you take action with your diet and make purer, cleaner choices by looking into a raw, organic, plant-based diet filled with fruits, vegetables, nuts, seeds, seaweeds, sprouts, flowers, fermented foods, herbs, superherbs, and superfoods (as described in my books *The Sunfood Diet Success System* and *Eating for Beauty*). Such a diet significantly reduces the toxic load, enhances the immune system, and helps achieve great strides toward clearing energy blockages, attaining wonderful health, and achieving vital longevity.

Here are the benefits of eating live food and avoiding cooked and processed foods.

🔖 Benefit #1: Living food is better for the environment.

When one eats a bag of corn chips, the wrapper goes into a landfill. When one eats an orange, the wrapper (peel) becomes compost. When one follows a raw-plant-food lifestyle, the amount of trash produced by that individual decreases to almost nothing. Test for yourself and see. Cooked food and pollution are directly related.

🔖 Benefit #2: Living food is easier on your immune system.

Swiss scientist Dr. Paul Kouchakoff discovered that if at least 50 percent of your meal consists of raw plants, then the body's reaction to digestion is much easier on the immune system.[5] Most people are activating their immune system with every single meal. This is because every single cooked meal stimulates the production of white blood cells. The body experiences this food as an attack on the immune system. Everything has to be "recoded" in order to be properly divided up and delivered throughout the body. When each meal is at least 50 percent raw, there is no such white blood cell response.

Most people don't realize that the very act of cooking food can introduce toxins, as the food's chemicals change during the heating process. In *Instinctive Nutrition,* Severen Schaeffer wrote:

> *The number of derivatives appearing at the end [of the cooking process] is extremely impressive; we are constantly discovering new ones: volatile alcohols, cetones, aldehydes, esters, ethers, nonvolatile heterocycles. The overall result is a mixture of derivatives with different chemical and biological properties: aromatic, peroxydizing, antioxidizing, toxic, some of them possibly mutagenic or carcinogenic. As an indication, at the present time in a fried potato we have identified more than 50 derivatives, most of them derivatives of pyrozenes and thiazole, but we know that in all, there are still 400 yet to be identified.*

> TIP Make sure to add a high-quality enzyme supplement to your diet. Do this regularly, with your meals and/or between meals. Enzymes will help you digest raw and cooked food, help your tissues remain young, assist you in losing weight, and help purify your body of toxins.

Benefit #3: Living food is rich in enzymes.

More than twenty years of experience have shown me that enzyme-rich foods (raw foods) and enzyme supplements (especially taken in large doses) do accelerate healing. In spite of controversies on the subject usually generated by pessimists, my experience compels me to inform you of the healing, youthening power of raw foods and enzymes.

Research shows that once food is cooked between temperatures ranging from 120 to 170°F, valuable nutrients and enzymes are destroyed. Enzymes have many important functions in the body. They break down food, assist the immune system, carry out functions of the metabolism, and help the body detoxify harmful substances. Enzymes help the body unlock nutrients. Enzymes are, in fact, vital to all life processes.

There are two classes of enzymes: metabolic and digestive. Metabolic enzymes operate in all the cells, tissues, and organs and are an essential part of every biological activity. Digestive enzymes are produced by and appear in the alimentary organs—that includes your stomach, pancreas, salivary glands, and to some degree your intestines. They help to digest carbohydrates, fats, and proteins.

Within these classes of enzymes are three main sub-categories. Amylases are enzymes that digest carbohydrates. Lipases are enzymes that digest fats. And proteases are enzymes that digest proteins.

Enzymes are small proteins. Some nutritionists mistakenly believe that enzymes are destroyed by stomach acid. However, protein cannot be broken down by hydrochloric acid in the stomach; therefore enzymes, especially plant enzymes, survive in our intestines. There they can be absorbed into our tissue system and can help us break down cooked-food particles, incompletely digested raw-food particles, as well as toxins that are caught up in our metabolism.

Enzymes are also present in their proper proportions in whole raw plant foods. These enzymes are there to assist the digestion of food. Many food enzymes are destroyed at 150°F (66°C). The dehydration of food below 104°F (40°C) keeps nearly all enzymes intact. Enzymes are heat-sensitive and therefore their loss is likely the primary reason cooked food affects us very differently from raw food. After a great deal of research, loss of enzymes was identified by Dr. Edward Howell (author of *Food Enzymes for Health and Longevity* and *Enzyme Nutrition*) as being the main reason humans age prematurely. Food-enzyme shortages sooner or later result in physical degeneration.

All our food comes naturally packed with enzymes. As long as that food is raw, natural, and intact, the enzymes themselves will help to predigest the food. For example, an apple comes complete with all the enzymes to help digest its apple self in our bodies. If we cook that apple, we remove those enzymes, and we end up having to use our own enzymes to do the job. When the digestive enzymes present in the body are insufficient, the body draws upon its reserves—the metabolic enzymes from the major and minor organs and glands—which weakens one's overall vitality. It takes ten metabolic enzymes to form one digestive enzyme!

To understand this more clearly, let's say we were on a diet of all processed food, everything is cooked, with no enzymes in anything. Our body then has to use digestive enzymes that are secreted by the pancreas, the salivary glands, and the liver. Once those digestive enzymes are depleted, the body starts drawing upon and sucking energy from the metabolic enzymes that are keeping all our cells healthy and happy. Because the draw on the metabolic enzymes is so high, we can see a cascading reaction later in life when someone goes into such an enzyme depletion that major vitality is sucked out, not in a year's time but literally in months.

One of the most enzymatically active locations that exists in Nature is to be found in the mouth of a child eating cooked food. If cooked food is eaten, the body attempts to adapt by increasing the enzyme content of the saliva in order to begin breaking down cooked food as quickly as possible. This adaptation will last as long as the body has enzyme reserves. As we age our reserves decrease; later in life they decrease significantly because we have cashed out our enzyme bank account.

The level of amylase in human saliva is approximately thirty times more abundant in the average twenty-five-year-old than the average eighty-one-year-old.[6] In contrast, whales and dolphins, who live in the perfectly balanced aquatic environment and eat only raw foods (like the rest of the two million species of this planet) have no difference in cell enzyme composition in young and old.[7]

Without the proper enzymes to break down our food, we begin to accumulate undigested materials in our system. This leads to weight gain, inflammation, stagnation, digestive distress, and fatigue. According to Dr. Bernard Jensen, the enzymes found in raw foods are codes that tell the food where to go in our bodies. For example, the enzyme erepsin that is found in cucumbers encodes for breaking down excessive protein in the kidneys.[8] Therefore cucumbers are excellent for kidney health.

Many herbs also work along enzymatic principles; thus, it is important that the herbs we consume are dried properly so that the enzymes remain intact. When we consume the powder of those dried herbs, we get a tremendous blast of enzymes in the form of food, thereby decreasing the amount of digestive enzymes we need, which decreases our draw upon metabolic enzymes. The next thing we know, we start building up our enzyme bank account—which is Dr. Howell's entire scientific point.

Every time we eat cooked food the body has to recode the food, or reidentify it, because the enzymes are missing. To recall the example about erepsin (the enzyme in cucumbers): that enzyme is like a code, and when the body sees that code it says, "I need to deliver this food to the kidneys!" If that code is missing because the food has been cooked, the body says, "Okay, we have some work to do to figure this out," and a new code has to be put on the food. What ends up happening is that the body has to send all sorts of signals and rearrange lots of different pieces. This is where mistakes can happen over time because food often gets sent to the wrong places. We can actually become malnourished because of this. This is critical, especially later on in life, because our primordial vitality or *jing* decreases, and cooked food actually drains us of increasingly more vital energy.

Raw food is a great source of enzymes. Whenever you eat raw food you are getting enzymes 100 percent directly from your food; but enzymes are also found in every cell of the human body. This is an important point. All cells have the potential to act as highly charged batteries, and each cell contains at least four thousand different enzymes. Most of us have not activated each of these four thousand enzymes within each cell because we do not have enough of the major and trace minerals in our diet. Minerals, when obtained through their whole-food complexes, especially their whole raw-food complexes, activate our cellular metabolic enzyme system. Trace elements and minerals are essential for the proper release and functioning of enzymes.

The goal is to increase the minerals and nutrition within each cell so as to activate every enzyme while simultaneously building up one's enzyme bank account with the visualized goal of increasing the electromagnetic charge in each cell, causing all cells to resonate in harmony. At the cellular level, this is truly the picture of perfect health.

Cooking or heating shifts the molecular structure of food to both slight and great degrees. These altered molecules are not the ideal building blocks for our tissues; however, since our body is always doing the best it can, if given nothing else it will incorporate these altered or cooked molecules into our bodily structure. Cooked and processed foods have an accumulative effect on our body because one's inherent enzyme bank account decreases over time in the effort to digest these enzyme-deficient foods. Once the body's enzyme bank account, or enzyme potential, is diminished beyond a certain threshold (usually having to do with the inability of the glands to produce the enzymes trypsin and chymotrypsin), the body wears out and inner vitality is lost.

Because we know that heating raw food destroys enzymes, this question often comes up: does freezing food destroy enzymes too? Here is what we found out. Freezing food destroys at least 30 percent, and up to 66 percent of enzymes. So, it is not a complete loss; enzymes remain to some degree. For example, frozen berries are still considered raw—they still have that raw "high" about them. When you eat frozen berries you don't feel your energy sag or notice any kind of depletion in the food; however, if you cook those blueberries, things change—the enzymes are lost—and they suddenly take on a slight "downer" vibe.

We know that enzymes are particularly beneficial for our health if they come from raw unfrozen plants (as opposed to animal sources or the body's endogenous enzyme stores). This is because plant enzymes initiate the most health-giving activity throughout all the various pH (acid and alkaline) conditions in the body. When we eat food we have an environment within our mouth of either an acidic pH or an alkaline pH. As the food goes down into our stomach we have an acidic pH, and as it continues into our intestine we have both acidic and alkaline levels of pH. The most desirable enzymes are those that survive all the way through our system, through both acid and alkaline pH.

When you take cabbage, put it in a crockpot, add acidophilus to it, and make raw sauerkraut, you will discover that there is a very high enzymatic activity present in the final product. This is because the good bacteria actually begins breaking down (digesting) the cabbage, and this process secretes enzymes. This is why fermented foods like sauerkraut are a very important part of a healing diet. They are rich in friendly bacteria and they supply tremendous amounts of enzymes directly into one's digestive system.

Going back to Dr. Howell's research, he presents a wealth of evidence in his books *Enzyme Nutrition* and *Food Enzymes for Health and Longevity,* demonstrating that all living creatures have a fixed enzyme bank account. He believed that we have a certain amount of enzymes, and if we wipe them out early, our life is going to end early. In his words, "Humans eating an enzyme-less diet use up a tremendous amount of their enzyme potential and lavish secretions of the pancreas and other digestive organs. The result is a shortened life span of sixty-five years or less as compared to 100 or more years. Also resulting will be illness and a lowered resistance to stresses of all types both physiological and environmental."

As opposed to Dr. Howell's view, my experience and research supports the view that by eating raw and living foods, and taking the right superfoods, superherbs, and supplements, you can actually rebuild your enzyme bank account and get your vitality back. In my opinion, nothing is fixed in this universe, and you can always get more out if you put in the intention, time, energy, and discipline.

Dr. Howell uncovered connections between enzyme deficiencies in the diet, eating cooked food, and a decrease in brain size and weight. Proper nutrition is the basis of mental power. The nutriment of the brain cells is derived from the blood corpuscles being perpetually suctioned in to nourish the brain cells by the delivery of rarified gases from the lungs. If the food stream is devoid of enzymes and impure, then the heart regulator valves become weak, the stomach disordered, the liver contaminated, the lungs congested, and the brain starved, drugged, and poisoned. When a body is in this condition, all the thoughts that germinate therein will be inappropriate to solve the problems that we are facing in our world today.

> **TIP** Add raw plant foods to your diet to increase enzyme activity. This includes raw fruits, vegetables, activated nuts, sprouted seeds, seaweeds, sprouts, flowers, wheatgrass and other grasses, herbs, superherbs, superfoods, and fermented foods. If I try to take something away from you, you are going to try to take it back. So let's simply add in the good stuff, and the bad stuff will naturally fall away when we are ready; that is the approach that works.

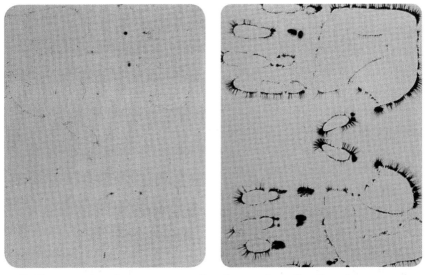

Kirlian aura imagery: the hands of a junk-
foodist on the left; the hands of a raw-foodist
on the right

Benefit #4: Living food is great for your "right brain."

There is a known connection between eating cooked food and a change in brain chemistry. This was recently confirmed by my friend Tony Wright, who broke the world record for staying awake (nearly twelve days straight). He has been a raw and living foods eater for more than fifteen years, and he discovered that eating cooked food not only changes brain size but also causes us to suffer from left-brain dominance (the left brain is the logical, analytical side of our brain). In comparison, the right brain is action-oriented and imaginative, the part that has fun and wants to go out and do new things. The right brain has been shown to not need sleep—only the left brain requires sleep, hence Tony Wright's ability to stay awake by avoiding left-brain activities.* It has been shown that living foods and enzyme-rich foods help us access our right brain and activate those energy centers.

*You can read about Tony's philosophy about the brain in his book *Left in the Dark*.

This might actually be one of the greatest discoveries in human history, because it indicates why the world is in the shape it is right now. Because the majority of the population is left-brained, we are not thinking in an imaginative way and have become too linear, too much in the box, and are therefore not really capable of solving problems at a level above the consciousness that created them. We have to get out of that place where we created the problem, which is all the cooked food we ate throughout all the history of civilization, and start getting back to the creative side of our brain by eating food that is rich in enzymes—raw and living foods.

The Benefits of Mineral-Rich Foods

When minerals are discussed I always correlate them with atoms. According to the conventionally accepted atomic theory, atoms are the basic material substances that we can understand as frozen clouds of energy of different, extremely small weights and sizes. With the Ormus minerals we also consider differing levels of materialization. (Ormus atoms in higher states of spin can actually lose mass and apparently move out of this dimension entirely.)

Early in my nutrition career, I was exposed to the importance of mineralization for health and longevity by my friend Don Weaver. Don is a soil remineralization agricultural scientist who focuses on using rock dusts and rock powders to remineralize soil and thus improve the quality of plant nutrition for humans and animals. Don gave me the book *Trace Minerals and Man* by Henry Schroeder, in which the author posits that trace minerals play a crucial role in complete nutrition and disease resistance.

The book *Minerals for the Genetic Code* by Charles Walters compiles the research of geneticist Dr. Richard Olree. As summarized by Walters on the back cover: "Radiomimetic chemicals, faltering nutrition, injury and—not least—an absence or marked imbalance of critical minerals can injure the chromosome by altering the chemistry of a gene so that it conveys misinformation (called point mutation) or by breaking the chromosome (called deletion). The cell may be killed, or it may reproduce the induced error."

Later, due to the urging of another soil mineralization scientist, Don Jansen, I read Dr. Maynard Murray's *Sea Energy Agriculture,* which precisely correlates the concept that plants become healthier and more disease-resistant when they are given access to a wider spectrum of mineral nutrients. Because the concept of longevity presupposes resistance to disease, the inference is clear: if mineralization improves the health of plants, then consuming mineral-rich foods will increase human longevity.

As reported in Valery Mamanov's book *Control for Life Extension,* raw foodist Sauren Arakelyan's work in extending the life span of chickens to world-record levels indicates that the mineralization idea is valid. Arakelyan's success can be attributed to utilizing three factors:

1. Eat mineral-rich food.

   All food eaten should be of a mineral-rich character, coming from healthy soil and water, such as organically grown vegetables, wild plants, and healthy animals.

2. Eat less food.

   Calorie restriction (the only well-known scientifically accepted method of extending life span) should be practiced. This, of course, becomes probable and possible only when mineral-rich food is eaten, because mineral-rich foods shut off hunger instincts by meeting our nutrition and mineral requirements.

3. Eat raw food.

   Raw food is more complete and nutritious. Raw foods are free of oxidative damage caused by heat and fire—the minerals in raw foods are intact and original. Interestingly, French scientist Louis Kervran's life work, summarized in the English-language book *Biological Transmutations,* indicates that oxidation reactions, reduction reactions, enzymatic activity, low-energy phenomena, and nuclear phenomena are able to change one mineral (atom) into another, thereby changing the "mineral character" of foods and substances.

The Three Categories of Minerals

As a result of compiling all the research I am aware of, along with my own laboratory studies, I have grouped the minerals that are required for excellent health, genetic integrity, and longevity into three categories: major minerals, trace minerals, Ormus minerals.

Major Minerals

These include carbon, iron, magnesium, nitrogen, phosphorus, potassium, sodium, silicon, sulfur, and good calcium. (Hydrogen and oxygen also fall into this list, even though they are not traditionally considered minerals. They are in fact atoms, and they fall into the definition of minerals I use in my writings and lectures.) Best sources of major minerals: organic raw or wild uncooked foods, organic superfoods, and organic or wild superherbs.

Trace Minerals

These include boron, chlorine, chromium, copper, fluorine, germanium, gold, iodine, manganese, molybdenum, selenium, silver, tin, vanadium, and zinc. Best sources of trace minerals: sea salt, seaweeds, or sea vegetables, organic superfoods, and organic or wild superherbs.

Ormus Minerals

These were rediscovered by David Radius Hudson around the year 1980 via his analyses of Arizona basalt rock. These minerals were known to European alchemists, Arabic alchemists, Vedic scientists, the ancient Egyptians, and the ancient Chinese. Evidence is present, though not conclusive, that civilizations in Mexico, Peru, and Bolivia were also aware of these strange mineral substances. Ormus minerals are atoms that do not fit into Mendeleev's Periodic Table of the Elements, or Walter Russell's Periodic Chart. They are typically metals in a hidden, infolded form; thus we identify them as Ormus copper, Ormus gold, etc. When oxidized or presented with specific types of high-energy environments, these Ormus elements can "pop" and become fully materialized as metals. Thus Ormus copper becomes copper, and Ormus gold becomes gold. Best sources of Ormus minerals: sea salts or sea vegetables, organic super-foods, organic or wild superherbs, and fresh spring water.

According to Hudson's research, all living things contain Ormus elements in quantities ten times greater than all trace minerals combined. Just like other minerals, certain animals and plants contain different amounts of Ormus minerals and concentrate them in different parts. The idea that has been presented by Ormus researchers is that we are not realizing our genetic potential for the use of these Ormus minerals—this means that we are not getting enough of these minerals.

Ormus minerals have a high affinity (like mother with baby) for hydrogen, spring water, salts, lava, fats/oils, polysaccharides, and silicon-bearing plants (horsetail, nettles, bamboo, etc.). It has been theorized that the nervous systems of mammals and the fast-growing annual antlers of

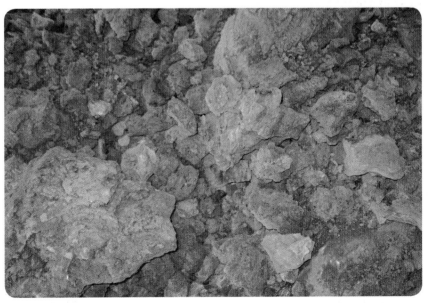

Ormus-rich volcanic rock

Cervids (deer, elk, reindeer, moose, etc.) are rich in Ormus, some of this theory being based on Hudson's research. It appears that what makes superfoods and superherbs "super" is their high fraction of Ormus minerals. Indicators continue to point to superfoods and superherbs as being critical components of a longevity strategy. Going beyond that, it appears that growing superfoods and superherbs with substances containing a high fraction of Ormus minerals (ocean water, dead sea salt, spring water, certain rock powders, biodynamic preparations, and other modalities) to increase the Ormus-bearing fraction of the constituents of those foods intuitively leads us to what may be the destiny of longevity nutrition.

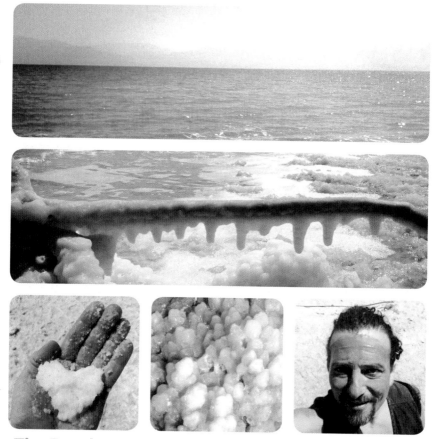

The Dead Sea: Its salt and clays contain Ormus minerals.

Ormus minerals are known to behave "consciously" or "intelligently," and they defy conventional approaches of analysis. For example, the spectroscopic signature form of mineral analysis misidentifies the Ormus minerals as aluminum, carbon, silicon iron, and/or calcium. The implication of the discovery of this mistake across the sciences is profound.

Ormus minerals are trapped more easily by alchemical phenomena (vortexing, implosion, clever use of magnets, simple chemistry tricks, etc.) and not by cutting, burning, poisoning, radiating, oxidizing, or any form of adding high-energy acids typically used by science.

A Word on Hydrogen

The most important atom or mineral for life is hydrogen. Hydrogen is the embryonic substance of the universe—it is the infant. Ormus minerals are the mother, oxygen is the father, and silicon is the grandmother or nanny who is always silently supporting and present.

Hydrogen is the basic building block of all other atoms. If we look at the word "hydrogen" closely, we see that it consists of two Greek root words, "hydro" (water) and "gen" (generator). Thus, hydrogen means generator of water.

Russian research on longevity indicates that water-carrying "heavy" hydrogen known as deuterium and tritium are radioactive, poisonous, and have an adverse effect on our longevity. Water exposed to nuclear reactions (depleted uranium, irradiated foods, nuclear power plants cooled by water, and nuclear explosions near water) becomes contaminated with deuterium and tritium. Russian research cited by Valery Mamanov indicates that periodic practices of alternate dry fasting (one day of consuming no food or water, followed by one day with only water, no food, then repeat) can reduce the presence of deuterium in the body and increase life span. In my opinion, nobody is fit to dry fast unless they are experienced with cleansing, detoxification programs, juice fasting, and water fasting.

Ormus gold may have applications for removing bad calcium via topical application. It is probable that most or all Ormus minerals have a role to play in longevity. It appears from field research and experience that Ormus gold behaves very much like DMSO (reactive liquid sulfur) in helping to soothe arthritic joint pain when applied topically. Some Ormus minerals appear to take up the same receptor sites as sulfur and silicon in our joints, and perhaps in other areas of metabolism such as the hair, skin, nails, cardiovascular system, and nervous system. Ormus gold may be involved in remineralizing teeth and bones. I have experienced the healing of a cracked broken tooth by topically dripping liquid Ormus gold on the tooth two to five times a day for several months. Additionally, Ormus gold appears to be a powerful antiviral but not an antifungal.

If you would love more information on the subject, I have written extensively on Ormus minerals in my book *Amazing Grace*.

The Benefits of Drinking Pure Water

The best sources of clean, pure waters (that are relatively free of bacteria) emanate from deep (sometimes new, sometimes ancient) volcanic aquifers and natural forest springs far away from civilization. Fresh spring water is the quintessential product of the Earth's natural hydrological cycle. Spring water captured in glass, that you bottle yourself at the source or purchase secondarily, is a great choice for drinking water. The best spring water is, of course, low in calcium and iron. You can test for the presence of calcium by boiling the water off in a pot and looking for white film residue on the pot surface.

Drinking spring water, especially fresh from the source, is one of the best ways to pull inflammation right out of our systems and de-stress our bodies. Stress is associated with over-heating, which is inflammation; because ice-cold spring water has the exact opposite type of energy (cooling), it balances us. Spring water is a natural anti-inflammatory with a high antioxidant potential.

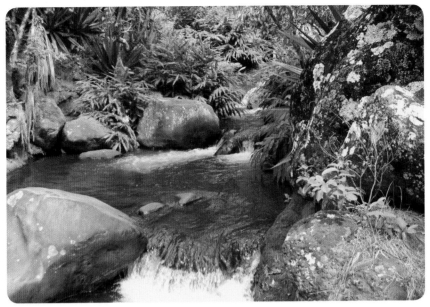

Pure, wild, spring water (Kalalau Valley, Kauai)

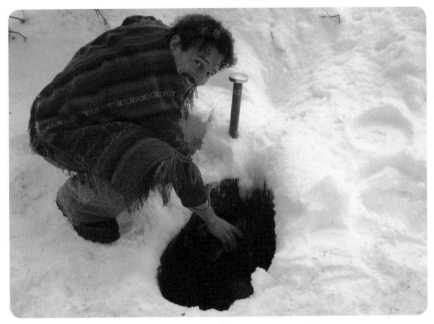

Real spring water never freezes at the source.

When we drink spring water collected fresh from the source, it typically has low surface tension (a low dyne count), and therefore it is absorbed directly into the body. The cells are able to absorb all the hydrogen ions present in the water (water = H_2O + Ormus + Silicon + Carbon), so the water barely reaches the stomach. When we drink water that feels heavy inside our body it means that the water is of a poor quality and high surface tension, as it did not directly absorb into our system.

Victor Schauberger was the first person to bring to my attention the idea that water can be "ennobled." He also taught me how all of life is about ennobling water in a dynamic interaction between the "heavens" and the Earth. I started to see that what is going on inside every tree, every plant, and every living organism is, ultimately, an ennobling of water. That organism is taking water into its own biology, its own consciousness, and is ennobling the water to reflect its view of the world. For example, a gecko's perspective of the world is clearly different than ours, and so the "consciousness" of the water gets to go through a wide range of life and collect infinite information.

When any living thing takes in water, whether a bee, a tree, or ourselves, the water gets to experience its perspective of the world. This is an interesting angle from which to approach life on Earth. When we look at water as a living thing that is having experiences just like we are, it helps us come into a relationship with water whereby we don't pollute our rivers, we don't pollute the aquifers, and we actually produce pure drinking water and spring water, consciously bottled in glass.

One of my personal goals is: "I drink the best water ever." I hold this very strongly as an ethic in my life, as water, to me, is sacred and to be respected as the most holy substance.

Dr. Masaru Emoto, whose work with water crystals has recently become very popular, wrote in his books how water immediately and literally reacts to our thoughts and intentions. I think Dr. Emoto's information is great; however, it was from Victor Schauberger that I first heard someone say that we need to go to a spring and drink the water directly from the spring source, because that is the real water that we

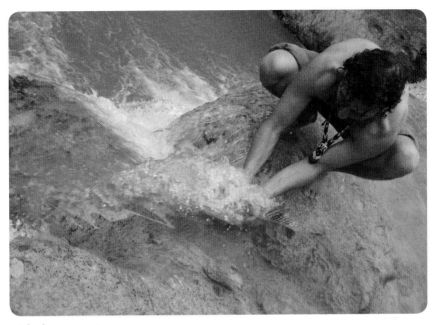

Living waters

want. If he had never said it, I would never have tried it. Eventually I did try it, and now, as a hobby, I am a wild cold-spring hunter.

At my house the water comes from a spring that is about 400 meters away. When I am not at home I am always on the lookout for fresh spring water sources to fill up at. It is such a gift to be able to drink fresh, natural water, the way the Earth produces it. When one has this kind of radiant living water in one's diet, it becomes much easier to fast and eat less in general, because the water is so deeply nourishing. See page 153 to read about the health concerns of regular tap water.

> TIP As a reminder, it is important to check the level of calcium present in your water. Boil it. The amount of scale (white film) left behind will indicate to you how much calcium is in your water.

Charging Water

Charging water means giving a "life pattern" or structure to the water at a microscopic level. The hydrogen molecules in water are closer together if the water is charged. This makes the water more polar (strongly electrical). The best ways to charge stored or dead water are as follows:

- Squeeze fresh juices into the water. Lemons or limes are excellent choices because they have incredible cleansing and mucus-dissolving properties. Citrus juice lowers the surface tension of water, thus increasing its absorbability.
- Add a blade of grass or a few green herbs and leaves to the water.
- Add some green superfood powders (you can add some honey, lo han guo syrup, yacon syrup, or stevia to sweeten up the taste).
- Add a few pinches of sea salt or Himalayan pink salt. These are some of the best choices for nonvegetable sources of salt. These salts each contain more than eighty different minerals in similar ratios as they appear in seawater. They are "raw" salts, thus they differ from coagulated table salt and most "kiln-dried" sea salts that have had their minerals oxidized away through heating.
- Add Dr. Patrick Flanagan's Crystal Energy. This product is known to lower the surface tension of water (lowers its dyne count) and increase the absorbability of the water.
- Add MSM powder crystals.
- Add TMG (betaine) powder.
- Place a crystal inside your glass of water.
- Put water in a glass jar outside under moonlight for the night (especially the full moon). Water reacts positively to moonlight.
- Run water through a magnetic vortex, water spinner/vitalizer, or vortrap (the tornado effect) to improve its quality and lower surface tension.
- Dr. Emoto has shown in his book *Messages from Water* that water responds to loving thoughts and even words written on a water bottle. Water quality seems to always reflect our actions and intentions. Try it for yourself!

> **TIP** When buying bottled water, always choose glass over plastic. Plastic leaches into the water (this is often detectable by taste) and is detrimental because it mimics estrogen hormones in our body, causing glandular imbalances and feminization in males and over-feminization in females. Obviously, select brands that are low in calcium and iron.

Well Water, Distilled Water, and Alkaline Water

Well water may be a great source of water, yet let us consider that it is being pulled up prematurely, before the water is ripe. Therefore it may actually contain too many sedimentary minerals such as iron or calcium. I recommend, for any high-calcium and/or high-iron well water sources, that they be filtered using a water softener purification system before they are bathed in or consumed.

A lot of people drink distilled water. Distilled water is not natural since Mother Nature utilizes evaporation, not distillation, to vaporize water most of the time. Distilled water is a disturbed and unnatural form of water. It is lacking in information and should be avoided. Most of the time distilled dead water that is bottled in plastic absorbs plastic.

The alkaline water (8–9+ pH) craze has become increasingly popular in recent years. Please be aware that some of the machines that produce alkaline water may have a number of challenges inherent in the way they work and the quality of water they deliver. It directly depends on how they are constructed and engineered. Therefore, please do your research before you purchase a machine. These challenges include the following:

- Alkaline water machines do not effectively soften the water, therefore they require pre-filter water softeners. Without a pre-filter water softener a wide variety of contaminants, including bad calcium and toxic chemicals found in municipal water, may enter into the final drinking-water product.

- Bad calcium (instead of pearl calcium or magnesium bicarbonate) is used to alkalize the water. Because calcium is alkaline does not automatically mean it is good for us.

- Natural cold spring water with a low total dissolved solids count (TDS count) is acidic because it is high in hydrogen (hydration potential). We want water the way that Nature presents it to us in spring water, with high levels of embryonic, rejuvenating hydrogen.

- Alkaline water usually contains more hydroxy free radicals (OH-) and increases oxidation damage to healthy tissue, thus speeding up aging.

- The actual water-structuring mechanism of the electrified platinum plates inside some of these alkalizing machines works along not-well-understood high-spin Ormus mineral physics. High-spin Ormus platinum atoms that are being sheared off the platinum plates may be the actual agent that is structuring the water. Our general understanding of this phenomenon is mostly a "shot in the dark" and we should only proceed with this technology when this area of physics is better understood.

- Many alkaline water machines lack effective pre-filters to clean up municipal tap water before alkalizing it. Municipal tap water is usually of such poor quality due to its content of low-spin elements, bad calcium, bad iron, radioactive tritium content, bad estrogens, diluted pharmaceutical drugs, and numerous other dangerous contaminants that it cannot be rejuvenated into healthy, healing, spring-like water based on our current technology.

TIP Be aware that dehydration can happen rapidly. An hour of intense exercise, or a four-hour airline flight, can cause us to lose up to a quart (liter) of water.

🍵 When and How Much Water to Drink?

We should ideally drink when our stomach is empty. Drinking water with food can dilute digestive fluids, leading to poor absorption and constipation. The best time to drink water is upon rising in the morning. Drink at least a half liter (16 fluid ounces) or more at that time. Feel free to experiment with adding several pinches of sea salt to your water to enhance the water's ability to hydrate you.

The typical recommendation to drink "eight to ten 12-ounce glasses of water" each day is excessive if one eats at least 80 percent juicy raw plant foods. But even if one eats 100 percent raw foods, drinking water each day is still very important. Straight water has flushing abilities that simply are not found in coconut water, fruits, and vegetable juices.

If one eats at least 80 percent raw foods, I recommend drinking a daily quantity of water based on the following ratio. Take one's total body weight (in pounds) and divide it by four. This number is then the number of fluid ounces of water one should drink in a day. For example, if one weighs 170 pounds and eats primarily raw plant foods, 170 divided by 4 is 42.5. A good daily intake of water for this person would be 42.5 ounces. (One fluid ounce is equivalent to approximately 30 milliliters.)

CHAPTER 2

The Essential Raw Plant Food Groups

Where to get started with raw foods? First, let's review the landscape. Listed below are the essential raw plant food groups. Shop and select from each group. Consider growing or wild-harvesting items from each food group. Add these groups or categories of foods into your daily regime!

A Note on Abundance

Let's look at this process as starting a new diet while avoiding implied limitations. This is not about deprivation—99 percent of all the food on Earth is raw plant food. Eating a natural diet is the ultimate freedom.

There is such a variety of raw plant foods on this Earth it is astonishing. Have you ever tried a black sapote, cherimoya, durian, eggfruit, elderberry, galia melon, habanero pepper, jackfruit, lemonade berry, loquat, lychee, mamey, mountain apple, pomegranate, prickly pear, saguaro cactus fruit, sapodilla, suriname cherry, or white sapote? Have you ever tried butter lettuce, drunken woman lettuce, chicory, dandelion, dinosaur kale, fennel, lamb's quarters, lemongrass, miner's lettuce, nopal cactus, sorrel, watercress, wild mustard, wild onion, or wintercress?

Obviously I have only just touched on the variety of edible plants that are out there. You could try a new fruit and vegetable every single day for the rest of your life and not even come remotely close to trying them all. There is too much abundance!

Fruits

A fruit is an edible product of a plant that contains the seed within itself for reproduction. Certainly fruits are the most enchanting of all food groups and an excellent quick source of energy. Fruits may be sweet, nonsweet, or fat-dominant. Fresh and in their raw form, they are a highly nutritious, delicious, and important food category for achieving and sustaining excellent health.

Fruits are fine sources of antioxidant color pigments and vitamin C. More and more we are seeing the truth about antioxidants: they are found within Nature's color pigments! Fruits also contain simple sugars such as glucose and fructose, which serve as fuel for the body. Simple sugars are used by each cell's power station—the mitochondria. The mitochondria create nucleotides (ATP, GTP) that, in turn, fuel the inside of the cell. Some people require more operational fuel than others, depending on their metabolism and how much they exercise (more exercise requires more fuel/fruit). The best source of carbohydrates (sugars) is organic fruits or wild fruits that contain seeds, as they contain living energy that is easily and quickly transferred into a form usable by our bodies.

Improving the quality of your carbohydrates improves the quality of your health and life. Eliminating refined sugar and white flour, then

> # TIP
> - Eat fruits that contain good, strong, viable seeds.
> - Eat fruits that are rich in minerals. Generally, the richer a fruit is in minerals, the better; this is usually detectable in the quality, flavor, texture, viability, and overall richness of the fruit.
> - Eat fruits in their perfectly ripe stage. A perfectly ripe jalapeño pepper is red. A perfectly ripe lime is yellow. A perfectly ripe eggplant is yellow.

replacing those with whole foods and natural fruits (with seeds) is the core of any sensible diet.

Sugar Content

The amount of sugar and type of fruit that I recommend consuming in the Longevity Now approach depends on the level of your health and how many infections your body is fighting.

If you are suffering from candida, cancer, severe viral outbreaks (shingles, hepatitis), or feel that your health is in a severely compromised state, I recommend that you stay away from sugar of any kind (including fruit) as much as possible, ideally avoiding sugar completely until better health is achieved. In general, unless you are heavily exercising, it is best to avoid large quantities of high-glycemic (sugar) fruits, as this can throw your body's blood-sugar levels out of balance. If you are active and don't have current infections in or on your body, you can eat more sweet fruit. If you are sedentary, select more low-sugar fruits instead (cucumber, tomato, bell pepper) and vegetables.

Great Low-Sugar Fruits

Excellent low-sugar fruits include:

- avocado (fatty fruit, excellent)
- bell pepper (not green; green peppers are harsh and unripe)
- bitter melon
- breadfruit (raw)
- cranberry
- cucumber (very healing)
- dragon fruit
- grapefruit
- jalapeño pepper
- lemon*
- lime*
- noni*
- okra (very healing for digestion)
- olives (not from a can)
- pumpkin
- serrano pepper
- sour apple
- squash
- summer squash
- tomatillo
- tomato
- zucchini

*breaks down calcification

Low-sugar, raw, high-water-content, lowfat, organic fruits—such as cucumbers, tomatoes, ripe red (not green) bell peppers, okra, etc.—help alleviate blood sugar disorders and substantially influence one's mental state, inducing a more balanced and positive demeanor with less moodiness and agitation. Nonsweet fruits are great snack foods and weight loss foods, as they contain low calories and high nutrients. Nonsweet fruits are low-stimulation foods. Eating a low-sugar diet (even low in natural sugars such as fruit, honey, etc.) creates a feeling of calmness and "lightness."

Berries—such as blueberries, raspberries, blackberries, cranberries, Incan berries, and goji berries—have a moderate sugar content but they also carry the benefit of not overstimulating the nervous system like higher-sugar fruits can. Spells of depression and mood swings are often associated with moments of low blood sugar and poor food choices. Eating mildly sweet fruits such as berries can help moderate blood sugar while avoiding the excessive release of insulin.

Fruits Can Be Excellent Fats!

Fats are the caloric bridge that carries one from a cooked-food diet to raw-food-based nutrition. Fats fill that empty space. They satiate hunger and provide plant-based raw calories. An appropriate intake of healthy fats and oils is what the body requires to function optimally.

The most digestible fats come from the oleaginous fruits (oily fruits) such as avocados, durians, and sun-ripened olives. They have a high water content and a simple structure, making them easy for the body to identify, metabolize, and assimilate.

The best fatty fruits (and their oils) include akee (a relative of the durian fruit that grows in West Africa and the West Indies), avocado, durian, and olives and their oil (stone-pressed if possible; cold-pressed is also good).

I recommend that you enjoy and experiment with eating these delicious, oily fruits, which will supply your body with the best possible form of mono-unsaturated fat and satiate cravings for cooked

Great Sugary Fruits

The best sugary fruits include the following:

- apple (breaks down calcification due to malic acid content)
- apricot
- berries of all types
- black sapote
- blackberry
- blueberry
- cacao fruit (chocolate fruit)
- cherimoya
- cherry (wild is best!)
- crab apple (breaks down calcification due to malic acid content)
- dates of all exotic types
- figs of all types (wild are best!)
- goji berry
- grapes with seeds
- Incan berries
- jackfruit
- loquat (they are close to the wild state)
- lychee
- mango
- mangosteen (the rind can be used medicinally)
- melon with seeds
- mulberry
- orange with seeds
- papaya (must be organic; all conventionally grown papayas are now genetically modified)
- passion fruit
- paw-paw
- pear (the wilder, the better)
- persimmon with seeds
- plum
- pomegranate (extremely strong fruit, resists hybridization)
- raspberry
- sapodilla
- white sapote
- all wild sweet fruits and berries

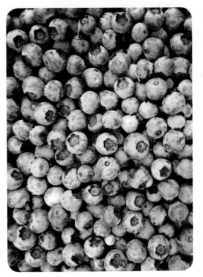

Blueberries are
The Best Ever.

and processed fatty foods. The idea that all fats/oils are bad for us is a complete hoax and a mistake. As with most anything, it is only when fat/oil is eaten in excess, especially in its cooked and therefore rancid form, that it overburdens the liver, clogs up the body, and contributes to less-than-excellent health. Listen to your body above all else and eat the balance of fat, carbohydrate, and protein that truly gives you the most energy and makes you feel the best.

The Pasteurization Scam

Be sure to drink unpasteurized fruit juices or juices in general. Flash pasteurization is a scam. Heat pasteurization destroys enzymes and therefore destroys food value. Heat pasteurizing is also an outdated technology. Adding one drop of 35 percent food-grade hydrogen peroxide will sterilize one gallon of any liquid while maintaining nutrient content. Also, recent innovations in pressure pasteurizations appear to preserve enzymes and maintain shelf stability of fresh juices.

Our paranoia about bacteria on fruits, vegetables, and nuts is completely absurd when the most contaminated foods in the world are flesh products (e.g., meat, fish, chicken). Flesh is sold directly on counters with billions of particles of bacteria on them, such as *E. coli* and salmonella. The flesh industry is so well subsidized that there is no way the government will allow a warning label to go onto that meat to alert people about bacterial infections. When we see these warnings on juices it is because juice companies are nowhere near as powerful as flesh companies, and therefore they cannot stop the regulation through lobbying and money.

Avoiding Hybrid and GMO Fruits

Hybrid foods are the result of crossed strains of a species (human-induced), and they are foods that generally will not grow or grow well in a natural environment. Seed quality and quantity are low among non-cultivated offspring, so although hybrids are created to be hardy and to yield well (among other characteristics), their descendants are not hardy in the wild. Hybrid foods and genetically modified (GMO) foods also spread weak and genetically contaminated pollen into their own species. These types of foods must be nurtured and protected by humans, or else they will be overcome by birds, insects, worms, fungi, and bacteria. As part of your longevity strategy, I recommend that you avoid hybridized and GMO foods, including seedless fruit as much as possible.

Hybrid fruit is not only unnaturally high in sugar, it is devoid of the proper mineral balance that all wild foods contain. Excessive hybrid fruit consumption leads to mineral deficiencies, dental damage, and bone density loss. Overconsumption of these foods causes the body to bring alkaline minerals from the bones into the blood to buffer the hybrid sugar, which is not completely recognized or defused by the liver and pancreas. The minerals and the sugar are then spilled off into the urine. So, over the long term, hybrid sweet fruit can overstimulate you, causing you to lose minerals.

I have noticed that hybrid foods are attacked by different forms of fungi than wild food. Hybrid foods are much more susceptible to early decay. For example, I have set seeded ruby-red grapefruits (from a fruit-foraging mission) outside on my porch to ripen alongside extremely hybridized yellow seedless grapefruits. The ruby reds (though not a wild strain) will last months out there as they ripen to perfection (citrus ripens best in the sun, on the ground). However, the yellow seedless grapefruits will be overcome by bright to dark green mold outlined by white. You will never see this type of mold attack a wild fruit.

Seedless foods are so hybridized they can no longer reproduce. The inability of hybrids to reproduce stems from a deficiency in the pro-creative cells. Seedless hybrids can lack a double set of chromosomes in their reproductive cells, and this leads to the inability to produce viable seeds.

The standard bananas we all know are hybridized foods. The black "seeds" found in the common banana are not seeds at all, but rather nonviable remnants of what should be semi-hard, pellet-size, walnut-tasting seeds.

Fruits to Be Careful With

Common hybrid fruits, grafted fruits, or fruits grown from cuttings include:

- apple (seedless or few seeds)
- banana (seedless)
- date (most varieties)
- grape/raisin (seedless)
- pineapple (seedless)
- citrus fruit (seedless)
- persimmon (seedless)
- watermelon (seedless)
- kiwi (their black seeds are not viable)

These foods are bred for certain genetic traits including sweetness, shelf life, climate hardiness, and durability instead of nutrition. Grafting has allowed excessively sugary fruit varieties to be crossed with hardier types of the same fruit tree. These weak strains are essentially artificial and loaded with sugar (however, if these foods have viable seeds they are okay, which indicates the hybridization has not led to loss in survivability). Hybrid sugars (excessive levels of fructose, glucose, and sucrose) are the favorite foods of all decomposing organisms, from nanobacteria to viruses to candida to cancer cells.

The solution to hybridized food? Grow your own food from heirloom seeds. Contact heirloom seed resources locally or through the internet and let the strongest survive. Nearly all seeds, edible plant varieties, and fruit trees are hybridized in various degrees; however, the key distinctions are maximum survivability and lower sugar content. Also, whenever possible, eat wild plants and fruits. Wild fruit is high in minerals, and always lower in sugar than commercial, chemical-laden, hybrid fruit.

Common fruits that are close to the wild state and extremely viable when grown from seed include: avocado, cacao, cherimoya, crab apple, guava, heavily seeded citrus fruit, jackfruit, mango, most melon varieties, most pepper or chili varieties, papaya, peach, tomato, tomatillo, white sapote, and others.

Fruit enthusiasts should seek out perfectly ripe fruit. Picked fresh, "from the tree right to me," is an unrivaled experience.

> TIP In order to get the most out of your fruit, eat all the way to the edge of the rind or eat the rind (with fruits that contain edible rinds) to get the maximum nutrition available. Melons contain most of their vitamins and mineral salts near the edge of the rind.

Green Leafy Vegetables

Western civilization's diet consists mostly of roots, seeds, and animal muscles. This is translated into a burger (the bun is seeds, the meat is a muscle) and french fries (roots). This is translated into a fancy steak (muscle), potato (root), and peas (seeds). The standard rice and beans dish is nothing more than seeds (acid-forming). Civilization's acid-forming root, seed, muscle diet is balanced by alkaline green vegetables and their juices.

Green leafy vegetables are probably the most important group of foods because they are so overlooked. Green leaves are the best consistent sources of alkaline minerals (good calcium, magnesium), are an excellent source of fiber, have many calming antistress properties, and are the best source of chlorophyll. Chlorophyll is a blood-builder and one of Nature's greatest healers. It is the pigment in plants within which photosynthesis takes place. It absorbs the vibrant sun energy and transforms it into plant energy. This energy is transferred directly to you when you eat chlorophyll-rich foods such as green-leafed vegetables. Eating green leafy food is a transfusion of sun energy to blood energy in the cardiovascular system. One could say chlorophyll is the blood of plants, just as hemoglobin is the blood of the human body. The difference between the two molecules is that chlorophyll is centered on magnesium, while hemoglobin is centered on iron.

Fresh juices filled with chlorophyll from green leafy foods (such as celery, parsley, spinach, kale, broccoli, etc.) and fruits (such as apples or pears to sweeten) are a wonderful way to begin and maintain a beautiful body for a lifetime. Our best and most reliable source of fiber, green leaves are transformed into the structure of the body. Be they green herbs or big leafy vegetables such as kale, green leaves should be an important part of the diet.

The Best Green Leafy Vegetables

- arugula
- bok choy
- celery (an excellent source of sodium)
- cilantro
- crane's bill
- collards
- dandelion
- dark green cabbage
- endive
- fennel (wild)
- kale (especially dinosaur kale)
- lamb's quarters (goosefoot)
- lettuce (all types)
- malva and mallow
- mustard (wild)
- parsley
- purslane
- spinach
- spring onion (green)
- sunflower greens
- radish leaves

All the building blocks necessary to construct and energize your body are present in plants. Out of the twenty-two amino acids found in the body, eight must be derived from food/bacteria (these latter are called "essential amino acids"). The body is capable of recycling and manufacturing the other fourteen amino acids. All eight essential amino acids are in abundance in raw plant foods, especially in green leaves and superfoods (spirulina, blue-green algae, bee pollen, maca, goji berries, and hemp seeds, to name a few).

Green-leafed vegetables are a great source of iron, with dandelion, parsley, and spinach being particularly high in good iron. Other than red meat and the blood of animals, greens along with spirulina, cacao, seaweeds, and tubers in the sunflower family of plants (Jerusalem artichoke, yacon) heal anemia. Other sources of iron include red-colored fruits such as cherries, berries, pomegranates, and red-flesh figs.

Green-leafed vegetables are always the best source of heavy alkaline minerals: calcium, magnesium, iron, etc. The alkaline minerals in greens balance the acid-forming minerals (sulfur, chlorine, and phosphorus) found in avocados, nuts, seeds, onions, garlic, flesh products, etc.

Green-leafy vegetation is also an excellent detoxifier of the liver, especially wild greens. The calcium, magnesium, and iron in deep green and wild green vegetation bind with heavy metals, chemicals, and chemical drugs and allow the body to wash them out as salts through the urine.

> **TIP** The habit of drinking fresh vegetable juices and blended green drinks daily is one of the fastest ways to transform your body and succeed in achieving Longevity Now. Remember, to utilize the nutrients in food, that food must first be turned into a liquid. Blending and juicing quickens the digestive process and delivers nutrients more swiftly to your bloodstream.

Oxalic Acid Content and Kidney Health

If green-leafed vegetables that are high in oxalic acid, such as beet greens, chard, lamb's quarters, rhubarb, and spinach, are excessively eaten raw or cooked (cooking does not destroy oxalic acid), then the oxalic acid can contribute to the accumulation of calcium oxalates in the body—especially the kidneys. This interferes with iron absorption, and eventually (if eaten in large quantities over a long period of time) leads to stone formations in the kidneys. Some people are devoid of the appropriate probiotic bacteria to digest oxalates and are, in addition, sensitive to oxalates; these folks should avoid oxalate-rich foods. If oxalic foods are eaten raw in small quantities, the oxalates in these vegetables are normally metabolized properly by the body and are actually good for the intestines. If one feels kidney pains three to six hours after eating oxalate-rich foods (even in the raw state), then they should be avoided.

Oxalic Acid Content of Selected Vegetables

Vegetable	Oxalic acid content (g per 100g)	Vegetable	Oxalic acid content (g per 100g)
parsley	1.70	eggplant	0.19
chives	1.48	cauliflower	0.15
purslane	1.31	asparagus	0.13
cassava	1.26	endive	0.11
amaranth	1.09	cabbage	0.10
spinach	0.97	chaga[†]	0.10
beet leaves	0.61	okra	0.05
carrot	0.50	onion	0.05
radish	0.48	pea	0.05
collards	0.45	potato	0.05
beans, snap	0.36	tomato	0.05
brussel sprouts	0.36	turnip greens	0.05
garlic	0.36	parsnip	0.04
lettuce	0.33	pepper	0.04
watercress	0.31	rutabaga	0.03
cacao	0.15–0.50*	cucumbers	0.02
sweet potato	0.24	kale	0.02
chicory	0.21	squash	0.02
turnip	0.21	coriander	0.01
broccoli	0.19	corn, sweet	0.01
celery	0.19		

*See page 36 of *Naked Chocolate,* by David Wolfe

[†]According to research done by scientist Ramiz Saad at Maxxam Analytics (Toronto, Canada)

This table was originally published in *Agriculture Handbook* no. 8–11, "Vegetables and Vegetable Products," 1984. All data from www.ars.usda.gov/Services/docs .htm?docid=9444, except where noted.

If one is dealing with calcium oxalate stones, acidic vitamin C (which is effective against calcium phosphate stones and magnesium ammonium phosphate [struvite] stones) will not be effective. Andrew Saul, in his book *Doctor Yourself,* recommends: taking B vitamins twice a day, at least 400 mg of magnesium daily, as well as buffered vitamin C (non-acidic ascorbate vitamin C).

TIP Root vegetables (garlic, onion, burdock, radish, etc.) typically have antifungal properties and are great for neurological health. Also, a traditional folk treatment for uncommonly painful kidney stones is to eat and juice radishes—especially black radishes. Three radish-filled vegetable juices a day are recommended when trying to eliminate kidney stones.

Mixing Fruits and Vegetables

If sweet fruits are eaten with cooked or steamed nonstarchy vegetables (asparagus, cauliflower, broccoli), the fruit should be eaten first. Sweet fruits should otherwise not be mixed with cooked or dehydrated foods due to the potential for fermentation and gas.

Sweet fruits may be mixed together and blended with green-leafy vegetables in order to create green smoothies. Watch for banana in these drinks as banana is starchier than most sweet fruits, ferments at a different rate, and could cause digestive disturbances. You may choose to remove bananas from your green fruit smoothies.

Low-sugar fruits and raw cruciferous vegetables may be eaten together (e.g., okra and cauliflower; cucumber and broccoli). Also, different types of low-sugar fruits may be mixed together (e.g., cucumbers, ripe bell peppers, and tomatoes).

Nuts

Nuts contain numerous oils and phytochemicals that protect the body against free-radical damage and physical degeneration. They are rich in the minerals phosphorus, magnesium, boron, zinc, and manganese, all of which are essential for bone health. All nuts are a good source of the antioxidant vitamin E, copper, folic acid, and the amino acid arginine, which is a secretagogue (human growth hormone precursor). Many nuts contain tryptophan, a compound that stimulates serotonin in the brain, which boosts relaxation. The fats in nuts are concentrates of anti-oxidant hydrogen. Nuts are rich in longevity-enhancing unsaturated fatty acids, especially in the form of the monounsaturated oleic and palmitoleic acids. They also contain polyphenols, a type of antioxidant compound found to be beneficial in reducing oxidative stress in the body. Nuts are rich in soluble fiber.

Nuts help moderate blood sugar (they contain no sweet sugars). When eaten in moderation, nuts have been found to be helpful in satisfying appetite. It is easy to overeat nuts, especially if you purchase them unshelled. Quantities should be kept to less than 2.0 pounds (0.9 kg) of nuts per week. Remember: if you eat too many nuts you will end up going nuts! It is recommended to rest one's body from nuts every couple of months for a week or two (sometimes several months). Nuts are rich in antidigestive factors (enzyme blockers such as phytic acid) and therefore should not be eaten consistently; these antidigestive factors are minimized by soaking nuts in pure water for six to twenty-four hours and then eating or preparing them through various strategies such as cooking or dehydration. Also, nuts contain high levels of arginine (which is a beneficial amino acid); yet if arginine-containing foods are not properly balanced with lysine (an essential amino acid from bee products, raw dairy products, pea protein, deer antler velvet, or L-lysine supplements), this can make one susceptible to infections.

Contrary to popular opinion, nuts are a fat-dominant food, not a protein-dominant food. Because nuts are so concentrated, they should always be eaten with or just before a large meal of green leafy vegetables and/or green superfoods.

Tree nuts are also potentially allergy instigating and mucus forming. If you eat too many nuts, you may find that your throat or inner ears become itchy and/or clear mucus flows from your nose. This is because nuts could be causing an allergy and are acid-forming in the body. A mucous discharge is a way for the body to dispel allergens and some acid-forming minerals to create a more alkaline internal environment. Sea salt can combat the allergens in nuts. Eating alkaline-forming green leaves counterbalances the acid-forming elements in nuts, thereby diminishing/eliminating mucous discharge.

The Best Raw Organic Nuts Ever

- almond
- brazil nut (they are always wild foods)
- cashew
- hazelnut
- macadamia nut
- pecan
- pili nut
- pine nut
- pistachio
- sacha inchi
- walnut

Raw nuts are a delicious, quick, and easy snack that you can add into your diet any time of the day. It doesn't take much effort to switch over from roasted-salted nuts to raw nuts, and you may even find that you prefer the noncooked taste and/or prefer preparing the nuts yourself! Try eating nuts on their own with a dash of sea salt, throwing them into salads, making homemade nut milks, adding to superfood smoothies, soaking and dehydrating (for added crunch), and creating your own trail mix by combining nuts with goji berries, cacao nibs, Incan berries, mulberries, hemp seeds, sunflower seeds, pumpkin seeds, coconut flakes, and whatever else you desire!

🍃 Soaking Nuts for Maximum Nutrition

Although raw nuts are an excellent choice to eat out of the bag, if you have weak digestion or eat too many at once, they can be somewhat difficult to digest and a strain on the pancreas and liver. This appears to be at least partially due to the enzyme inhibitor phytic acid, which is Nature's way to ensure dormancy before sprouting. To neutralize this acid and gain the maximum nutritional benefit and digestibility from nuts, it is best to soak or sprout them in water before eating (as previously mentioned). Doing so stimulates the process of germination, releasing the vitamin C content and increasing vitamin B content and carotenes (precursors of vitamin A).

Soaking nuts also breaks down into simpler sugars the complex sugars and starch responsible for intestinal gas. Almonds and walnuts require a soaking time of between 12 and 24 hours. Pecans and cashews require only 6 to 12 hours. Specific soaking times for different nuts can

---

The Doctrine of Signatures *Revealed* in Walnuts

In *New Foods Encyclopedia,* Rebecca Wood wrote:

> *The thin, outer green husk, which is removed before the walnuts are marketed, is likened to the scalp. The walnut's hard shell is like a skull. The thin envelope inside, with its paper-like partitions between the two halves of the nut, is like the membrane. The convoluted nut itself represents the human brain's two hemispheres.*

Walnuts obviously look like brains. They are rich in antioxidants, vitamin E, vitamin B6, linoleic acid (omega-6 fatty acids), and in the case of freshly cracked walnuts also rich in alpha-linoleic acid (omega-3 fatty acids). Walnuts nourish the nervous system, which is directly related to the health, happiness, and effectiveness of the brain. (For more information on how to medicinally use the walnut fruit (black walnut hull) see the section on Triple Herbal Treasures on page 242.)

be found online, but the general rule is to soak them to the point of being slightly soft. Never soak any nut for longer than two days or it will go rancid.

Once they have finished soaking and are softened, rinse the nuts in water and add them directly to a superfood-superherb smoothie or some other blended recipe. Alternatively, you can dehydrate them at 115°F or less, or dry them in the sun. For a real treat, season with your favorite sea salt and/or herbs and spices. Be sure to fully dehydrate nuts before storing them.

Brazil Nuts

Brazil nut trees *(Bertholletia excelsa)* are a powerful, enormous evergreen species that is indigenous to the Amazon jungle. Brazil nut trees are not cultivated—they grow wild. Attempts at domestication have been unsuccessful. Because they are a wild food, they still have all their original wild vigor intact. These nuts have a rich, creamy flavor. They make a fantastic, healing nut milk.

Brazil nuts contain sulfur-bearing amino acids (methionine and cysteine), giving them strength-building, liver-supporting, and tissue-repairing properties. They are best known for being the number-one plant source of the mineral selenium. Rumors of Brazil nuts' selenium concentration vary widely. Some say their selenium content is not true; others say that Brazil nuts contain up to 2,500 times as much selenium as any other nut. My review of the science indicates that Brazil nuts are a reliable source of selenium, yet not all Brazil nut samples are rich in selenium; they vary because they are a natural wild food. Selenium is a powerful antioxidant that has been proven to protect against thyroid disorders, viruses, and cancer. Only three of these nuts a day may provide one with enough selenium to affect the thyroid.

Like all nuts, Brazil nuts are an excellent source of healthy oils, protein, and fiber.

Hazelnuts

Hazelnuts (*Corylus americana, Corylus avellana, Corylus* spp.) are nutritional powerhouses, exhibiting the highest folate content of any tree nut. This essential nutrient, also known as vitamin B9, has been studied for its positive effect on the cardiovascular system, and it is especially important for pregnant women because it helps to reduce the incidence of neural tube birth defects. The folate in hazelnuts may also help lift depression.

In addition, hazelnuts have the highest proanthocyanidin content of all tree nuts. These healing antioxidant compounds concentrated in plants have been studied for their ability to reduce blood clotting. Proanthocyanidin together with the high folate content may provide a powerful boost to our cardiovascular health. In addition, proanthocyanidins help to lower the risk of urinary tract infections. All these potential health benefits combine with a satisfying crunch and a smooth taste to make raw hazelnuts one of the best snacks ever!

The Best Raw Not-Milk Ever in Five Minutes or Less!

1 cup almonds (or Brazil nuts, hazelnuts, hemp seeds, cashews, etc.)

3 cups spring water

1 medjool date *or* 1 tbsp sweetener of your choice (raw honey, maple syrup, birch syrup; or stevia or another nonglycemic "sweetener")

½ vanilla bean (optional)

Place nuts and water in a blender and blend on high speed until nuts are completely broken and nut milk is created. If you want a vanilla flavor, add half a vanilla bean into the blender with the nuts and water. Strain the contents of the blender through a fine sieve or nut milk bag into a bowl or jug. You can save the leftover pulp to add to a dessert recipe, or compost.

Rinse blender and add back the strained nut milk. Add sweetener and blend. (Note: For a creamier, richer flavor, you can include a teaspoon-sized scraping of coconut butter when adding in the sweetener.) Taste for sweetness and add more if desired.

Seeds

Seeds contain explosive phosphoric compounds that create the potential for the quick growth of a young plant. All seeds are acidic in nature, with some being less acidic than others.

In general, seeds are more digestible than nuts. Even so, if they are not eaten fresh from below the plant or tree, you still might consider soaking seeds in water and/or sprouting them for 3 to 12 hours to disarm their phytic acid and enzyme inhibitors. Enzyme inhibitors keep nuts and seeds in their dormant state until conditions are right for growth. If eaten in the dormant state without being activated by soaking (to help with digestion), seeds can, in those with compromised digestion, burden the pancreas and sit "heavy" in the stomach.

Soaking nuts and seeds makes them more alkaline. However, they cannot be classified as truly alkaline until they sprout and grow green leaves.

Eating seeds in moderation with green-leafed vegetables and herbs will prevent excessive acidity. A strong digestive tract, strengthened by months and years of clean eating, should be capable of digesting calorically valuable nuts and seeds with little difficulty.

The best seeds are those that contain a reasonable ratio of fat to protein. A good edible seed should contain no more protein than 2 parts fat to 1 part protein (2:1 ratio). These include chia, hemp, pumpkin, sesame (used to make tahini), sunflower, poppy, and especially young coconut (a coconut is actually a seed).

The Best Seeds Ever

- chia seed
- coconut butter/oil (see super-foods section)
- flax seed (a complete protein, yet controversial for their phytoestrogenic and cadmium content)
- hemp seed and hemp butter (complete protein)
- milk thistle seed (excellent for the liver—try added to salads, or as a seed milk blended with water and then strained)
- pumpkin seed or raw pumpkin seed butter
- quinoa (great nutritious seed that could be sprouted, yet in my opinion, should be cooked)*
- seed oil (cold-pressed)
- sesame seed or raw black tahini
- sunflower seed
- young coconut

*Careful for those sensitive to oxalic acid; quinoa contains oxalic acid.

The seeds that we call "grains" and "legumes" are protein-dominant, not fat-dominant.

Raw legume sprouts, such as mung beans, kidney beans, lentils, and soybeans, can drain the body of water because they carry subtle toxins. This is why we have traditionally cooked legumes; cooked and then fermented them (e.g., soy products); or made extracts of them (e.g., mucuna powder). If legumes are eaten, nutritionally the best legumes are wild jungle peanuts. Peanuts are loaded with niacin (vitamin B3), which assists in mental wellness and detoxification of the brain. Peanuts also have a higher ratio of fat to protein than other legumes.

Hemp Seeds

Hemp *(Cannabis sativa)* is an extremely adaptable plant believed to have originated in Central Asia. Although usually a meter or two in height at full growth, hemp can exceed a height of five meters!

Hemp is a tough plant. It can be grown in practically any ecosystem, in any part of the world. Hemp does not require any of the pesticides

The Problem with Soy and Many Grains

Because soybeans are such hybridized foods (so far out of the natural wild state), and because most are genetically modified (more than 90 percent of the soybeans grown in North America), I do not endorse them or products made primarily from them, such as soy milk, tempeh, soy cheese, soy burgers, etc.

Research offered by Mary Enig (a nutritionist representing the Weston A. Price Foundation's unconventional view on the importance of saturated and other types of fats and oils in the diet) indicates that more than two servings of soy per week can influence hormone metabolism. Soy is known to be thyroid-suppressive, meaning it can cause glandular imbalances and make hypothyroidism worse.

Grains (especially hybridized, weak seeds) do not metabolize cleanly when cooked. Cooked grains, and to some degree sprouted grains such as oats, rice, and wheatberries, may leave behind a gummy protein residue (e.g., gluten in wheat) that will cause digestive irritation if overeaten over a long period of time. Wheat today contains too many exorphins and gliadins, which act as opiates in the body, causing addictions.[1]

If one enjoys eating grains, they may be eaten uncooked and unsprouted in their hard, natural state in the way that the Roman soldiers ate them. Use ancient grains, not present-day hybrid grains such as wheat. After a few moments of chewing, they soften and become quite edible. Raw grains mix well with grasses and wild greens. Be careful, as grains eaten in this state contain amylase inhibitors that typically create digestive distress if any sweet food (e.g., fruit) is eaten within several hours following a raw grain meal.

If one is to sprout or cook grains, the best ones are quinoa and millet (not true grains). They have a higher ratio of fat to protein than other grains, although they are still protein-dominant. Quinoa and millet are also closer to the wild state than most domesticated foods (meaning they will revert to their wild state very quickly to survive outside a farmer's fence line).

or herbicides that are used to keep weak plants alive. Only eight out of nearly a hundred known common crop pests may cause problems for hemp, and these can be dealt with by natural means. Hemp also naturally suppresses weeds, due to its rapid growth and the development of a canopy. On top of all of this, the hemp plant produces a superfood as a seed.

How to Eat Hemp Seeds

Hemp seeds are great eaten alone as a snack. They also can be sprinkled on salads, blended to add richness and flavor to superfood smoothies and salad dressings, and can be easily added to fresh juices and raw chocolate (cacao) confections too. Hemp seeds are richer in protein and more filling than most salad seeds such as sunflower and poppy seeds.

Whole unhulled hemp seeds may be soaked in water, if desired, to lower enzyme inhibitors typically found in seeds. They can then be sprouted, deshelled, and eaten (use a mortar and pestle to crush the slightly soaked hemp seeds, then use a metal strainer to separate away the shell particles), or the hemp seeds may be crushed into a milk, strained, and drunk. I personally enjoy them both ways.

For an excellent book of healthful hemp recipes, check out *The Galaxy Global Eatery Hemp Cookbook.*

The Nutritional Power of Hemp Seeds

The hemp seed is a complete protein source, and the oil from hemp seeds has the highest percentage of essential fatty acids of nearly any seed on Earth. Hemp is one of very few plants to contain significant amounts of omega-6 (linoleic acid and GLA) and omega-3 (ALA). The oil fraction of the overall hemp seed normally contains about 80 percent of these essential polyunsaturated fatty acids, with omega-6 and omega-3 in the ideal ratios of approximately 3:1 or 4:1. The specific, average, perfect ratio of omega-6 to omega-3 is 3.38, closely approximating the 3:1 ratio recommended by America's leading dietary fat and oil expert Udo Erasmus, and the 4:1 average ratio recommended by the World Health Organization (WHO), Sweden, and Japan for the human diet.

TIP Consuming hemp seed with raw organic coconut oil is recommended, since coconut oil appears to increase the effectiveness of the omega-3 fatty acids in hemp seeds.

Hemp seed is the only known food (other than chia seed) to contain this ideal ratio. Fish oil, krill oil, algae oil, and flax seed oil are rich in omega-3, but not omega-6. Almost all the commonly consumed nuts and seeds are rich in omega-6, but not omega-3.

As a point of interest, the omega-3 content of hemp seed increases when the plant is grown in the higher latitudes of the northern and southern hemispheres. The cooler the climate, the higher the human need for polyunsaturated fatty acids, especially omega-3s, which are well-represented in not only hemp seed but also in cold-water fish, marine phytoplankton, krill, flax seeds, walnuts, noni seeds, sacha inchi, blue-green algae, and many other interesting sources. Omega-3 fatty acids also protect us from overexposure to the sun, which occurs in the extreme northern or southern hemispheres in the summer due to the longer days.

Hemp seed, like spirulina, contains the super anti-inflammatory essential fatty acid known as gamma linolenic acid (GLA), which has been shown to inhibit the formation of inflammatory prostaglandins (short-lived hormones) and fatty arachidonate metabolites of digestion. GLA is also known to help balance hormones. This means that hemp seed may positively improve premenstrual syndrome (PMS) symptoms including mood swings. A deficiency of GLA has been shown to cause women to become oversensitive to their own prolactin hormone, causing breast pain.*

Hemp seed typically contains more than twenty trace minerals. Hemp seed naturally sprouts late in the season (during the autumn),

*For more on prolactin hormone, read Dr. Sara Gottfried's *The Hormone Cure.*

lowering its phytic acid content and increasing enzymes, making the seed even more digestible. Hemp seed is exceedingly easy to thresh (extricate from the plant's grip), making it extraordinarily useful to non-machine agriculture. Hemp seed's essential fatty acid and protein profile provides a healthy alternative to fish, which is becoming more inedible with rising mercury and PCB contamination. Hemp seed is considered by leading researchers and medical doctors to be one of the most nutritious food sources on the planet. The hardiness and nutritional power of the hemp seed could significantly address the planet's protein needs and starvation problems.

As our exposure levels to artificial chemicals, pesticides, chem trails, and radioactive materials continue to increase, more and more people are becoming interested in eating low on the food chain, as opposed to eating conventional animal products such as meat, large ocean fish, crustaceans, and conventional dairy that are high on the food chain where toxins and calcium-forming organisms accumulate. This means eating more and more plants.

It's becoming harder to ignore the side effects of eating animals, such as excessive calcification, increased risk of every major disease, and weight gain; the increasingly poor quality and taste of the flesh foods; and the artificial chemicals (pesticides, injected hormones, animal vaccinations, etc.). As a result, millions of people are seeking refuge in a more humane and sustainable diet. This means vegetarian, vegan, and raw-food sources of protein and fat. One of the best sources of plant protein and fat is found in hemp seed.

In terms of its nutrient content, shelled hemp seed is 35 percent protein, 47 percent fat, and 12 percent carbohydrate.

Hemp seeds contain all the essential amino acids and essential fatty acids necessary to maintain healthy human life. No other single plant source has the essential amino acids in such an easily digestible form or possesses the essential fatty acids in as perfect a ratio to meet human nutritional needs.

Packed with 33 to 37 percent pure digestible protein, raw hemp seeds with all their original life-force energy and enzymes intact are one of

The Importance of Essential Fatty Acids

Essential fatty acids (EFAs), found in high doses in hemp seed, are considered "essential" because our body does not manufacture them independently, nor can they be efficiently created from other fats or oils in our diet. The presence of essential fatty acids in our diet is now considered a critical aspect of maintaining great health for a lifetime.

Essential omega 3 fatty acids are powerful antioxidants that protect our skin from excessive sun exposure. They also play an important role in improving our immune system, due to their commonly noted anti-inflammatory properties. They help us burn excess fat by delivering easily available, easily digestible energy. They help to carry and remove toxins from the skin, intestinal tract, kidneys, and lungs. Omega 3 fatty acids nourish and feed the brain and eyes, which are made up of a large fraction of omega-3 fatty acids. They also lubricate our cardiovascular system, reducing the threat of heart disease and stroke.

Nature's richest sources of complete protein. Only plankton and algae, such as spirulina and AFA blue-green algae, exceed hemp in protein.

Approximately 47 percent of each hemp seed is composed of "good fats," with an ideal balance of omega-3 (alpha-linoleic acid) and omega-6 essential fatty acids (linolenic acid and gamma linolenic acid). Hemp seed is also an outstanding source of monounsaturated omega-9 fatty acids, which are considered a healthy energy source and a quality beautifying oil.

The carbohydrate content of shelled hemp seed is 11.5 percent and its sugar content is 2 percent. Of the shelled hemp seed carbohydrate, 6 percent is in the form of fiber. The fiber content of hemp seed flour is the highest of all commercially grown seeds. In addition to containing the basic human nutrient groups, hemp seeds have a high content of vitamin E (three times higher than flax) in the form of alpha-, beta-, gamma-, and delta-tocopherol and alpha-tocotrienols.

Hemp seed is a good source of brain-building, liver-supporting lecithin, a lipid substance (fat-oil) composed primarily of choline and inositol. It is found in all living cells as a major component of cell membranes. The term "lecithin" is derived from the Greek word "lekithos," meaning "egg," as lecithin was first discovered in eggs.

Hemp seed is one of the few seeds that contains chlorophyll. Present inside each hemp seed are infant green leaves that will eventually open and grow as the seed sprouts.

The THC found in various concentrations in the hemp genus is now well known to be medicinally useful to individuals with chronic pain and nausea, such as cancer patients. THC-rich hemp also is supportive of helping those with glaucoma[2] (as it relaxes eye tension/pressure) and multiple sclerosis[3] (as it relaxes stiff and spastic muscles).

Hemp seed, unlike commonly available animal protein, is a pure, raw source of complete protein. It never needs to be cooked to kill bacteria, so all its vital components remain intact. In addition, hemp seed protein can be more readily absorbed than animal protein because it can be easily blended into water, beverages, smoothies, shakes, salad dressings, etc., without coagulation or heat. Hemp seed, like chia, is easy on the digestive system.

Hemp seed protein delivers a balanced array of eighteen amino acids. An important aspect of hemp seed protein is a high content of arginine (123 mg/g protein) and histidine (27 mg/g protein), both of which are important for growth during childhood; and also a high content of the sulfur-containing amino acids methionine (23 mg/g protein) and cysteine (16 mg/g protein), which are needed for proper enzyme formation. Sulfur-bearing amino acids help the liver and nervous system detoxify poisons. They also improve the immune system, as well as one's physical strength, flexibility, agility, complexion, luster of hair, and speed of healing. They support the functionality of the liver and pancreas.

Hemp Seeds and Immunity

Edestin is a plant globulin, which are simple globular proteins constructed entirely from amino acids. Nearly all antibodies, enzymes, hormones,

The Importance of Healthy Proteins

Amino acids are chemical units of "building blocks" that make up protein. Protein builds muscles, ligaments, tendons, organs, glands, nails, hair, body fluids, and nearly all aspects of microscopic cellular machinery. Protein is essential to the growth of bones. Proteins themselves can act as neurotransmitters or precursors to neurotransmitters, enabling all our cells to receive and transmit messages. Next to water, protein makes up the greatest portion of the body's weight. Protein is not just useful for building muscle and strength, it is also useful for endurance, balanced blood sugar, balanced brain chemistry, neurological health, rapid healing, building strong bones, detoxification, and nearly every other aspect of healthy living.

The challenge we face is that "high-protein" animal foods are becoming more and more difficult to obtain. High-protein wild game is rarer and rarer, and factory-farmed beef, chicken, and fish are lower in protein and higher in fat and toxins. Factory animal farming is environmentally, emotionally, and psychologically dysfunctional, the impact of which is making us all aware that we must move away from toxic and inhumane sources of protein.

hemoglobin molecules, and fibrogin (which converts to the blood-clotting agent fibrin) are globular proteins and can be constructed out of edestin.

Of the fraction of the hemp seed that is protein, 65+ percent consists of globular edestin. This is the highest concentration found in the plant kingdom. The word "edestin" comes from the Greek word *edestos,* which means "edible." Edestin is considered by many scientists to be the most edible and easily digestible form of protein in the food chain. The other 35 percent of the protein in hemp is albumin, which is also considered one of the more easily digested forms. Edestin and albumin are "soft" broad-spectrum proteins that are hypoallergenic (low in allergy-forming reactions within the population). Many people are allergic to common high-protein foods such as whey and soy.

Globulins are divided into three classes: alpha, beta, and gamma globulins. Alpha and beta globulins are super transporters that carry protein and information from one part of the body to another via the blood. They cart the raw materials required to build new tissues as well as replace injured tissues. Gamma globulins work on the immune system and are divided into five classes of antibodies called immunoglobulins. All are formed to combat specific cell-invading microbes. These globulins are responsible for both the natural and acquired immunity that a person has to fight against foreign microbes. They are essential to a healthy immune system.

Gamma globulins comprise the first line of defense against infection. They are antibodies programmed by white blood cells and replicated by white blood cell clones known as plasma cells. These gamma globulin antibodies destroy antigens (microbes) such as viruses, bacteria, toxic fungi, and cancer cells, as well as toxins, dead tissue, and internal waste debris. Antibodies are custom-designed to neutralize or disintegrate only one specific type of antigen. The antibodies circulate in the lymph fluid and the blood (sometimes for years) awaiting near-contact with the antigen they are made to destroy. Once they come within the vicinity of the antigen, the antibody initiates the release of a cascade of corrosive enzymes that pulverize the antigen surface.

One white blood cell can give birth to hundreds of clone plasma cells in just a few days. A mature plasma cell produces about two thousand antibodies every second during its few days of life. The body's ability to resist and recover from illness depends upon how rapidly it can produce massive amounts of antibodies to fend off the initial attack. This is how we develop and acquire immunity. If the globulin protein starting material is in short supply, then nutrient transport is impaired and the army of antibodies may be too small to prevent the symptoms of sickness from setting in.

Hemp seed is the world's best source of globulin-building materials—edestin. Eating hemp seeds will ensure that the immune system has the reservoir of globulin resources necessary to transport raw materials and support the immune system and immune response.

Chia Seeds

Chia seeds *(Salvia hispanica)* are an indigenous Native American staple food. Historically, chia seeds were considered to be nearly as important as corn to many Native American tribes. Chia seeds are an excellent source of omega-3 fatty acids, complete protein, antioxidants, and fiber. The small, ornate seeds can be mixed into superfood smoothies, raw puddings, sprinkled on cereal, eaten as a snack, or added to salad. The nut-like flavor is very pleasing.

To prepare chia seed puddings, instead of simply eating or blending the seeds, soak them in water for ten minutes. This will cause the seeds to secrete a demulcent anti-inflammatory gel. *Voila!* Instant pudding. You can then add honey, berries, slippery elm bark powder, marshmallow root powder, or any number of digestive-system healing ingredients to this pudding and eat one, two, even three times daily, depending on your health needs.

Chia seeds are similar to flax in composition but are easier to digest, with no phytoestrogens. They have higher zinc and lower cadmium levels than flax. Chia seeds are gluten-free and do not come from GMO crops. Chia has a much longer history of being used as a staple food than does flax.

Seed and Nut Oils

Many plant fats are cold-pressed to create wonderful oils such as olive oil, hemp oil, borage seed oil, primrose oil, chia seed oil, etc. Cold-pressed oils retain more sensitive elements and delicate flavors than heat-processed oils do.

Raw or cold-pressed fats and oils are one of the best foods to include in our diet because they beautify the skin, lubricate the joints and intestines, strengthen cell membranes, and restore fat-soluble nutrients to the tissues.

There is a dramatic difference between raw fats/oils and cooked fats/oils. Cooked fats/oils are not miscible with water. Since we are a

Continues

Continued

water-based life-form, this presents a challenge to our digestive system and liver. Cooked fats/oils (especially polyunsaturated seed oils such as safflower oil, canola oil, sunflower oil, soybean oil, and cotton seed oil) tend to break down improperly. They lead to cardiovascular plaque formation, calcium overgrowth, easier viral replication, tendencies toward acne and other common skin disorders, liver stagnation, porous cell membranes, body odor, and nutritional deficiencies. Cooked fats/oils (especially polyunsaturated seed oils) are fattening and their over-consumption results in many health challenges.

Close inspection reveals that animal foods advertised as being low in fat are still high in fat. Consider that lean ground beef provides about 54 percent of its calories in the form of fat, while 51 percent of the calories from chicken come from fat, as do 40 percent of the calories of salmon. Thus, supposedly lowfat, high-protein foods are still calorically high in fat. The best way to avoid a high cooked-fat diet is to abstain from all cooked-oil products and high-fat animal products.

The quantity of raw fats/oils eaten should be limited to what an individual can handle based on his or her metabolism. Generally, it is a good rule to eat fats (especially raw nuts and seeds) with green leafy salads for ease of digestion. Excessive intake of fats and oils, even raw fat and oils, can lead to facial pimples and a general feeling of lethargy due to overburdening the digestive organs.

Note that eating fats such as avocados, macadamia nuts, olives, olive oil, and coconut oil can help "cool" or "cut" the spicy sulfurous elements found in hot peppers, onions, garlic, arugula, radishes, and watercress. Fats help digest spicy sulfur compounds. The opposite is also true (spicy sulfur compounds help digest fats). Sulfur compounds cause fat to disperse in the bloodstream, preventing it from clumping (agglutinating) in the blood.

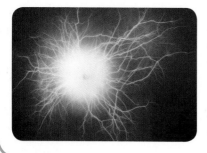

A Kirlian image of olive oil

Seaweeds

A very important food category that we should be aware of for a healthy future on Earth is the seaweeds. These ocean vegetables were popularized in the Western world after the discovery of nuclear power and realization of the toxicity of radioactive elements. High in minerals, seaweed has the ability to detoxify these compounds in the human body, which was discovered when the people in Hiroshima and Nagasaki (Japan) who were seaweed eaters survived the radioactive fallout from the nuclear attacks. In particular, they ate kelp.

Seaweeds are rich in life-giving nutrients drawn in from the ocean and sun. They help remove heavy metals from the body, are an excellent source of numerous trace minerals, provide all eight essential sugars (glyconutrients), and decrease the risk of cancer. Seaweeds benefit the entire body and are especially excellent for the thyroid (high iodine), immune system, adrenals, and healthy, balanced hormone production.

Seaweeds can be contaminated by nuclear waste in the oceans. Purchase your seaweeds from the southern hemisphere or from near-Arctic sources. You can test your seaweed for radiation with a Geiger counter.

In addition to those listed below, other types of incredibly great seaweeds include hijiki, bladderwrack, whole-leaf sea lettuce, alaria, wakame, sea palm, and arame.

Kelp

Kelp *(Fucus vesiculosus)* is an especially rich source of potassium, iron, iodine, vitamin B6, riboflavin, and dietary fiber. It also contains a natural substance, glutamic acid, that enhances flavor and tenderizes fibrous foods. Phytochemicals in kelp have been shown to absorb and eliminate radioactive elements and heavy metal contaminants from our bodies.

Kelp (like cacao and chlorella) is extraordinarily rich in minerals, including alkaline minerals such as good calcium and magnesium. Sufficient mineralization from proper nutrition has been known to normalize and calm behavior. A lack of proper mineral nutrition has been implicated in practically every symptom of poor health and emotionally extreme behavior.

The iodine and other minerals in kelp increase the mineral content of all the organs, allowing them to function more effectively, which includes being able to readily throw off toxins and rejuvenate. Also, kelp helps replace toxic minerals with healthy minerals (e.g., radioactive iodine with healthy iodine). The iodine in kelp helps restore thyroid function, allowing one to lose weight swiftly.

Kelp contains polysaccharides in the form of carrageenan, which has antiviral properties and is particularly effective at fighting herpes.

Nori

Nori (*Porphyra* sp.) is a dark, red-lavender seaweed. Nori has the highest protein content of any seaweed, and it contains valuable enzymes that help break down bad calcium deposits. Nori is high in vitamins A, B1, and B3 (niacin), and trace minerals. Nori is perhaps most celebrated due to its delicious flavor.

Dulse

Dulse *(Palmaria palmata)* is a red seaweed with flat, fan-shaped fronds. An excellent source of protein, iron, and trace minerals, dulse also contains iodine and manganese, which activate enzyme systems. Dulse with avocado is a treat few can resist.

Irish Moss

Irish moss *(Chondrus crispus),* which is actually a seaweed, imparts a smooth, creamy texture to raw sauces, spreads, and any other raw creation imaginable. Like all sea vegetables, Irish moss is a wild food high in minerals and long-chain sugars known as polysaccharides. These long-chain sugars have been studied for their benefits to the immune and digestive systems. Irish moss contains a large portion of polysaccharides in the form of carrageenan, which is responsible for this useful plant's gelling and thickening properties. As mentioned in the kelp section, carrageenan has antiviral properties and is particularly effective at fighting herpes.

To use it, raw Irish moss is rinsed and soaked for 24 hours, causing it to expand to three times its original size. Blending it with water or nut milk creates a thick liquid, ready to impart its unique gelling properties to any recipe that may benefit from extra body or a smoother texture.

Fresh, raw Irish moss is a truly wild food. It is found all around the shores of Ireland and Great Britain and can also be harvested along the coast of Europe including Iceland, the Faroe Islands, and from the western Baltic Sea to southern Spain. It is found on the Atlantic coasts of Canada and recorded from California to Japan.

By soaking and then adding Irish moss to blended concoctions, you can turn your favorite chocolate smoothie recipe into a healing raw chocolate mousse. Irish moss contains demulcent gels that heal the digestive tract with their anti-inflammatory power. Create smooth,

How to Prepare Irish Moss

1. Rinse fresh, raw Irish moss under cold, pure, running water to remove all traces of sand and salt. Not cleaning the Irish moss properly may lead to a slight "seaweed" or brackish taste in recipes.
2. Soak fresh, raw Irish moss in an airtight container, completely covered with water.
3. Leave soaking for 24 hours before using.

Once a batch of Irish moss is soaked, it will keep in the fridge for seven to ten days. Do not rinse or change the water during this time, as this may wash away some of the carrageenan that is activated through the soaking process. Similarly, for best results, avoid rinsing fresh, raw Irish moss after it has been soaked. In general, 1 ounce of fresh, raw Irish moss, after soaking, will gel 1 cup of liquid. Oversoaked Irish moss will have a transparent look and will be much larger in size. The gelling effect can still be obtained, but in this case you may have to almost double the amounts called for in recipes.

creamy, delicious raw ice cream that can help soothe your digestive system. Experiment, and watch your creativity blossom with the newest addition to your healing kitchen!

Irish Moss Raw Vanilla Ice Cream

2 cups raw, organic cashews

3 cups pure spring water, or a combination of spring water and young coconut water

1 cup soaked Irish moss, drained

2 tbsp raw, organic honey

1 vanilla bean (whole), cut into small pieces

3 pinches of sea salt

1 cup coconut oil

Blend cashews and water to a milk using a blender or food processor. Strain with a nut milk bag and reserve the pulp for another recipe. Blend 1 cup cashew milk with the Irish moss until completely smooth. Add all other ingredients in order, slowly adding the coconut oil last. Pour into a freezer-safe container and freeze overnight. When ready, scoop and enjoy with fresh fruits or raw chocolate sauce.

Sprouts

Sprouts are one of the most nutritious foods on the planet. You can buy sprouts at your local health food store or grow them on your own for pennies! Sprouts are rich in vitamins, minerals, amino acids, and live enzymes. They are also an excellent source of fiber and chlorophyll.

In the way I classify things, there are two different types of sprouts: seed/legume sprouts and green sprouts (grasses). Seed/legume sprouts are in the first stage of sprouting. These sprouts are protein-dominant foods. As the sprout matures, it begins to form green leaves of one type or another. It then becomes a green sprout and falls into the green-leafed vegetable category. So, for example, sprouted sunflower seed is a seed sprout, but as it grows its green leaves and turns into a sunflower sprout, it becomes a green sprout.

Seed/legume sprouts include:

- chickpea sprouts
- pea sprouts
- quinoa sprouts
- sprouted sunflower seed
- sprouted wheatgrass/kamut grass/spelt grass
- soaked wild jungle peanut
- sprouted wild rice

Green sprouts fit into the category of essential chlorophyll foods. For most people, sunflower greens are the best sprouts of all because they are the "softest" and most nourishing for the body. Green sprouts include:

- alfalfa
- barleygrass blades
- buckwheat sprouts (in moderation)
- mung bean sprouts
- pea shoots
- radish sprouts
- sprouted broccoli
- sunflower greens
- wheatgrass blades

Be careful not to eat too many buckwheat sprouts—they contain fagopyrin, a neurotoxin. When eaten in moderation these toxins have no effect; in excess they are toxic. If you are overeating this type of sprout, you are increasing the toxin load in your body, leading to photosensitivity of the skin, foggy thinking, confusion, and even potential numbness in the nerves.

Seed sprouts are not essential in the diet. However, if they are eaten occasionally, they can be beneficial because high-quality seeds contain many trace minerals and available amino acids. Also, seed sprouts are therapeutic, as they are very high in enzymes and help reverse an enzyme-deficiency situation. If overeaten or miscombined (with avocado, for example), seed sprouts may create digestive distress. Before eating, legume seed sprouts should typically be cooked in order to destroy all the leguminous toxins they naturally contain.

Grasses

For healing power and natural highs, nothing beats wild grass juice in flavor or nutrition. Wild grass from a pollution-free zone of your local neighborhood can be collected with scissors and a paper bag. Bring home your prize and juice it—add fresh cucumber and celery juice, along with fresh lemon or pineapple juice. A small dose of microalgae (spirulina, blue-green algae, chlorella, marine phytoplankton) blended into the potion adds even more flair.

Wild grass and more original forms of grass are superior to weak hybridized wheatgrass seed strains. If you want to grow your own grass, know that seed quality counts—seek out the best-quality seed stock available. Other grass seeds (kamut, rye, barley, oat) tend to be of a higher quality than wheatgrass.

In general, grass juice is an excellent addition to any healing program. Grass blades are one of the best natural sources of MSM, good calcium, and mineral salts, and, if grown in fully mineralized soil, are the only land-produced food with the potential to absorb and contain all ninety-plus known food minerals.

Every animal takes in plant food directly or indirectly and concentrates it. So, for example, a zebra is physically nothing more nor less than concentrated grass, and the lion that feeds on the zebra is also simply concentrated grass. Metaphorically speaking: there is nothing in the zebra that was not in the grass, and nothing in the lion that was not in the grass. A steak is actually concentrated grass. Whether we like it or love it, we are composed of concentrated plants.

Grasses come in two main forms:

- Fresh young or mature grasses

  Young grass is five to twelve days old. Consuming young grass has detoxifying powers. Mature grass is thirteen to twenty-six days old. Chew on or juice the mature blades before they have flowered. Mature grass has anabolic, body-temperature-increasing, body-building, strengthening, high-energy powers.

- Grass powders (dehydrated and powdered grasses)

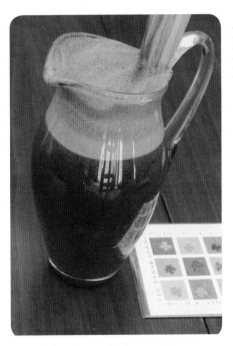

Wild grass juice blended with fresh organic celery-cucumber-pineapple juice and AFA blue-green algae

To make grasses taste more palatable, you may use the dried, powdered grasses (mixtures of powdered barleygrass, wheatgrass, etc.) in fruit or coconut water smoothies. These powders will allow you to get the minerals without resisting the taste. On an interesting note, oftentimes very young children will prefer the taste of dried, powdered grass to typical green vegetables. Powdered grasses are also good for traveling, as they are a highly concentrated and convenient way to get nutrition into your body without taking up a lot of space and weight. You can add them to juice, superfood smoothies, blend them into homemade salad dressings, or even sprinkle them on top of salads. (Try this with chlorella and spirulina as well!)

Superherbs

In addition to the powerful herbs listed in this section, the following are also excellent: reishi, chaga, ant, rhodiola, ginseng, schizandra berry, astragalus, asparagus root, tulsi, and ashwagandha. All of these are covered elsewhere in this book; use the index to locate and read about them.

Pau d'Arco

Pau d'arco *(Avellanedae* or *Tabebuia impetiginosa),* sometimes known as *lapacho,* is the inner bark of a majestic flowering Amazonian tree that grows up to 30 meters in height. Its base can measure up to 3 meters in circumference.

Indigenous people noticed that the pau d'arco tree does not rot quickly, even when it is long dead. Pau d'arco bark contains intrinsic chemical factors that fight fungus and mold, even in some of the wettest, most fetid environments on Earth. This was likely why indigenous people started using the tree to make their tools out of (including their bows), and the bark to fight fungal conditions.

Pau d'arco is a wonderful herb with many documented properties, including the following:

- improves toxic blood-related conditions, such as acne, hepatitis, environmentally produced allergies and asthma, and poisons attacking the liver
- stimulates the immune system to such a positive degree that it has been traditionally used as a primary treatment for viruses, such as flu, herpes, and hepatitis
- as a systemic antifungal, works to eliminate candida and candida-type problems
- inhibits free-radical-induced cell mutations, especially those within the blood or skin
- decreases the spreading of mutated cells and the formation of new malignant growths

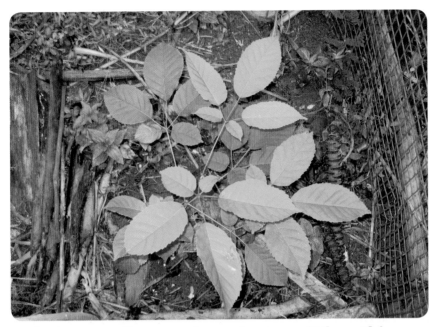

A baby pau d'arco or lapacho tree. When this tree is mature, the bark may be used medicinally.

◉ helps balance blood sugar levels, thus reducing the amount of insulin needed by diabetics

Pau d'arco teas make a fantastic base for cacao drinks. Simply add cacao beans or nibs and blend. Pau d'arco tea has a naturally sweet taste, yet contains no sugar. Pau d'arco is a great herbal base for all teas. Experiment with mixing it with other herbs. Also, adding some form of sweetener (such as raw yacon root syrup, stevia, honey, fruit, etc.) makes a wonderful tasting beverage. Please note that the more sweetener that is used, the less effective the pau d'arco.

You can make 1–2 liters of tea with 10 grams of pau d'arco. One may add 3.5 grams of the herb cat's claw to the pau d'arco tea to make a traditional Shipibo Peruvian tea. You can also add chanca piedra (known to assist in the elimination of kidney stones).

Note: As with many potent herbs, an excessive amount of pau d'arco tea may cause cramping, nausea, or intestinal upset—although this is rare. However, there have been no reports in the scientific literature of any danger in ingesting pau d'arco tea. It has been in human use for thousands of years.

Pau d'Arco Tea

10g pau d'arco

3.5g cat's claw

20g goji berries

3g chanca piedra

1 raw vanilla bean

Steep the herbs in hot water (150–170°F) for an hour or longer. This makes 2 liters of healing tea and is extraordinary hot, warm, or even when chilled.

Vanilla Bean

From the exquisite blooms of the vanilla orchid come the pods that yield one of the world's greatest flavors. Vanilla beans (pods) are the cured dried fruit of the only fruit-bearing orchid. Although there are about 150 species of vanilla orchids, only a few are used commercially.

Vanilla is one of the oldest and most valuable of all spices. It is best known for its flavor-enhancing and aromatic qualities and uses.

Among the purported health benefits of vanilla known by ancient peoples was its potential to act as an aphrodisiac. In the eighteenth century, it was recommended by physicians in the form of an infusion (drink) or tincture to increase male potency.

When purchasing vanilla, look for beans that are hand-cultivated without pesticides or synthetic fertilizers, and cured only in the sun and in wood boxes. Avoid vanilla extracts, especially artificial vanilla extracts, because when vanilla is processed into this form it may be cut with tonka beans which have blood-thinner qualities (and actually may endanger the lives of those on blood-thinner medication).

Use vanilla in favorite raw creations, including chocolate drinks, smoothies, and desserts. If you have a NutriBullet or another powerful blender, you can snip (with kitchen scissors) small pieces of the whole bean right into your blended creations (the beans, flavor, and nutrition are maximized this way). Try adding half a vanilla bean to any tea recipe along with other herbs for a delicious and smooth taste. Another way to use vanilla is to split the bean open lengthwise, scrape out the thousands of tiny black seeds, and add them to your culinary creations. Nothing compares to using whole, raw vanilla beans when you want real vanilla flavor!

Chaparral

Chaparral *(Larrea tridentata)* is a desert-growing plant believed by native peoples of the Sonoran desert ecosystem to be the first of all plants and the most powerful of all medicines. It contains numerous potent medicinal substances, the most well known of which is NDGA (nordihydroguaiaretic acid). Chaparral's active ingredients are found in its stems, leaves, and flowers. Typically, the stems, leaves, and flowers of chaparral are soaked in water for an hour or more. Or it is prepared by soaking the chaparral in warm coconut oil for 24–48 hours. A cold chaparral tea water can then be taken internally or applied topically to the skin or hair. The coconut oil extraction can be applied topically after the chaparral leaves have been strained out.

Chaparral is noted for its ability to ease arthritic pain, fight cancer, reduce inflammation, and fight viruses. As an antiviral, chaparral is one of the most powerful anti-herpes substances ever found. In fact, chaparral-infused coconut oil makes for an innovative antiviral sex oil that when used with nonlatex condoms is a good strategy to prevent disease transmission.

Special note: Chaparral contains a wide range of medicinal antioxidants and compounds. Chaparral is liver- and kidney-toxic to some people. If this herb calls you, investigate its interesting properties.

🌿 Mucuna

Mucuna pruriens has long been used in Ayurvedic and Amazonian herbal systems to treat nervous system disorders, low sex drive, and infertility. Mucuna has also been used as a carminative, antihypertensive, and antihypoglycemic agent. The word "mucuna" is derived from the Amazonian Shipibo tribe's word *mucunan.*

I categorize mucuna as an antistimulant that should be taken with stimulant-containing foods or beverages (i.e., coffee, yerba maté, cacao, etc.). The cacao-mucuna stimulant-to-antistimulant relationship is one of the oldest known, dating back thousands of years. Historically, cacao shamans always had in their possession cacao and mucuna during their travels and would concoct cacao brews with whatever else was available locally.

Mucuna is best known for containing a very powerful neurotransmitter precursor called L-Dopa. L-Dopa is an amino acid that converts into dopamine and provides mucuna with most of its antistimulant action. Dopamine is required for proper functioning of the brain. Dopamine is depleted by stress, stimulants, legal and illegal drug abuse, and alcohol. L-Dopa is known to be the most important nutrient for those suffering from Parkinson's disease.

Experimental studies show L-Dopa also helps in the reduction of cholesterol and blood sugar levels.

L-Dopa may support the body's ability to produce health-giving hormones. As dopamine is carried into the brain, it naturally optimizes the production of other hormones, including testosterone, which leads to an increased sex drive and improved sexual performance for both men and women.

Due to its high levels of L-Dopa, some people who are sensitive to L-Dopa may be limited in their use of mucuna. For these cases, I recommend switching to another antistimulant superherb—reishi mushroom.

Mucuna also contains nervous system–supporting neurotransmitters, including serotonin and 5-HTP.

Benefits of *Mucuna pruriens:*

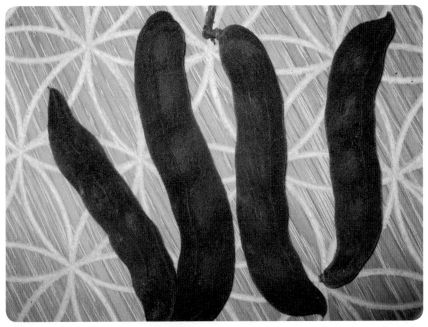

The ripe black mucuna seed pod (hairless variety)

- better sleep (promotes deep sleep)
- reduces body fat, and decreases cellulite and wrinkles
- stimulates muscle growth
- improves skin texture and appearance
- helps maintain bone density
- increases lean muscle mass
- improves sense of well-being
- enhances libido and sexual performance
- increases energy levels
- favorably modulates blood lipids
- improves adrenal and kidney health—builds jing energy
- strengthens the immune system
- provides L-Dopa, which converts to dopamine

Look for cold water–extracted mucuna powder or simply experiment with the whole mucuna bean.

Sacha Jergùn

Sacha jergùn *(Dracontium loretense)* is one of the main herbs in traditional Amazonian medicine: the root is dried and mixed with other herbs as tea or pulverized and mixed with other herbs. This perennial herb, which grows wild in the Amazon basin up to the lower elevations of the Andes Mountains, earned "sacha" (part of its name) from its effectiveness in combating snake venom.

The active elements of sacha jergùn are found in the tuberous off-white-colored root. In addition to being one of the best herbs in the world for liver support and rejuvenation, sacha jergùn activates and improves the effectiveness of the herbs that it is used with. It provides the key that unlocks the potential of many of the extraordinarily rich herbs of Amazonia. Sacha jergùn can be used with any combination of herbs to help improve immunity, cleanse the body, and restore optimal health and well-being.

Raw sacha jergùn powder is in a form that may be easily mixed into any juice, smoothie, or other beverage. This herb has traditionally been used in cold-water infusions, therefore no special preparation is required. Sacha jergùn mixes easily into cold water and has a mildly sweet taste. Try mixing it into a smoothie with raw cacao beans to increase the antioxidant and heart-opening effects of the raw chocolate.

When choosing sacha jergùn, look for sustainably harvested and wildcrafted products.

Horsetail

The great philosopher Rudolf Steiner recognized and recommended two herbs more than any other: horsetail and nettle. Whether or not you are familiar with the body of work that Steiner brought to the Earth, listening to Steiner and taking action with these herbs is highly worthwhile. This is because horsetail has a high Ormus mineral content in general and silicon in particular (See the Ormus discussion on page 42). Silicon is essential for hair, skin, fingernail, and connective tissue health.

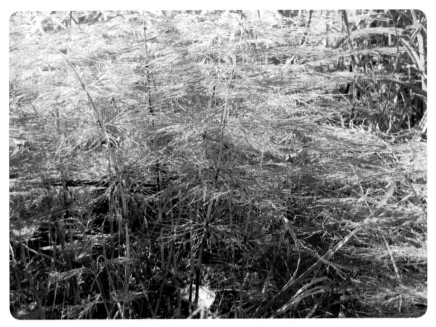

Horsetail

Horsetail *(Equisetum arvense)* is known to promote the following:

- helps to repair cartilage, bones, and connective tissues
- cleanses the kidneys
- functions as an anti-infective and astringent to the urinary system
- helps expel toxins from the body
- acts as a very powerful antifungal

Note: Do not use fresh horsetail continuously over the long term, as the fresh herb contains a vitamin B1 inhibitor. The material must be dried in order to deactivate its vitamin B1 inhibitor. The best way to use horsetail is as a dried herb that is added to tea.

🍃 Nettles

Stinging nettle *(Urtica dioica)* has a long medicinal history. In medieval Europe, diuretics and remedies for joint problems were made from stinging nettle. Nettle leaf is also known to be an excellent source of the bone-building mineral silicon.

Stinging nettle leaf and root have been used for hundreds of years (at least) to treat disorders of the muscles and joints, eczema, arthritis, gout, and anemia. Today, more and more men are using nettle root to treat prostate problems during the early stages of an enlarged prostate (called benign prostatic hyperplasia or BPH). It is also useful against urinary tract infections, kidney stones, and hay fever (allergic rhinitis), and it can be used in compresses or creams for treating joint pain, sprains, strains, tendonitis, and insect bites.

Nettle leaf and root have been shown to relieve pain, have mild anti-inflammatory effects, and to lower blood sugar levels. Active compounds in stinging nettle leaf may serve as an expectorant (meaning that it can loosen and break up a cough) and have antiviral properties.

Nettle root is a natural aromatase inhibitor. This means that nettle root—particularly the alcohol extracts of the herb—inhibits the conversion of health-enhancing androgens into toxic estrogens. In men, nettle root's inhibition of the enzyme aromatase endows it with prostate-protective qualities. Nettle root also shows promise in generating hair growth and slowing male pattern baldness.[4]

Stinging nettle is the name given to common nettle, garden nettle, and hybrids of these two plants. Originally from the colder temperate regions of northern Europe, Asia, and perhaps America, this shrub now grows all over the world. Stinging nettle grows well in nitrogen-rich soil, blooms between June and September, and typically reaches over a meter in height.

The leaves are heart-shaped, finely serrated, and tapered at the ends. Underground, the branching roots put off multiple shoots.

The entire plant is covered with tiny stinging hairs, mostly on the underside of the leaves and stem. Each of these stinging hairs is pres-

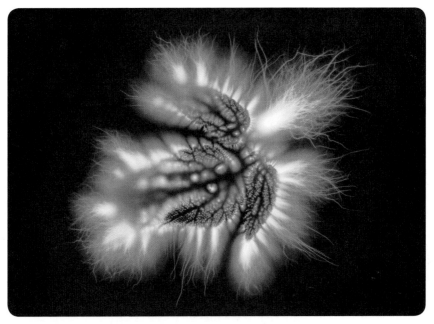

A Kirlian image of wild nettle leaves

surized with an explosive sting potential. These needles can sting the skin, leaving pains of various sorts that may last hours; yet amazingly, our mouth environment will deactivate a sting in under 30 seconds, making nettle leaves edible.

Nettle is available as dried leaf or root, as leaf and root tinctures/extracts, and in encapsulated form.

Prepare nettle tea by adding dried leaves or dried root to pure spring water. Heat the water containing the herbs for 30 to 50 minutes without boiling. Drink three to four cups of nettle tea a day.

Nettles are known to:

- improve resistance to pollens, environmental pollutants, and molds
- nourish and tone the veins to help prevent blood clotting
- contain anti-inflammatory properties
- cleanse the blood of toxins and eliminate waste in the kidneys and liver

- contain large amounts of nutrients, especially iron, good calcium, silicon, and potassium
- promote alkalinity
- help remove uric acid
- prevent calcification in the kidneys and joints
- fight arthritis and arthritic pain
- curb appetite
- improve energy levels
- fight candida and internal digestive infections
- help tone tissues, muscles, arteries, and skin
- increase bone mineralization due to its silicon content
- lowers allergic responses and improves resistance to allergies

Super Bone Formula Hot Chocolate

1 liter horsetail and nettle tea (rich in silicon)

2 tbsp raw cacao powder (rich in magnesium)

3 tbsp raw cacao nibs (rich in magnesium)

1–2 tsp maca

2000mg reishi mushroom powder (mycelium)

1000–2000mg carob or pearl powder (this is good calcium)

Blend the tea with the remaining ingredients. If you drink this Super Bone Formula Hot Chocolate most days of the week (and yes . . . you can drink this more than once a day), stay connected to the grounding technologies (see page 307), and do weight-bearing exercise, you can rebuild healthy bones. To amplify the effects of remineralization even more, use your internal hormonal power as outlined in Chapter 5.

Yerba Maté

Yerba maté *(Ilex paraguariensis)* is a traditional medicinal herbal beverage that was introduced to the world by the Guarani Indians of South America. It has been celebrated for centuries as "the drink of the gods" and is enjoying rapidly spreading popularity worldwide by people seeking a healthier alternative to coffee, without the side effects.

Yerba maté (pronounced "yerba mah-tay") contains stimulants and is inappropriate for those with overly sensitive body types, such as people prone to excessive anxiety and those with adrenal fatigue or a vata constitution.

The leaves of the yerba maté tea provide twenty-four vitamins including vitamins A, C, E, B1, B2, B3, B5, and traces of other constituents of the B complex. They also contain the following minerals: good calcium, manganese, iron, selenium, potassium, magnesium, and phosphorus. In addition, yerba maté contains fifteen amino acids and many powerful antioxidant properties.

There are 196 volatile (or active) chemical compounds found in the yerba maté plant. Of those, 144 are identical or similar to those found in green tea. Maté contains stimulating xanthines including: caffeine, theophylline, matteine, and theobromine; some of these well-known compounds are also found in coffee and cacao (chocolate).

Yerba maté contains eleven polyphenols. Polyphenols are a recently discovered group of compounds that act as powerful antioxidants. Polyphenols may strengthen an organism's natural defenses and protect it against cellular destruction (e.g., lycopene in tomatoes, flavonoids in blueberries, and epicatechins in cacao). In addition to polyphenols, yerba maté leaves contain saponins, which are phytochemicals that have been found to specifically stimulate the immune system and thus aid the body in protecting against disease.

Yerba maté is known to:

- boost the immune system
- control the appetite
- stimulate clarity and focus

🛡 increase energy
🛡 help reduce stress
🛡 combat fatigue
🛡 aid elimination; fight constipation

The xanthine content helps yerba maté to activate or amplify the medicinal properties of any herb(s) that it is mixed with.

The word "maté" derives from the Quechua word "matí" for the gourd *(Lagenaria vulgaris)* that is traditionally used to drink the infusion in South America. To re-create this traditional brew, fill your cup an eighth to a quarter of the way full with the dried, tea-cut yerba maté leaf, then pour hot or cold water over the herb. After allowing it to steep for a few minutes, the infusion may be sipped with a filtered straw, or strained through cheesecloth or a nut-milk bag. This can be repeated many times over until the beverage is nearly flavorless. Yerba maté may also be brewed with a traditional drip-percolating automatic coffee maker, or with a reusable tea dunker. Enjoy the delicious, smooth, rich flavor of this extraordinary beverage.

🍃 Chuchuhuasi

Chuchuhuasi *(Maytenus aelivis)* is the bark of a giant Amazonian climax rainforest tree that can exceed a height of 30 meters. Amazonian herbalists ritualistically strip reasonable sections of the bark in order to avoid seriously injuring the trees.

Chuchuhuasi tea (made from the bark) has excellent anti-inflammatory properties that help alleviate arthritic joint pain and most types of back pain. In Chinese medicine it would be considered a yang jing herb. Chuchuhuasi's other extraordinary healing abilities include: fortification of the immune system, relief of tension, adrenal support, and enhancement of sex drive. Chewing or drinking a tea of the bark is an effective treatment for arthritis, diarrhea, menstrual irregularities, and an upset stomach.

Chuchuhuasi bark tea has a gentle effect on the digestion and metabolism and can be consumed daily by itself or with other teas and/or superfoods to create super-tonic beverages. Chuchuhuasi tea is a great herbal base for all teas and has even been added by shamans to ayahuasca beverages. Experiment with mixing chuchuhuasi bark and pau d'arco, cat's claw, and chanca piedra, as well as other herbs, to make unique antinanobacterial, antiviral, antifungal teas.

Chuchuhuasi tea makes a fantastic base for cacao drinks, a combination that has been consumed in the Amazon for countless centuries. Simply add cacao beans or nibs, as well as 1,500 milligrams of anti-inflammatory mangosteen powder, and blend. This can provide needed joint pain relief by creating healthy tissue at the source of the problem. One may further add 2,500 milligrams of MSM powder (after the tea is made) for even greater anti-inflammatory power.

Try adding some form of mineral-rich natural sweetener (such as yacon root syrup, jerusalem artichoke syrup, and/or dark honey) in order to make this blended anti-inflammatory drink and other chuchuhuasi-based healing beverages more flavorful.

You can make 2 liters of potent tea with 5 grams of chuchuhuasi. You can add 10 grams of pau d'arco and/or 3.5 grams of cat's claw to the chuchuhuasi bark tea to make a traditional Amazonian-style super-healing tea.

Note: There have been no reports in the scientific literature of any danger in ingesting chuchuhuasi tea. Anthropological evidence suggests that chuchuhuasi bark tea has been in human use for thousands of years.

Superhero Tea

10g pau d'arco

1 vanilla bean (whole)

5g cat's claw

2 oz goji berries

5g chanca piedra

10g nettles

5g chuchuhuasi

10g horsetail

Steep the herbs in hot water (150–170°F) for an hour or longer. That means you will have to keep some low flame or heat on the water continuously for the duration. This makes 3 to 4 liters of potent tea.

These herbs are 100 percent medicinal. They effectively fight off mental and physical stress, as well as combat fatigue in the body. They fortify our immune system, build up energy, break down calcification, build healthy bone, rebuild our stress defense shield, increase longevity, and make us feel calm and relaxed.

Chamomile

Chamomile *(Matricaria recutita)* is one of the most widely used flowers for herbal tea. Chamomile tea is so popular that it can be found in the tea aisle of almost any grocery story in the Western world. Its reputation as a medicinal plant to treat common ailments is as old as medicine itself. Revered by herbalists for thousands of years, chamomile has been used to relax the nerves and encourage sleep, treat anxiety, promote longevity, and improve digestion.

Chamomile possesses antispasmodic, anxiolytic, anti-inflammatory, antidiabetic, and antimutagenic effects. Chamomile has sped the healing time of wounds in animals. The essential oil of chamomile has potential as an antiviral agent against herpes simplex virus type 2 (HSV-2) in vitro.

Chamomile and its relatives in the Asteraceae family contain chrysin and apigenin—both known natural aromatase inhibitors. That means that chamomile varieties help stop the age-related conversion of healthy androgen hormones into unhealthy estrogens. This property indicates that chamomile varieties can be used to guard against reproductive cancers (breast, prostate, ovarian, testicular, etc.).

Chamomile can be drunk as a tea and it can also be used topically. Chamomile is an excellent addition to salves and lotions, and it is often used to treat skin inflammation, burns, eczema, insect bites, cuts, and scratches. One can gargle with chamomile tea to relieve a sore throat. It can also be used as a mouthwash to prevent gum disease.

Chamomile has a wonderful scent and when added to a bath can reduce stress, soften the skin, and induce calmness.

The most common way to ingest chamomile is by making a tea: For one cup hot water add two teaspoons dried flowers. Steep covered in hot water for 10 to 20 minutes. Chamomile flowers are entirely edible in their raw form and make for a healthy and delicious addition to salads.

TIP For a chamomile bath, use one cup fresh or dried herb tied in a linen bag. Place the herbs in the tub with hot water and let them soak for 10 minutes. Avoid adding soap to the bath, as it will coat your skin and not allow the chamomile to penetrate.

Fermented Foods

Fermented or cultured foods have a very high enzymatic activity and thus have been used by natural health pioneers such as Dr. Ann Wigmore and Donna Gates to accelerate healing and disease recovery.

The process of fermentation in foods involves "friendly" bacteria (like acidophilus and bifidus) eating up compounds in the food, therefore helping it become more digestible. Once the fiber in the food has been broken down, it takes on a bit of an acidic quality, which helps our stomach produce more stomach acid for digestion. Digestive power is going to determine how much nutrition we actually absorb and are able to utilize from the food we are eating.

Raw fermented foods help promote the growth of healthy bacteria in the digestive tract, including the colon. Friendly bacteria cannot be underestimated because they are an integral part of our immune system. They also help us alleviate constipation, fight candida, absorb nourishing micronutrients, and create feelings of well-being. If we are missing certain nutrients or minerals in our diet, the friendly bacteria can actually produce them (including vitamin B12). In addition to creating vitamins in the body, raw fermented foods can help us absorb minerals that we would not normally be able to absorb.

It appears that the excretions (enzymes, antiviral/antifungal agents, fatty acids, amino acids, essential sugars, vitamins, trace minerals, etc.) of the great probiotic bacteria (*Lactobacillus acidophilus, Bifidus infantis, Lactococcus thermophilus, L. salivarius, L. plantarum, Enterococcus faecium,* etc.) play a pivotal role in keeping us healthy, modulating immunity, and rejuvenating our body. In the future we will see more and more health products that consist of concentrated excretions of probiotic bacteria that have been given superfoods and superherbs as their food medium.

Fermented foods may be eaten with green leafy vegetables to calm digestion. Raw fermented foods combine well with cooked and/or dehydrated crackers.

Instructions for creating fermented live-food dishes may be found in nearly all the raw-food recipe books available, including books by Dr. Ann Wigmore. Donna Gates also provides fermentation/culturing strategies in her *Body Ecology Diet* book as well as in her other writings.

My own investigation into extreme longevity and longevity science indicates that fermented and/or cultured foods of one sort or another (live cheeses, sauerkrauts, etc.) play a role in keeping the body young. This may have something to do with the fact that the human body

---

The Best Fermented Foods Ever

- raw cultured vegetables (sauerkraut, kimchi, etc.)
- kombucha (when homemade, or made from a high-quality strain)
- *jun* (bacterial culture used to make beverages that originated in Tibet)
- fermented cheeses (dairy, nut, seed, etc.)
- cultured coconut water
- cultured milk from cow, goat, or from nuts/seed

contains more bacteria than it does cells, and that the DNA of the bacteria in our bodies actually outnumbers our own DNA—indicating that we live symbiotically with bacteria.

Raw Cultured Vegetables

> Raw cultured vegetables have been around for thousands of years, but we have never needed them more than we do today. Rich in lactobacilli and enzymes, alkaline-forming, and loaded with vitamins, they are an ideal food that can and should be consumed with every meal to help replenish our inner ecosystems.
>
> —DONNA GATES, *THE BODY ECOLOGY DIET*

Cultured foods improve digestion because they are already predigested. This means that even before they enter your mouth, the friendly bacteria have already converted the natural sugars and starches in the vegetables into lactic acid, a job your own saliva and digestive enzymes would do anyway.

Cultured foods increase longevity. By eating fermented vegetables, you maintain your own enzyme reserves, improve your digestion, and are able to use more energy to eliminate toxins, rejuvenate your cells, and strengthen your immune system. That all adds up to a longer, healthier life.

Cultured foods help us control cravings because they contain live bacteria such as acidophilus that naturally fight back candida yeasts that influence us to eat the sugars they crave. They are ideal for appetite control and thus for weight control, because they lessen cravings for carbs and sugars that are found in bread, pasta, dairy products, and desserts.

Cultured foods are cleansing. Raw cultured vegetables help restore the body's homeostatic balance, especially if it is in a toxic condition.

A note on pasteurized sauerkraut: Most of the sauerkraut sold in grocery stores is pasteurized and heavily salted (and usually not with healthy sea salt!). The process of pasteurization (heating) destroys living enzymes and essentially "cooks" the food. When purchasing pre-made sauerkraut, look for the words "living" and/or "raw" on the label. You can also make your own sauerkraut at home—look in raw-food recipe books and online for instructions.

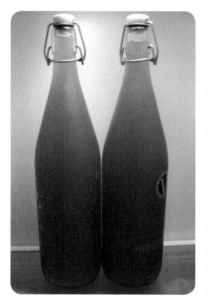

Homemade kombucha

Kombucha

Kombucha is a naturally fermented beverage made from black tea and some concentrated form of sugar. Kombucha has been used for thousands of years to help stimulate the metabolism, support the liver, and maintain a healthy immune system. Recently kombucha has become even more well known for its abilities to spark natural detoxification processes and replenish vital organic acids and enzymes required by the body for optimal performance.

Kombucha contains beneficial bacteria in the form of *Lactobacillus acidophilus,* as well as dozens of other probiotic strains that help promote a healthy digestive system—the primary gateway through which nutrients enter our body, and one of the last lines of defense against microbes that can deprive us of life energy. Thus, the health of the digestive system is intimately linked to the strength of our immunity and our natural, vibrant beauty.

When kombucha first enters the digestive system it coats the stomach with digestive enzymes and live probiotic organisms. These healing elements of the live kombucha culture immediately begin breaking down many of the toxic chemicals, undigested foods, and wastes produced by pathogenic bacteria that interfere with our normal digestive processes. Kombucha works to break down these harmful substances before they can enter the blood stream, converting them into a form that may be easily excreted by the body.

The probiotics in kombucha actively detoxify the digestive system, producing organic acids and B vitamins that speed the cleansing process and create a cascade of rejuvenating effects throughout the body.

The boost of probiotic strains provided by kombucha helps to flush out harmful bacteria and pathogens by regulating the level of acidity in the digestive tract. As long as the kombucha is ripe (not too sweet or sugary) and as long as the kombucha culture agrees with us, regularly consuming live probiotics in the form of kombucha is part of an excellent strategy for attaining longevity and transforming our health and beauty from the inside out.

> **TIP** Most kombucha products sold in stores are not entirely ripe; therefore, they have too much sugar, caffeine is still present, and basically, they only slightly aid digestion and health (if at all). These kinds of unripe, store-bought kombucha products should not be drunk more than three or four times a week. These unripe drinks should be avoided by those with weakened immunity, adrenal exhaustion, and sugar sensitivities.
>
> When ripe, the flavor of kombucha is sour/sweet, with a fermented, vinegar-like, champagne taste. The nature of ripe kombucha may be especially health-giving. My recommendation is to make your own kombucha at home.

Pineapples are a rich source of bromelain enzyme and are great for making kombucha drinks.

The Amazing Enzymes and Nutrients in Kombucha

Ripe kombucha contains the following key digestive enzymes and nutrients (among others):

Enzymes

- **bromelain:** Originally isolated from pineapple, this potent enzyme helps to break down protein in the foods we eat, while also acting as an anti-inflammatory affecting all areas of the body. Bromelain has traditionally been used to reduce the specific symptoms of calcium-induced inflammation associated with osteoarthritis, and it may also be used to relieve discomfort related to nasal congestion, sore throats, and sports injuries.

- **papain:** Present in large amounts in papaya (especially if unripe), papain is a powerful digestive enzyme that also works to break down and help digest protein. The beneficial actions of papain propagate throughout the whole body. Preliminary results have shown that this enzyme may assist in the treatment of degenerative and inflammatory conditions of all types.

Organic Acids

- **glucuronic acid:** Toxic substances bound by glucuronic acid are made water-soluble and can be excreted by the body. Made in large quantities by a healthy liver, glucuronic acid helps to slow the progression of viral infections and has been shown to promote the dissolution of gallstones and to inhibit the proliferation of candida yeast infections.

- **hyaluronic acid:** This organic Ormus mineral containing acid helps to lubricate and cushion the joints by forming a gel-like substance that holds cells together. This may lead to an increase in the body's mobility and flexibility, and may help to reverse some of the effects of aging on the skeletal system.

- **lactic acid:** A major element of raw, live kombucha, lactic acid helps prevent the growth of putrefactive bacteria in the large intestine. It also promotes oxygenation of the blood and major organs, and helps to establish a normal pH in the body.

- **malic acid:** Instrumental in the body's detoxification process, malic acid helps to cleanse the body of toxic substances, undigested foods, and environmental pollutants.

- **chondroitin sulfate:** A fundamental Ormus mineral substance contained in multiple components of the cartilage, bone, and blood vessels, chondroitin sulfate helps to maintain these bodily structures by binding to foreign substances and eliminating them from the body, keeping the tissues safe and healthy. Chondroitin sulfate has been studied for its beneficial effects on arthritis.

- **tannic acid:** This organic acid exhibits antibiotic and antiviral properties. Working together with lactic acid, tannic acid helps to regulate the body's pH, leading to a more efficient immune response.

- **usnic acid:** This organic acid exhibits potent antibacterial and antibiotic properties, helping to keep the immune system healthy and removing toxins from the blood. Usnic acid also acts as an anti-inflammatory and displays analgesic (pain-relieving) action.

B Vitamins

The B vitamins work together as a family of water-soluble nutrients to help the body create energy, maintain optimal organ health, and ensure that all cells operate with a fluid, vibrant energy that reflects our overall well-being. Given the interrelationships among the B vitamins, it is clear that these nutrients are best taken all together in their naturally occurring forms (not laboratory-made supplements), such as we find in ripe kombucha, other fermented/cultured foods, in bee pollen, in royal jelly, and in blue-green algae.

- **B1:** Thiamine plays a key role in helping the body create energy from the foods we eat. This vitamin has been studied for its beneficial effects in relieving symptoms of osteoarthritis, atherosclerosis, and other calcification diseases.

- **B2:** Riboflavin figures prominently in the hydrogenation process that releases energy from carbohydrates, proteins, and fats. It has also been shown to play a supportive role in maintaining the health of the mucous membranes and eyes.

- **B3:** Niacin dilates capillaries and helps to stimulate blood flow and the exchange of dissolved gases in the body. It may contribute to alleviating the symptoms of arthritis. A direct relationship has been made between a deficiency of niacin and neurological challenges including schizophrenia, depression, and addictions to tobacco.
- **B6:** Pyridoxine helps create energy. It facilitates reactions in which amino acids are absorbed and assimilated. It also assists with the formation of blood cells and is required for the function of more than 60 known enzymes. Vitamin B6 helps to protect the skin and, together with vitamin B2, supports optimal eye health. Due to poor nutrition, vitamin B6 is likely the most deficient vitamin in the Western diet.
- **B9:** Folic acid is vital for the growth of the beneficial bacterium *Lactobacillus casei.* Folic acid assists in the formation of proteins in the body for genetic material, and it is essential for the efficient production of red blood cells by the bone marrow.
- **B12:** Cobalamin is only needed in minute amounts, yet it is often found to be deficient in the body due to the sterilization of the food chain. Vitamin B12 is essential for the normal functioning of all cells in the body, particularly blood and bone marrow cells. Vitamin B12 reduces dangerous homocysteine, a substance that potentiates calcification. Many people who begin supplementing with vitamin B12 report a significant improvement in mood and a boost in mental clarity.

Superhero Fizzy Drink

1 cup kombucha

1 piece raw, fresh aloe vera gel (4" x 2" x 1")

3 tbsp honey (Noniland honey works great!)

1 vanilla bean (whole)

2 tsp MSM powder or Opti-MSM flakes

1 tsp camu-camu powder

1 pinch cayenne

1 piece fresh ginger root *or* powdered ginger to taste

4 cups fresh purified water

Combine the ingredients in a blender or food processor on high until completely liquefied, and enjoy! This sweet, tangy beverage is best imbibed within several hours after blending to gain the full effect from the live kombucha probiotics.

Superfoods

Superfoods are the best building blocks we can use to create a powerful foundation for longevity. They catalyze incredible physical and mental health, helping us to develop a youthful radiance that is unparalleled. Superfoods lead to increased levels of energy that are inconceivable to those living on a poor diet.

These amazing foods mineralize the body, eradicate toxins, eliminate fatigue, boost the immune system, and enhance one's absorption of valuable vitamins and nutrients. All this ensures the body's ability to successfully fight off calcification and its progeny: infections, inflammation, chronic aches and pains, viruses, fungi, and harmful bacteria. These organisms and adverse conditions have no opportunity to become established in a healthy inner ecosystem.

> **TIP** Please be underwhelmed with all of this information. The beauty of the Longevity Now approach is that by incorporating just one or two new concepts into your diet, you will begin achieving the results you have been looking for.

Superfoods are powerful and transformative. They work. And they are so simple, so easy, and so fun to eat! How hard is it to add cacao (chocolate) to your diet? Or the delicious goji berry? These foods taste great and are so good for you!

Remember, you are what you eat. The technology behind the diet section of Longevity Now is intended to bring you from zero to superhero. Build a body out of the best foods ever so that the body can build health that lasts forever. We have the potential to live free from arthritis, inflammation, joint problems, heart problems, wrinkles, cancer, cysts, and other unwanted conditions.

Incorporating powerful superfoods into our diet at whatever level we can right now is a health investment. The more we rely on Nature's abundance, the better the results we will achieve with Longevity Now.

Following are some of the top superfoods you can find. Those interested in exploring the subject of superfoods more in depth should read my book *Superfoods: The Food and Medicine of the Future.*

Marine Phytoplankton

Marine phytoplankton contains raw nucleotides (ATP, GTP) that the body can easily convert into energy. This food is loaded with protein, chlorophyll, and long-chain omega-3 fatty acids.

Cacao

This nut, from which all chocolate is made, has an incredible nutrient profile rich in magnesium, chromium, vanadium, iron, manganese, antioxidants, PEA, anandamide, soluble fiber, theobromine, etc. University research cited in my books *Naked Chocolate* and *Superfoods* indicates that the more cacao one ingests, the longer one lives. Jeanne Calment, the longest-lived person and woman (according to official records) in Western history, who made it to 122 years and 164 days, ate a kilo of chocolate a week.[5] Cacao is relatively low in oxalic acid too.

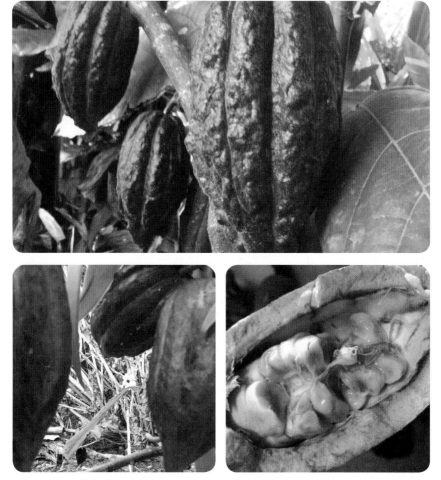

Fresh cacao pods. Notice the cacao beans (nuts) inside. All chocolate comes originally from this fruit.

Goji Berries

These are the most nutrient-rich fruit on the planet; they are loaded with protein, antioxidants, and polysaccharides. Goji berries help us produce more human growth hormone, thus making us younger. They also contain an extraordinary content of the eye-health-improving carotenoid zeaxanthin. Recent research indicates that goji berries can help protect the eyesight of the elderly.[6] Ranked number one in Chinese medicine, with its five thousand years of history and its cornucopia of more than eight thousand food/herbs, goji berries should be a staple food for any longevity specialist. According to Taoist tonic herbalist Ron Teeguarden, a great respect for goji berries is the one thing that all the longest-lived Chinese herbalists had in common. Teeguarden mentions this consistently at his live lectures on longevity.

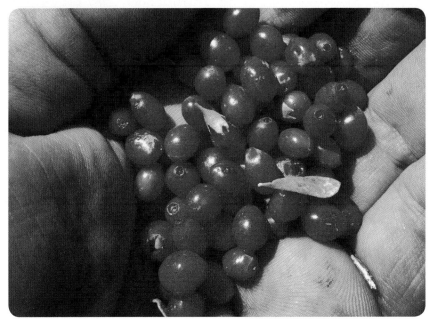

Fresh, wild Arizona goji berries

Maca

This is a powerful, creamy-textured, super-root powder adaptogen. A true adaptogen, maca helps us adapt to stress of all different types. It also increases vigor and vitality, and it acts (via the hypothalamus) as a subtle aphrodisiac. Maca is known to increase sperm count in all mammals tested and to double fertility rates in female mammals. Maca increases body heat and oxygen uptake. It acts as a hormone precursor that's useful in building a healthy endocrine system. Though not a complete protein, maca contains seventeen or eighteen amino acids and is 10 to 14 percent protein by dry matter weight. Native to the Andes region, maca was valued as currency during pre-Incan times.

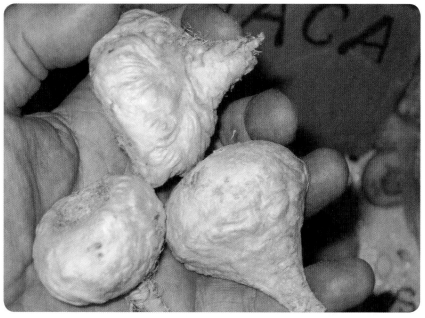

Fresh maca root

Spirulina

This single-celled blue-green algae delivers high-quality complete protein, DNA/RNA, and blue stem-cell-producing phycocyanin. Spirulina ranges from 65 to 70 percent protein, making it the highest-protein-content human food on Earth. Spirulina was a staple food of the Aztecs in Tenochtitlan (present-day Mexico City) and probably was utilized by prior civilizations in the Valley of Mexico, including the Toltecs.

AFA Blue-Green Algae

This contains mood-improving PEA as well as phycocyanin. Like spirulina, when ingested this blue pigment causes stem-cell production in the human body. AFA blue-green algae is a wild food harvested from Klamath Lake, Oregon. It is an excellent source of nearly all B vitamins; the major minerals including good calcium, magnesium, and iron; as well as the trace minerals: chromium, copper, manganese, and zinc.

Chlorella

This helps boost the immune system, assists in detoxifying the body of mercury and heavy metals, rebuilds the blood with chlorophyll, and is rich in good, absorbable calcium. Chlorella is the highest chlorophyll-content food in the world at 10 percent chlorophyll.

Bee Products

These comprise another great superfood category. Bee venom has been known to spontaneously (directly and/or homeopathically) reverse arthritic conditions and other calcification challenges. Unless you have an allergy to bees, getting stung by bees is healthy for you.[7] *National Geographic* magazine reported remission of the calcification condition known as *ankylosing spondylitis* following a scorpion sting (Holland, Jennifer S. "The Bite that Heals: Scientists are unlocking the medical potential of venom." *National Geographic,* February 2013) Many venoms and poisons (such as bee venom, scorpion venom, the Amazonian Kambo frog medicine, and others) activate the immune system and may improve longevity. Bee pollen rejuvenates us at the cellular DNA level with Ormus minerals, enzymes, B vitamins, complete protein, and polysaccharides. Honey is Nature's richest source of live, healing enzymes. It is also rich in high-spin forms of hydrogen and thus is hydrating.

Royal jelly rejuvenates and regenerates the body, thereby inhibiting the aging process. Royal jelly is an extraordinary source of folate or folic acid. Propolis has demonstrated anti-inflammatory properties and been helpful in treating chronic conditions such as arthritis.

> **TIP** Because of its natural synergy with vitamin B12 and its extraordinary content of folate (vitamin B9), bee pollen is often eaten just before consuming vitamin B12 supplements.

Noni

This tropical fruit native to Polynesia is high in sulfur, Ormus minerals, and hydrogen, which are key antiaging elements, largely because sulfur, Ormus minerals, and hydrogen all help to remove bad calcium and repair damaged tissue.

Coconut

This is a phenomenal resource for our immune system because of its antiviral, antifungal, and antimicrobial saturated medium-chain fatty acids. Of course, the natural electrolytes in its delicious water are also of note.

Aloe Vera

This contains incredible healing properties within its polysaccharide gel compounds that help improve the immune system, aid digestion, repair skin cells of all types, and facilitate the safe and effective elimination of toxicity from the body.

Açaí

The açaí berry, native to South America, is super-rich in antioxidants that help produce stem cells and reverse aging. Açaí causes the spontaneous destruction of 86 percent of leukemia cells in vitro.

CHAPTER 3

Foods to Avoid

During the course of your developing relationship with the concepts in *Longevity Now*, I highly recommend that you completely abandon all of the additives, beverages, foods, and food categories discussed below. They are contributing to the problem, not the solution. Regularly consuming one, two, three, or all the items below can result in any number of problems including indigestion, inflammatory responses in the body, decreased production of good calcium, and incomplete digestion (which can lead to toxicity in the liver).

Alcohol

Alcohol abuse is completely destructive. It is the most widely abused drug in the world. Alcohol has a toxic effect on the body and causes deficiencies of B vitamins and other nutrients. Alcohol also impairs judgment and can lead to irresponsible behavior such as drinking and driving, which results in car accidents, injuries, and death. The quantity of alcohol that a person drinks is one of the top three factors associated with longevity; the more drinking, the greater the risk of premature death.

Some of the negative effects of abusing alcohol include:

- rapid water loss
- depletion of electrolytes
- depletion of, and interference with, absorption of vitamins B6 and B12
- niacin (vitamin B3) deficiency, the symptoms of which are diarrhea, dermatitis, and dementia
- decreased ability to store vitamin A
- zinc deficiency

- liver damage that can end in cirrhosis of the liver
- malnutrition, because alcohol interferes with the absorption and storage of essential nutrients

Alcohol, if used at all, should be revered as an alchemical sacred substance that may be utilized to extract the active components in herbs, superherbs, and/or superfoods. Alcohol can extract and stabilize key nutrients and deliver them internally or topically.

Artificial Colorings

Up until the 1950s, natural plant- and vegetable-based compounds were used to add color to foods. For example, pale red colors could be achieved from beets, crimson reds could be achieved by cochineal insect dye, green could be achieved from chlorophyll, and yellow and orange could be achieved from extracts from a number of plants and spices, like saffron. After WWII, the chemical industry grew rapidly. They saw the potential to make money by creating human-made chemicals to add to food to enhance its coloring. They convinced the food industry to use chemical-based colors because they were more convenient, cheaper, and had an unlimited shelf life.

As a result, more and more foods are filled with artificial food-coloring ingredients that contain chemicals from highly toxic sources. These chemicals can cause serious diseases and mental disorders in humans. The majority of artificial food coloring ingredients are made with petroleum and are a derivative of petrochemicals and coal tar. These chemicals should under no circumstances be ingested by humans or animals—yet several artificial food-coloring products are added to many different foods and sold in the marketplace.

The FDA and EPA do not require detailed testing of these chemicals for the effects they might have on human beings. Still, it is being recognized more widely that artificial colors and dyes that are used to enhance the appearance of foods, drugs, and cosmetics may, in fact, produce dangerous consequences after prolonged use.

There are five dangerous food colorings that are still in foods today and are linked with cancer in animal testing:

- Blue 1 and 2: These artificial colorings lurk in candy, baked goods, pet foods, and beverages. They have both been linked to cancer in mice.
- Red 3: This artificial coloring is sprayed on cherries (not just canned cherries, but *fresh*, conventional cherries, to enhance the color), fruit cocktail, baked goods, and candy. It has caused thyroid tumors in rats.
- Green 3: This artificial coloring has been linked to bladder cancer. It is often found in candy and beverages.
- Yellow 6: This artificial coloring, which is one of the most widely used, can be found in sausage, gelatin, baked goods, candy, and

Other Substances to Avoid

As you embark on transforming your health, I highly recommend that you also avoid the following.

- Sugar and excessive fruits or sweeteners: Excessive sugars of all types cause demineralization and feed calcium-forming organisms, viruses, candida, bad bacteria, unwanted guests, and mutated cells.
- Recreational drugs: Chemical and heavy-metal contamination within legal and illegal drugs is common. Natural superfood and superherb highs are better anyway.
- Tobacco: Chemical tobacco is contaminated with 800 additives containing 4,000 different chemicals and is not a longevity substance. Chemical tobacco differs dramatically from natural-dried, organic, homegrown tobacco. Centenarians who smoke tobacco smoke their own natural-dried, organic tobacco, which retains tobacco's longevity properties without dangerous artificial toxicity.
- Caffeine: If coffee causes you anxiety and overstimulates your system, yet you like the pick-up, then curtail coffee habits as best you can by drinking yerba maté instead. Contrary to popular belief, chocolate (raw cacao) is a poor source of caffeine.

beverages. Studies show that Yellow 6 is linked to tumors of the kidney and adrenal glands.

Artificial Flavorings

> Natural and artificial flavors are now manufactured at the same chemical plants, places that few people would associate with Mother Nature. Calling any of these flavors "natural" requires a flexible attitude toward the English language and a fair amount of irony.
>
> —ERIC SCHLOSSER, *FAST FOOD NATION*

Artificial flavoring is a human-made creation used in processed food because over-processing destroys flavor. When you drink freshly made juice it needs no added flavors. But by the time apple juice, for example, has been pasteurized, filtered, etc., the original flavor has been lost.

Most processed foods contain artificial flavors and colors that have been made in giant chemical factories. There are now more than two thousand approved chemicals that don't have to be described on food labels because they are considered to be "closely guarded trade secrets."

When you see the word "flavor" listed in the ingredients, it means those flavors have been made in a laboratory. Even the words "natural flavors" don't necessarily mean that the flavor is coming from a natural source. These "natural flavors" could actually contain exactly the same chemicals as artificial flavors.

Eat organic foods that have no artificial flavoring or coloring and enjoy the delicious, authentic flavors that Mother Nature intended!

Artificial Sweeteners

Aspartame

Aspartame is a Monsanto-made, synthetic chemical that is now consumed by more than 100 million people in the Unites States. It is 180 to 200 times sweeter than sucrose (table sugar). More than twelve hundred products contain aspartame, including soft drinks, pudding, cereal, hot chocolate, yogurt, gum, fruit drinks, breath mints, and frozen foods. The FDA approved aspartame in a dry form in 1981 and then as a low-calorie additive to carbonated beverages in 1983.

Aspartame is made up of three main ingredients: phenylalanine, aspartic acid, and methyl alcohol (also known as wood alcohol). The latter is considered a deadly poison even when consumed in small amounts. It can cause serious damage to the tissues, blindness, and even death. Common complaints ascribed to aspartame products include severe headaches, diarrhea, rashes, extreme fatigue, memory loss, depression, change in personality, and convulsions.

The research on aspartame over the years has also indicated that it contributes to the formation of formaldehyde in the brain, causes frontal lobe deterioration, and is very likely the most dangerous food additive to go into mass production in recent decades.

I strongly recommend that you avoid any food with aspartame in it and that you help your family stay away from this very dangerous food additive or "pseudo-sweetener." This means read your food labels. Look for dangerous ingredients and avoid purchasing anything that contains them.*

Excellent Alternative Sweeteners
STEVIA

Stevia is a now widely used sugar substitute originally from the Andes that has a pseudo (false) sweetness. This makes stevia one of the great herbs of the world because it contains no sugar whatsoever that could re-invigorate an infection or disable the immune response.

Stevia is available in numerous forms: the straight herb (in dried leaves), concentrated liquid products, and powdered forms. There are many flavored stevias available that are delicious added to superfood smoothies, salad dressings, and desserts.

*For more information on the dangers of aspartame, read *Aspartame (NutraSweet): Is It Safe?* by H. J. Roberts, MD.

XYLITOL

Xylitol looks, tastes, and feels exactly like refined granulated sugar; however, chemically speaking, xylitol is not actually a sugar, but a sugar alcohol or polyol. Unlike other sweeteners such as sorbitol, fructose, and glucose, the xylitol molecule has five, not six, carbon atoms. As a five-carbon sugar, xylitol has antimicrobial properties, whereas six-carbon sugars can cause bacterial and fungal overgrowths.

Xylitol is naturally found in some fruits and vegetables and especially in various trees, such as in birch sap. Xylitol is also found in humans and animals, as an intermediate byproduct of carbohydrate metabolism. Xylitol is actually so natural that our bodies constantly produce 5–15 grams of it per day, under normal metabolism conditions. The natural presence of xylitol in plants, food, and humans suggests that consuming xylitol (in reasonable quantities) is safe for our health. Commercially obtainable xylitol is not a raw, whole-food product; however, xylitol itself is a natural substance.

Xylitol was discovered almost simultaneously by German and French chemists in the 1890s. In the former Soviet Union it had been used for decades as a sweetener for diabetics. In China, xylitol has been used for various medical purposes. In 1983 the Joint Expert Committee on Food Additives, under the auspices of WHO and FAO, officially pronounced that xylitol is a safe sweetening additive. The FDA agreed to this fact in 1986. (The World Health Organization is the public health branch of the United Nations, and the Food and Agriculture Organization is also part of the UN. The Food and Drug Administration is an agency of the U.S. government.)

Note: When choosing xylitol products, I recommend using only birch-derived xylitol, as opposed to corn-derived xylitol.

YACON ROOT (POWDER AND SYRUP)

A healthy, nonglycemic, natural, raw, organic, low-calorie sweetener, yacon syrup is fresh-pressed from the yacon root, a plant native to the subtropical Andean highlands and tropical foothills of Peru, where it has been enjoyed for centuries.

Yacon is both naturally low-calorie and low in mono- and di-saccharides (containing less than 1 gram per serving of the sugars that rapidly elevate blood sugar levels). Yacon is a distant relative of the sunflower, with edible tubers and leaves. It is commonly grown and consumed from Colombia to northwest Argentina; in recent years this easy-to-grow, important agricultural crop has spread as far as New Zealand and Hawaii.

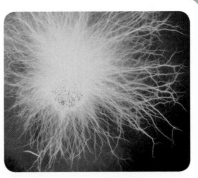

A Kirlian image of yacon root

Yacon is a prebiotic, which means it regulates and nourishes friendly intestinal flora.[1] Because of this quality yacon is great for digestion, stimulates positive colon health, and helps with the absorption of potassium, good calcium, magnesium, and other minerals. Its high antioxidant value makes yacon beneficial in reducing free-radical damage, especially in the small intestine and colon.

Though packed with sweetness, the sugar in yacon is mainly fructooligosaccharide (FOS), which cannot be absorbed by the body. In fact, the root of yacon is the world's richest known natural source of FOS. Most other roots and tubers store carbohydrates as starch—a polymer chain of glucose. Yacon stores carbohydrate as FOS—a polymer chain composed mainly of fructose. This FOS can be considered a subgroup of inulin because it has a similar molecular structure, but with shorter fructose chains.

Yacon helps manage cholesterol and triglyceride levels within the body, as well as normalize fat-oil metabolism in general. Yacon also contains glyconutrients and helps boost the immune system in ways similar to the great superfood aloe vera. Yacon is ideal for low-calorie, low-sugar detoxification and weight-loss diets, and it is a perfect food and low-glycemic sweetener to utilize as part of your longevity strategy.

Continues

Continued

> *How to use:* Use yacon syrup as you would honey or maple syrup on foods, in recipes, and to sweeten beverages and elixirs. Yacon syrup has very little influence on the curve of glucose tolerance and is dramatically less glycemic than other natural sweeteners.
>
> The Universidad Nacional Mayor de San Marcos in Peru tested the effects of yacon syrup on blood glucose levels in 2004. Participants (sixty nondiabetic men and women between the ages of twenty and sixty) fasted for at least eight hours before ingesting various sweeteners. Three groups were given different samples of yacon; one group was given bee's honey; another group was given maple syrup; and the last was given anhydrous glucose. The groups ingesting yacon syrup had the least blood sugar variance as measured before and after. These results showed that yacon had very little effect on glucose levels, while other sweeteners showed an immediate significant rise and a slow decline back to normal.

High-Fructose Corn Syrup

High-fructose corn syrup (HFCS) is a sweetener and preservative used in many processed foods. It is made by changing the sugar in corn starch to fructose.

HFCS was developed by the Japanese in the 1960s. Since that time it has been used by food manufacturers seeking a sweeter and cheaper alternative to sugar. High-fructose corn syrup extends the shelf life of foods, thus making it a popular ingredient in a long list of products that includes soda, salad dressing, ketchup, breakfast cereals, and many processed foods. Check for yourself by reading food labels. You might be surprised by how many foods contain high-fructose corn syrup. These types of empty sugars are high in calories and low in nutritional value and minerals. High fructose corn syrup also directly feeds certain types of infections (e.g., digestive candida infections, cancer) and infectious organisms such as harmful bacteria, viruses, fungi, and parasites.

According to the Mayo Clinic, HFCS is the leading ingredient after carbonated water in soda. Women who drink at least one regular soda a day are 85 percent more likely to develop type 2 diabetes than those who drink less. HFCS also leads to tooth decay. If you were to put a baby's tooth in a glass of soda, it would dissolve completely.

High-fructose corn syrup may be disguised under the name "crystalline fructose," which is contained in Glaceau Vitamin Water and other energy drinks.

Research by the U.S. Department of Agriculture (USDA) reveals that high-fructose diets shorten the life span of laboratory mice from the normal two years to a mere five weeks.

In my opinion, high-fructose corn syrup is one of the most destructive drugs in the world. It is more destructive than cocaine and alcohol. High-fructose corn syrup is a danger button that gets constantly pushed in everybody who eats fast food, junk food, processed food, and conventionally grown food. Chronic consumption of high-fructose corn syrup has been known to cause blood sugar disorders, mood swings, and hypoglycemia. It can also cascade into type 2 diabetes, anxiety, and

---

How to Reduce High-Fructose Corn Syrup in Your Diet

- Read food labels. If the food contains high-fructose corn syrup, avoid it!
- Use sweeteners that are healthier for you, like stevia, yacon, raw unprocessed honey, xylitol (from birch), and maple syrup.
- Avoid drinking soda.
- If you are going to eat canned fruit, eat the kind that is canned in its own juices instead of heavy syrup.
- Make your own organic juices instead of buying the processed kind. Fresh-squeezed orange juice and apple juice are great-tasting and healthy! Experiment with delicious fruits such as citrus, mango, and pineapple in order to create exotic combinations that taste great, satisfy your cravings, and are chock-full of nutrition.

more severe mental disorders. On top of this, high-fructose corn syrup feeds all pathogenic organisms.

Let's be smart. Let's ennoble ourselves to genius level and avoid toxic food ingredients.

Please keep in mind that all real sweeteners that contain sugar of any kind (including fruit sugar and honey) can feed internal infections. A critical consideration in any healing diet (especially when fighting internal infections such as candida and cancer) is how to retain a low sugar intake. This is important because consistent sugar intake (even if natural) can disable the immune system and directly feed the infection(s). By cutting off the food supply of the infection(s) while simultaneously allowing the immune system to properly respond, you allow the condition to start to heal.

Other Sweeteners to Avoid

In addition to aspartame (NutraSweet) and high-fructose corn syrup, watch out for these unhealthy sweeteners:

- barley malt syrup/sugar
- beet sugar (syramena)
- brown rice and rice syrup
- brown sugars
- crystalline fructose
- date syrup/sugar
- demerara
- dextrose
- evaporated cane juice
- fruit concentrate
- maltodextrin
- maltose
- molasses
- powdered sugar
- rapadura
- sucanat
- turbinado
- white sugar

A Note on "Raw" Sugars

Not all sweeteners are created equal. In fact, many of the sweeteners that are considered "healthy" are still highly processed and cooked. The term "raw" is not officially standardized in the food industry; therefore, just because something is labeled "raw" does not necessarily mean it has not been heated. For example, sweeteners like rapadura, sucanat, turbinado, and evaporated cane juice are often referred to as "raw"; however, in this case it just means that they are slightly less refined than standard white sugar. To make these sweeteners, the sugarcane plant is crushed to release its juice, which is then heated to create a thick, dark molasses that contains sugar crystals. These sugar crystals are the "raw" sugar. When these sugar crystals are refined further and the molasses is separated out, then white sugar is created.

Conventional Meat

Eating conventional meat is one of the biggest contributors to calcification conditions in the body. Consistently consuming more than 100 grams of protein per day over decades of time contributes to calcification conditions from gout to arthritis to coronary plaques. Red meat and chicken may even contain extremophile nanobacteria that can survive being cooked.

Conventional factory-farmed animals (and "free-range" livestock animals) are not drinking purified water. They are drinking water from contaminated sources, mostly well-water and municipal water systems. Not only do they consume the chemicals present in the water, they may also be ingesting great quantities of calcium and nanobacteria present in these poor-quality water sources. This bad calcium shows up in the flesh (meat) of the animals after slaughter and can contaminate us if we consume this kind of food.

Conventional Produce

The toxic pesticides used in conventional farming (for example, the deadly compound methyl bromine) have all been linked with a wide range of health problems such as cancer, sarcoma, male infertility, birth defects, chronic fatigue syndrome, autism, Parkinson's disease, heart disease, chronic allergies, and asthma, just to name a few.

Conventional produce may contain genetically modified organisms (GMOs). Genetically modified or GMO foods contain genes from other life-forms including plants, bacteria, bugs, animals, and fish that have had viruses injected into their gene structure under the pretense of "improving" them as a food. The exact potential health effects of tampering with Nature's original food are unknown. I suggest you do research on GMOs and make a well-informed decision as to whether you want this food in your body. Some animal studies indicate and some researchers now believe that consuming genetically modified food can cause cancer.[2]

Compared to organic, conventional produce has fewer vitamins (especially vitamin C), antioxidants, phenolic compounds, and essential minerals (calcium, magnesium, iron, phosphorus, chromium, etc.). Organic produce is the first step in finding edible produce; once you go organic then you proceed to grow your own chemical-free food and also to forage for wild food.

The most pesticide-contaminated conventional fruits and vegetables are strawberries, bell peppers, spinach, American cherries, peaches, Mexican cantaloupe, celery, apples, apricots, green beans, Chilean grapes, and cucumbers.

According to the EPA, the least pesticide-contaminated conventional fruits and vegetables are avocados, onions, sweet potatoes, cauliflower, brussels sprouts, bananas, plums, and broccoli.

Diet Soda

There is nothing "diet" about diet soda, which has been shown to double the amount of cortisol that the body produces, which causes an inflammatory response. Cortisol is an inflammatory stress hormone that is antagonistic to our healthy androgen hormones (progesterone, testosterone, DHEA, thyroid hormone, vitamin D3). This inflammatory response causes us to retain water and toxins because our body cannot flush them out properly. Therefore, diet soda actually causes weight gain, not weight loss.

Diet soda has aspartame as one of its main ingredients. We have already discussed why this human-made synthetic chemical is harmful to the body. One more fact to point out regarding aspartame is that it is unstable and breaks down in the soda can. It decomposes into formaldehyde, methyl alcohol, formic acid, diketopiperazine, and other toxins. Also, the aspartame in diet soda suppresses serotonin and makes us crave carbohydrates!

Like alcohol and coffee, diet soda is implicated in dehydration, despite being liquid. Many health challenges such as constipation are related to being dehydrated. Most chronic conditions hang in there because the person is chronically dehydrated.

Diet sodas are known to contain excitotoxins that literally cause brain cells to explode. Diet soda is one of the worst concentrates of phosphoric acid, which can dissolve a child's tooth right on the spot. Diet soda has no nutritional value, contains known toxins and poisons, and damages health.

A True Story

Our vegetable oil bus stopped running one day while we were touring Atlanta. We discovered that the problem was corrosion on the battery terminals. We used soda pop to remove the battery acid build-up on the terminals of our bus. It pulled the corrosion right off the batteries and our bus ran without any problems from that moment forward!

Fast Food

The fast-food industry has added every chemical legally allowed to addict people to this food. In fact, if you eat fast food and then you stop eating it, you actually go through withdrawal symptoms. It's a drug. Not only that, the level of preservatives is so high in fast-food burgers these days that the product does not even break down by bacterial action or mold if stored in a cupboard or closet.*

The rise of the fast food industry plays a critical role in why our country is plagued with obesity. Fast food is everywhere: in big cities, small towns, shopping malls, the airport, the bus station, schools, and even hospitals! There are 31,000 McDonald's worldwide—and almost 14,000 of them are in the United States.

Fast food has become cheaper and easier to buy at the ubiquitous outlets. In 2004, Americans spent $124 billion on fast food. That same year, *The American Journal of Preventive Medicine* published a study showing that the percentage of fast-food calories in the American diet had increased from 3 percent to 12 percent over the previous twenty years. And now it's already another decade down that greasy road.

Fast-food culture was introduced to other countries around the world in the 1980s. In countries like Japan and China, people have abandoned traditional healthy diets in favor of fast food, and as a result the rates of obesity and other diseases have soared there as well.

Not only is fast food everywhere, but fast-food companies encourage the consumer to eat more by supplying over-size burgers, extra-large servings of fries, and super-size buckets of soda. Products like the Whopper, Big Gulp, and Super Size meals pack a whopping amount of calories, refined sugars, and rancid fats. Let's take a closer look:

- The Double Gulp soda at a 7-Eleven store holds 64 ounces of soda—that is half a gallon! It contains the equivalent of 48 teaspoons of sugar.

---

*For an alarming look at fast-food burgers, see the video on YouTube called The World's First Bionic Burger, www.youtube.com/watch?v=mYyDXH1amic.

- A typical hamburger at a fast-food restaurant weighs 6 ounces. In 1957, it weighed 1 ounce.
- According to one nutritionist, your average fast food meal is more like three meals.
- The average meal at a McDonald's has 1,550 calories.

Fast food is a global phenomenon that is simply not good for us. We're eating more food that is not nutritious. Most fast-food meals are high in rancid fats, refined sugar, empty calories, cooked starch, refined salt, dozens of different pesticides, heat-resistant nanobacteria, and GMO ingredients, and low in plant fiber and essential nutrients. Because fast food lacks nutrients and minerals, after we eat it we are not satisfied. That makes us hungry for more soon after.

Children are particularly at risk from over-consumption of fast foods. Fast-food chains spend more than $3 billion every year on television advertising, exposing our children to an onslaught of appeals. In what is known as "cradle-to-grave" advertising strategies, they intentionally focus on kids so they become lifelong customers. Researchers have found that children can often recognize a company logo like the Golden Arches before they can recognize their own name.

In one year the typical American child watches more than forty thousand TV commercials. About half of these ads are for junk food: fast food, candy, soda, and breakfast cereals. This means that your child sees a junk-food ad every five minutes when watching TV.

To further motivate children to eat fast food, companies have Happy Meals with free toys. One fast-food chain gives away more than 1.5 billion toys every year. Almost one out of every three new toys given to American kids each year is from a fast-food restaurant.

In order to combat these calculated advertising strategies, it is paramount to educate our children on healthy eating habits that are easy, fun, and delicious. By teaching children how harmful fast food is and how to eat healthier, we are empowering them to make the right choices.

Here is the bottom line: fast food undermines our longevity potential and health, and it damages the Earth.

Obesity: A Killer

Fast food has been linked to the easily observed increase in obesity among people of all age groups. Obesity has reached epidemic proportions in the Western world, particularly in children. Here are some startling statistics to consider:

- 65 percent of American adults are overweight.
- 30 percent of Americans are obese.
- According to the American Obesity Association, 127 million Americans are overweight, 60 million Americans are obese, and 9 million are "morbidly obese"—this means they weigh 100 pounds more than they should.
- In the last twenty years, the rate of obesity has doubled in children and tripled in adolescents and teens.
- As of September 2004, 9 million American kids between the ages of six and eighteen were obese.

Obesity-related illnesses will kill around 400,000 Americans in 2013 (as I write this book)—almost the same as smoking. Americans have gotten so big that their coffins have to be supersized!

Illnesses caused by obesity include high blood pressure, heart disease, breast cancer, colon cancer, gout, arthritis, asthma, diabetes, and strokes.

In 2003, the Centers for Disease Control and Prevention reported that one out of three kids born in the U.S. in the year 2000 will develop type 2 diabetes. The life of a ten-year-old child who develops type 2 diabetes will be, on average, between seventeen and twenty-six years shorter than that of a healthy child. Diabetes can lead to heart attacks, strokes, blindness, kidney failure, and nerve damage in the lower legs that may result in amputation (82,000 of these cases occur every year). Diabetes is currently the sixth-highest cause of death in America.

Genetically Modified Food

Genetically modified foods are made from genetically modified organisms (GMOs) that have had their DNA altered through viral genetic engineering. Genetically modified food was first introduced in 1994 with the commercially grown, genetically modified Flavr Savr tomato, engineered to be more resistant to rotting by the California company Calgene.

An estimated 60 to 70 percent of all foods on supermarket shelves today contain genetically modified ingredients, with that percentage higher for processed convenience foods such as soda, soup, crackers, condiments, and candy bars. According to the U.S. Department of Agriculture, by the time you read this, 85 percent of the soybeans planted in the United States and up to 45 percent of the corn will be genetically engineered. If you are eating foods that contain vegetable oil, soy products (like soy burgers), or any foods that are made with corn starch, corn syrup, corn oil, or soy derivatives, then there is a good chance that you are putting food that's been genetically modified into your body.

The frightening thing is there's no way to know for sure.

The government has not implemented regulations that require producers of GMO foods to tell consumers that a food has been genetically altered or that it contains GMO ingredients. What's more, under current laws biotech companies don't have to inform the FDA or perform human testing before introducing a new genetically engineered food product. As a result, GMO foods are flooding the marketplace, and millions of unsuspecting consumers are purchasing and consuming unlabeled genetically modified foods. Don't be one of them! See below for tips on how to avoid eating GMO foods.

How are foods genetically modified? Genes (genetic codes) determine the production of specific proteins within each organism. Due to advances in technology, scientists are now able to select a genetic sequence from organisms such as plants, animals, or even microbes and insert that material into the permanent genetic code of another organism.

For example, a gene found in flounder that enables these fish to survive in cold water was transplanted into tomatoes so that they would

How to Avoid Eating GM Foods

- Eat organic. The Organic Food Production Act stipulates that food labeled organic cannot contain any genetically modified organisms.
- Eat superfoods and superherbs, as these are not contaminated with GMOs.
- Buy local. Shop at farmers' markets where you can buy direct from local growers. Ask them how they treat their crops.
- Avoid eating processed foods. Many processed foods include derivatives of corn, soy, and canola that more than likely come from genetically modified plants. Buy whole foods such as fruits, vegetables, nuts, seeds, seaweeds, and sprouts instead.
- Read food labels. If ingredients come from corn, soy, or canola, put the food back on the shelf. Look for labels that say, "This product does not contain genetically modified organisms."
- Get involved. Demand that proper labeling for genetically modified foods be required.

The following foods are currently being used and/or tested by the biotech industry in field trials in an attempt to create gene-altered varieties:

- Fruits: apples, bell peppers, cherries, cranberries, grapefruit, kiwi, melons, olives, papayas, pears, persimmons, pineapples, plums, squash, strawberries, and tomatoes
- Grains: barley, corn, oats, wheat
- Legumes: lentils, peas, soybeans
- Vegetables: cabbage, carrots, cauliflower, cucumber, lettuce, mustard, onions, potatoes, radishes, sweet potatoes, watercress
- Nuts and Seeds: chocolate, coffee, flax, peanuts, sunflowers, walnuts

become resistant to frost. Genes from soil bacteria are transferred into foods such as corn and canola so that they repel insects. Other examples of our tampering with Mother Nature include potatoes that contain bacteria genes, "super" pigs with human growth genes, and fish with cattle growth genes.

These genetically modified creations are being patented and released into the marketplace without scientists or consumers having any idea about what the long-term effects will be upon the environment, ourselves, and our children's health. Multiple studies reveal that genetically modified foods can pose serious health risks to humans, domesticated animals, wildlife, and the environment. The effects on humans can include dangerous transformation of the DNA of our friendly bacteria, resistance to antibiotics, suppression of the immune system, and even cancer.[3] The impact on the environment includes the contamination of nongenetically modified life-forms from contact with GMOs used in agriculture, as well as other forms of biological pollution (such as GMO salmon escaped from fish farms), all of which could completely throw off Nature's delicate balance. As just one instance, this has already happened in Hawaii with GMO papayas, which have contaminated wild papayas.

The bottom line is: We need at least a century of research on GMO products before we allow GM organisms into the environment. How much do we know about genetics, anyway? DNA was just discovered sixty years ago. We need to seriously contemplate the implications of what tampering with Mother Nature could cost us. We might destroy elements in our ecosystem permanently by introducing untested genetically modified foods and organisms. I suggest that you join the fight against genetically modified foods. The most powerful way to do that is to avoid purchasing GM products.

Hydrogenated Oils

Hydrogenated oils are used in the food industry for the sole purpose of prolonging the shelf life of processed foods. Many European countries have either banned hydrogenated and partially hydrogenated oils altogether or have implemented future dates for their elimination from foods. This is because of undeniable evidence from scientific studies that directly link rancid fatty acids (hydrogenated and partially hydrogenated oils) found in processed foods to the development of diabetes, cancer, and cardiovascular disease.

How to Avoid Hydrogenated Oils

Read your food labels. If they list hydrogenated or partially hydrogenated oils, do not buy the product!

Buy foods that use organic ingredients and contain raw, cold-processed olive oil, coconut oil, hemp seed oil, and/or chia seed oil. Use these same oils when preparing your own meals.

Avoid the following foods that are almost always made with partially hydrogenated oils:

- bread
- breakfast cereals
- cake, biscuit, cornbread mixes, pancake mixes, frostings
- cakes, cookies, muffins, pies, donuts
- crackers
- corn chips, potato chips
- frozen bakery products, toaster pastries, frozen snack foods, waffles, pancakes
- frozen burritos
- frozen entrees and meals
- frozen pizza
- instant mashed potatoes
- lowfat ice creams
- margarines, shortening
- microwave popcorn
- most prepared frozen meats and fish (such as fish sticks)
- noodle soup cups
- peanut butter (except fresh-ground)
- pasta mixes
- sauce mixes
- taco shells
- whipped toppings

Be aware that fast-food restaurants and chains use a lot of pre-prepared foods. These are loaded with hydrogenated and partially hydrogenated fats. Try to eat in restaurants that prepare your food from scratch—these establishments are less likely to have foods containing hydrogenated and partially hydrogenated oils. Italian, Greek, Spanish, and other Mediterranean restaurants usually use healthy oils such as olive oil.

Hydrogenated oils are rancid and often contain trans fatty acids. It is this type of oil that gets into the fatty tissue of your body, disrupts your brain chemistry, causes neurological disorders, wreaks havoc on your skin, and creates a multitude of serious health conditions. If you are serious about your health, please avoid these oils as much as possible.

Moving away from hydrogenated oil and moving on to raw, living oils and fats is one of the most powerful, transformative experiences you can have in your life. This is one of the reasons folks report such marked improvements in their health by switching to a raw-food-based diet.

Microwaved Food

The Russians did an enormous amount of research on microwaving, equal to the Americans. As in the West, they used microwaves to vibrate water molecules, making the water radioactive. Sometime in the 1970s they completely abandoned it because it was too dangerous. Microwaving food is not only destructive to whatever is in the microwave, but the appliance bleeds a lot of its dangerous EMF (electromagnetic frequency) field out into the local environment. That is why you cannot look into a microwave and this is why you have to stand at least six feet (two meters) away from a working microwave.

If you live in an apartment and you have a microwave, unplug it and use it as storage for plastic bags or other recycled goods. What I did with my old microwave is literally use it to store some of my alchemical products because they need to be protected from EMF fields. There's a lot of shielding that's been put into microwaves! As long as that microwave is sitting away from electrical outlet plugs and is unplugged itself, it will actually shield some of your health food products and keep them in good shape for a long period of time.

Monosodium Glutamate

Monosodium glutamate (MSG) is a byproduct of soybean chemistry. It is an excitotoxin. In 1997 Dr. Russell L. Blaylock published a great book called *Excitotoxins: The Taste That Kills*. In it he describes how excitotoxins cause your brain cells to explode. No one wants exploding brain cells—that means no MSG. MSG is just another example of a "flavor-enhancing" chemical that is being added to the many foods and drinks that average people consume on a daily basis.

Strong scientific evidence suggests that substances like MSG can cause brain damage in children, adolescents, adults, and the elderly. This is because the ingesting of excitotoxins such as MSG affects the development of a child's nervous system. It has also been determined that excitotoxins can be passed from mother to child and damage the developing brain of the baby.

Many excitotoxins are human-made, but others exist in Nature, such as glutamate. They are all amino acids that function as neurotransmitters. The function of a neurotransmitter is to send messages to the brain. Glutamate is one of the most common neurotransmitters found in both the brain and the spinal cord. When glutamate rises above a critical level it becomes a deadly toxin that affects the brain cells and the nerve cells connected to them. For example, if one is eating high concentrations of glutamate in one's diet, the brain cells are exposed to this substance, become excited, and rapidly fire impulses over and over again until they reach a state of exhaustion. The cells then die, as if they were "excited to death." Thus the moniker "excitotoxin."

Why You Should Avoid Nonstick Cookware

Nonstick cookware came into being as Teflon-coated cookware, and now it's time for it to go the way of the dinosaur. Teflon is used in the industry because nothing breaks it down. You don't want any Teflon getting inside your body! Teflon is extremely toxic, and it is now being implicated in a number of health conditions. Give it away, throw it away, get rid of it. If you use Teflon and any of the particles chip off and get into your food, or react into your food (which now is known to be happening), you could be exposed to a very serious carcinogen. I recommend you remove all nonstick cookware from your home. At 680°F Teflon pans release at least six toxic gases, including two carcinogens, two global pollutants, and MFA—a chemical lethal to humans at low doses.

Since around 2005, the multibillion-dollar "perfluorochemical" (PFC) industry, which underpins such world-famous brands as Teflon, Stainmaster, Scotchgard, and Gore-Tex, has flooded the market with toxic, nondegradable products. The PFC family is characterized by chains of carbon atoms of varying lengths, to which fluorine atoms are strongly bonded, creating virtually indestructible chemicals that were, until recently, thought to be biologically inert.

A flood of disturbing scientific findings since the late 1990s has clearly demonstrated that PFCs consist of highly toxic chemicals that contaminate human blood, wildlife, and the environment. Research scientists are especially concerned because unlike any other toxic chemicals, the most pervasive and toxic members of the PFC family do not break down in the environment under normal circumstances. Major companies like 3M and DuPont are getting away with contaminating the entire planet's remotely foreseeable future as they falsely assure the world's population that they are exercising responsibility with respect to public health and the environment. And PFCs are just the tip of that iceberg. . . .

For the best cookware ever, look for brands that use 316-T stainless steel (e.g., Saladmaster), because this type of stainless steel never outgases toxic metals or heavy metallic ions. Borosilicate is another type of non-outgassing, safe cookware material (e.g., Pyrex).

Pasteurized Dairy Products

Dairy is a multibillion-dollar industry in North America. We are raised to believe that pasteurized cow's milk is the perfect food, containing essential nutrients such as "calcium" that are necessary for our health and well-being. We are taught that there are adverse consequences if we do not drink milk—bones become weak, we lose our strength, and we will suffer from conditions such as osteoporosis, even though the evidence indicates that the more conventional dairy products we consume, the greater our calcification problems will be.

Consider that common conventional dairy products may be:

- pasteurized
- homogenized
- hormonally altered
- contaminated with genetically modified foods fed to the cows
- contaminated with viruses that have been linked to diabetes (type 1)
- contaminated with pus
- contaminated with blood
- contaminated with bad calcium (chalk) in order to keep a rich, white color
- contaminated with tap water (containing chemicals, bad calcium, and bad iron)

In 1995, Europe banned the use of hormones in farm animals because of the link to cancer in humans. Contaminated conventional dairy products may also be linked to calcium infections that manifest in our bodies as bone spurs, varicose veins, scleroderma, arthritis, strokes, diabetes, kidney stones, gallstones, and liver stones.

Preservatives

The function of preservatives is to increase the shelf life of food (prevent it from going bad), to improve the appearance so food looks more attractive, and to enhance the flavor of food so that it becomes addictive. Unfortunately, by loading up the Western diet with preservatives, we have created food that is nutritionally bankrupt. Many of these preservatives are not even required to appear on labels; therefore, average consumers are ingesting chemicals that they have no idea have been linked to cancer, allergies, liver and kidney damage, migraines, and birth defects.

Preservatives are so potent that they can keep a hamburger looking "fresh" for years without any decomposition taking place. Preservatives prevent oxygen and microbes from entering into the food and breaking it down. Eventually, as preservatives break down, they actually form carcinogenic byproducts that end up being more toxic and harmful than the preservatives themselves.

The following common preservatives should be avoided because of their known toxicity or because their short- and long-term effects are unknown (though suspected of being dangerous).

Eating fresh, whole foods is the best way to stay away from these harmful preservatives and chemicals. If you are still eating processed foods, please read the effects of preservatives listed below. If you see them listed on an ingredient label of a product you are about to purchase, pass on it instead.

Potassium Bromate

A preservative used to increase volume in breads and white flour, potassium bromate breaks down rapidly and is not considered harmful; however, some types of bromate compounds have been linked to causing cancer in animals and even trace amounts in bread can pose a risk to humans. California requires a cancer warning on the product label if potassium bromate is listed as an ingredient.

Potassium Sorbate

Potassium sorbate is a common, mildly toxic preservative used to prevent mold and yeast in foods such as cheese, wine, dried meats, yogurt, baked goods, and dried fruit products. Usually the toxicity of potassium sorbate is associated with dosage. Higher dosages can lead to allergic reactions, nausea, and diarrhea.

Propyl Gallate

Propyl gallate is a preservative used to prevent fats and oils from spoiling, often used in conjunction with BHA and BHT. It is frequently found in vegetable oil, meat products, potato sticks, chicken soup base, chewing gum, cosmetics, hair products, adhesives, and lubricants. This toxic preservative has been linked to cancer in animals.

How to Avoid Preservatives

- Avoid processed foods, most of which are filled with toxic preservatives that undermine our good health. Avoid them completely.
- Read food labels. If any of the above preservatives are listed on the product or food, avoid it.
- Eat organic. Preservatives are not contained in organic, whole raw foods.
- Use natural products. Cosmetics, shampoos, soaps, lotions, creams, etc., contain harmful preservatives too.
- Try to use natural products that use organic, natural ingredients and no harmful chemicals and preservatives. A good rule of thumb is: if you cannot eat it, then avoid putting it on your skin.

Sodium Benzoate

Sodium benzoate is a common, mildly toxic preservative that can be found in the following foods: soft drinks, fruit juices, margarine, confections, pickles, and jams. Benzoic acid is actually a superior preservative (and exists naturally in certain foods such as berries), but it lacks the solubility in liquids possessed by sodium benzoate. The biggest problem with sodium benzoate is that when it is combined with potassium benzoate (in the presence of vitamin C) the carcinogen benzene is produced.

Sodium Nitrate

Sodium nitrate is used to preserve the flavoring and coloring of meat products, commonly found in the following foods: bacon, ham, smoked fish, corned beef, hot dogs, and lunch meats. Studies have linked ingesting sodium nitrate to various types of cancers. According to Christine Gerbstadt, MD, MPH, RD, LDN, and a spokesperson for the American Diabetic Association, "Under certain high-temperature cooking conditions such as grilling, it transforms into a reactive compound that has been shown to promote cancer."[4]

Sulfur Dioxide

Sulfur dioxide has been known to contribute to respiratory illness in children and the elderly, and can aggravate existing heart and lung diseases. Sulfur dioxide is a known skin irritant and by logical deduction may irritate the inner skin cells of our digestive organs.

Sulfur dioxide in the environment contributes to the formation of acid rain that damages trees and crops, and makes soils and lakes acidic. This acid rain is even eroding old sculptures and architecture.

Sulfur dioxide is used on almost all nonorganic dry fruits. It is an unnatural preservative that is rarely tested for, although my company tests for it on products. For example, sulfur dioxide is used on nonorganic goji berries to keep them preserved. Out of fifteen goji berry brands taken off the shelf, twelve failed the sulfur dioxide test. I know that the people who actually manufacture and package those goji berries don't even know that they are being sprayed with sulfur dioxide. How does this happen? It happens because the conventional farmers don't tell them, and the brokers that sell to them don't tell them.

This is why I believe strongly in buying only organic products, growing your own food, and foraging your own food: because things like sulfur dioxide slip by the consumer and end up in our bodies.

Soy

> Soy foods contain trypsin inhibitors that inhibit protein digestion and affect pancreatic function. In test animals, diets high in trypsin inhibitors led to stunted growth and pancreatic disorders. Soy foods increase the body's requirement for vitamin D, needed for strong bones and normal growth. Phytic acid in soy foods results in reduced bioavailability of iron and zinc, which are required for the health and development of the brain and nervous system. Soy also lacks cholesterol, likewise essential for the development of the brain and nervous system. Megadoses of phytoestrogens in soy formula have been implicated in the current trend toward increasingly premature sexual development in girls and delayed or retarded sexual development in boys.
>
> —SALLY FALLON, MARY G. ENIG, PhD, AND MIKE FITZPATRICK, PhD,
> *MYTHS AND TRUTHS ABOUT SOY FOODS*

Soy is in a staggering number of foods these days including: soy flour, soy milk, tofu, soy protein isolates, texturized vegetable protein (TVP), soy oil, edamame (whole soybeans), and fermented soy products such as tempeh and miso. Adding to this list are all the processed items that are made from these soy products including soy meats, soy cheeses, and soy ice creams, among others. Soy flour and soy lecithin are often found in chocolate bars, cereals, cake mixes, granola bars, and a whole host of other items.

Soy has experienced a backlash in recent years. In addition to the benefits of its vegetarian protein, soy has been shown to cause a host of health problems that range from cancers to brain atrophy to immune and endocrine system disorders, thyroid disorders, infertility, breast cancer, and other types of cancer.

The research that favors soy as being good for the hormones and estrogen is inconclusive. There's research on both sides of the equation. Mary Enig's research indicates that soy can influence and disrupt natural hormone levels, even in children.[5]

I suggest you do your own research. At the very least, consume less than two servings of soy per week in order to keep your phyto-estrogen exposure to a minimum—even better, avoid soy altogether. By the time that you read these words, more than 90 percent of the soy products produced in North America will be genetically modified. We have no idea what the effects of genetically modified food are over a period of, say, five years or ten years, let alone generations. Genetically modified foods have nothing to do with what's natural or normal; we know that soy, in its natural form, even if it's not genetically modified, is toxic—it is actually poisonous. Remember that genetically modified soy lecithin (present in almost every conventional chocolate bar product) is fat-soluble and gets into the brain and nervous system.

In Asian cultures, soy was traditionally cooked and then fed to bacteria in order to detoxify it; the bacteria would convert it into reasonably useable nutritional compounds, to form the basis for miso, for example.

There's nothing that you need in soy protein. There's nothing you need in soy isolates. There's nothing in soy oils that your body requires that you cannot get from a superior source, namely superfood protein sources and superfood fatty acid sources. So soy is essentially irrelevant in terms of your body's needs.

Table Salt

I recommend only sea salts and/or rock salts (from within the Earth). All processed table and/or common salts should be avoided. Amongst salts we tested in our lab, table salt (sodium chloride) tested the highest in bromine, a semi-toxic halogen vaporous mineral.

Common salt usually begins as a rock salt. From there, all the trace minerals are cooked and processed off and sold to chemical companies. The remaining material is ionically rebonded into a sodium chloride salt with few trace elements. This artificial salt is then used as a preservative in nearly all processed and packaged foods. Americans consume five

Alternatives to Using Table Salt

- Read food labels. Any ingredient that has the word "sodium" in it is adding salt to your diet. Sodium nitrate is a form of salt that is often found in processed and preserved foods. When mixed with urea and stomach acid, sodium nitrate becomes a carcinogen.
- Avoid fast food. Fast food is loaded with toxic sodium.
- Avoid processed foods. These always contain a high-toxic salt content. Eat high-potassium raw foods such as fresh fruits, vegetables, nuts, seeds, sprouts, and wheatgrass in order to flush your system of toxic salt. Vegetables like celery have natural salt in them that can help you manage a no- to low-salt diet. At some point, when you are flushed of toxic salt, it is recommended to add sea salt back into your diet for minerals, nervous system health, hydration, and overall metabolic balance.
- When eating out at a restaurant, the common salt in your meal can be high. Ask the wait staff to prepare a no-salt meal for you.
- Appeal to your craving for salt without adding a lot of sodium to your diet. Use other spices to put some zest into your meal. Instead of reaching for the salt shaker, add pepper. Experiment with herbs. Try chopping garlic or adding spices like cinnamon, nutmeg, oregano, and rosemary. Fresh squeezed lemon or lime on food can add a lot of flavor to your meals.
- Add sea vegetables, which are usually coated with sea salt, to your diet. Sprinkle kelp or other seaweeds on your food. They taste delicious and are an excellent source of minerals.
- Make sure sea salt, Himalayan rock salt, or a full-spectrum salt is used in whatever you are eating once you start using salt again. If it just says "salt," on the label, avoid it.

hundred million pounds of this type of salt a year. Processed table salt is in everything from baby food to cereals like Cheerios, potato chips, candy, and pet food.

Processed table salt is a harmful condiment that, when consumed in excess, has been shown to have an adverse effect on human health. Table salt ingestion can lead to high blood sugar, heart attacks, hypertension, strokes, and kidney failure. This poor-quality salt can also cause water retention and contribute to inflammation.

The correct types of salts, especially sea salt, are holy and sacred. Claiming that all salt is terrible because of the sins committed by the common table salt industry is like claiming all food is terrible because Big Macs exist. Salt has an illustrious history within all cultures. Salt was used by the Egyptians to embalm bodies. Mark Kurlansky's book *Salt: A World History* delivers an extraordinary series of tales about salt, the Latin root of which is *sal.* For example, the Roman army was paid one week of the month via their needed supply of salt. This was part of their salary, or "salt pay."

Once you have detoxified your body (over a period of months or even years) of common table salt using a raw-food diet strategy (with low or no salt), then the Roman salt pay makes more sense. We are so saturated in salt that we don't realize how important salt is for health, hydration, and survival until we eat raw food and avoid all salt. Animals in Nature are never looking for potassium, they are looking for salt. This is because every natural animal's raw diet is high in potassium, which is antagonistic to sodium. Natural salts are the best mineral supplements and as essential to life as water.

Tap Water

Clean, safe water is essential to all noble life-forms and is the most important element of a healthy body. Water is a universal solvent. It carries nutrients to every cell in our body and flushes out harmful toxins. We are a water-based life-form. The first step in getting the body chemistry in proper order is to become well hydrated with the best water (and sea salt) ever. See page 46 for information on how to drink the best water ever.

Being well hydrated increases the strength of the immune system and maintains the health of the skin and organs. Proper hydration is essential to keeping us clear, bright, and beautiful. Hydration is the main factor that keeps one's tissues "juicy."

Finding a pure water source in today's polluted environment requires being able to think outside the box or plastic bottle. Unsafe water is not just a third-world problem. Finding water that is safe to drink can be even more difficult in industrially developed countries. Research from all directions continues to show that most tap and well water in the U.S. is not safe for drinking due to heavy industrial, pharmaceutical, radioactive (tritium), and environmental pollution. We have created a situation in which all sources of our drinking water, including municipal water systems, rivers, lakes, streams, and wells, contain some level of contamination. Even ice core samples from high mountains and polar regions show contamination.[6]

Although many of the contaminants that are found in drinking water do not exist at levels high enough to cause immediate illness, low-level exposure to many of them typically causes severe calcification illnesses over time.

A December 2009 U.S. government study found many states with consistent violations of maximum contaminant limits; a dozen states had more than 11 percent of their systems demonstrating such problems.[7] According to the EPA, tap water contains more than 700 organic chemicals that are suspected cancer-causing agents. Public water systems do not test for most of the carcinogens and other dangerous chemicals that are being found.

Common pollutants present in our tap water include:

- arsenic
- bad calcium (insoluble, lacking electrons)
- bad iron (rust)
- copper
- cyanide

- lead
- nitrates
- organo-phosphate residues
- pesticide run-off
- petrochemicals
- phosphates
- radon
- strontium
- toilet paper (yes, that's correct; in fact, used toilet paper residues are the most common pollutant of tap water)
- tritium (radioactive heavy hydrogen)
- uranium

In his book *Extreme Toxic Times: How to Escape on Your Own Two Feet*, Dr. Howard Fisher states that government sources list four categories of drinking water pollution:

- chemical byproducts (which are present due to the reaction of the disinfectants with organic or inorganic materials in the water)
- disinfectants and coagulants (which are left over from treating the pathogen load present in the water)
- natural pathogens
- organic, inorganic, or radioactive chemicals

Please keep in mind that not only are we drinking from contaminated water sources, we are also bathing in them. Do you have a water filter on your shower or bathtub? If you don't, then your skin, which is the largest eliminative organ in your body, is soaking in all those poisonous chemicals. All the toxicity that is present in the tap water is being delivered directly to your skin cells and perhaps deeper into your body.

Completely avoid drinking tap water in any form. It is dangerously undermining any prospect of health. People are more and more dehydrated and toxic. They are not flushing anything out, but adding to the problem and not the solution (pun intended).

Either get a filter or become a filter!

CHAPTER 4

Detoxification

Raw plant foods, superfoods, medicinal herbs, fresh spring water, laughter, bliss, joy, positive thoughts, hope, and unconditional love all exist in the same frequency range. Tuning into this frequency range raises the overall vibration of your energy field, causing anything that is vibrating at a lower frequency, such as fear, pain, doubt, cancer, ugliness, depression, toxins, parasites, bad calcium, and so on, to eventually percolate out and be ejected from the body. This process is known as detoxification.

Detoxification is the process, and the symptoms that coincide with, the body cleansing itself of wastes and poisons. These toxins can include metabolic waste, heavy metals, pathogenic organisms, volatile organic compounds, distressed emotions, spiritually stuck energy, and other energies. Though every tissue and organ is able to go through its own detoxification, it is the liver, kidneys, lymph fluid, skin, brain, gastrointestinal tract, along with the entire immune system, that are the key facilitators of this process.

Detoxification transforms us yet also challenges us. As we embark and continue into this process, remember that we do not need to focus on perfection, just progress. Old habits die hard, but they do die. Some shifts happen immediately while others take time. The path may be relatively easy or it may be challenging, but it is always worth it.

By decreasing the pathogen, viral, and nanobacteria load in our bodies, we improve our physical and mental energy and acuity. The Longevity Now approach enables us to step into higher-energy states where we feel a deeper joy in being alive, a deeper sense of well-being, a return of laughter and the big four letter word, H-O-P-E, where we feel that things are turning a corner and going in a positive direction.

To be able to handle the metabolic change that occurs during this shift, we need to begin where we are and move at our own pace. As we progress, we can consistently increase that pace. Small commitments lead to large commitments. Minor victories lead to major victories. An object in motion tends to stay in motion, whether it is a train, a car, an emotion, a habit, or a belief. One step leads to another. Each triumph brings you one step closer to realizing the goal of eternal youth and beauty.

There are different ideas about the nature of detoxification. I believe that two key factors are at work when we detoxify:

- Chelation by replacement: This is when lower-quality nutrients are displaced by purer, higher-energy equivalents.
- Removal of toxins (artificial substances, parasite waste products, natural waste products of metabolism): hardened, mucous, sludge-like waste matter and all types of "excess" substance.

> **TIP** Be aware that certain unhealthy foods and lifestyle cravings present themselves when we are tired, such as at the end of a long day. Be prepared. Go to sleep early if necessary. Drink a glass of pure spring water with a twist of fresh lemon and a pinch of Celtic sea salt. Be persistent; break the old cycles and soon the desire will disappear. Cravings are always temporary.

A brief list of prominent detoxification tools:

- detox products that remove artificial environmental toxins: fulvic acid, MSM (pine resin), zeolites, shilajit, EDTA, clay, and Patrick Flanagan's Crystal Energy (Chapter 6)
- the general strategy and application of the Longevity Now approach: to dissolve and remove parasites and their waste products (bad calcium)

- herbal detox systems: Triple Herbal Treasures and herbal cleansing systems—these are designed to remove hardened mucoid plaque from the small intestines
- fasting: Juice fasting (usually centers on alkaline green vegetable and beet juice); blended fasting (no solid food, this fast usually centers on detox lemonades and raw green soups); water fasting (should be done with spring water); dry fasting (alternate days of dry and water fasting have been shown in Russian research to reduce dangerous deuterium or heavy hydrogen levels in the body, thus increasing longevity)
- a thinned-down raw detox diet (with low fat, low sugar, and high fiber/alkalinity): This type of diet—an Ann Wigmore–style detox diet—should be done temporarily and not as a maintenance diet.

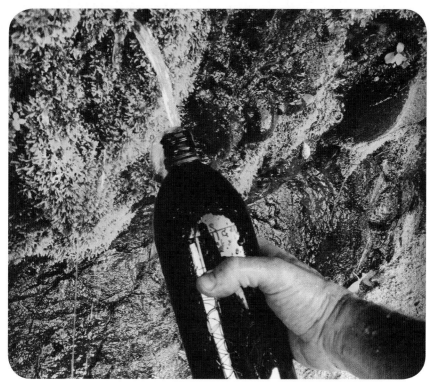

Drink fresh, living spring water while fasting.

- sauna (hot/cold water therapy): This can include traditional American-European Water Cure, Russian *banya* therapies, Finnish saunas, variations of Ayurvedic *panchakarma,* etc. The idea behind these therapies is that heat expands your tissues and cold contracts them; in the dynamic between heat and cold, the body is purified and detoxified, like the squeezing of a sponge.

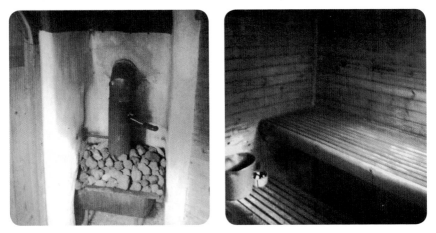

A traditional wood-fire sauna

- a lymphatically activating exercise program (inversion-oriented yoga, rebounding, etc.)
- enemas and colonics (it is important to pull the plug and let all wastes drain out semi-regularly)
- deep-tissue bodywork (Romi Romi, Rolfing, etc.): See part five of the Longevity Now decalcification system.
- grounding and zapper technology: Zappers draw toxins right through the skin to the negatively charged electrode on the zapper. Being grounded by touching the Earth directly or via grounding technology alters the exchange of gases excreted when we breathe. This may take several months of consistent grounding in order to normalize. This indicates that by being grounded, we are detoxifying substances that we typically cannot excrete. Bad

hormone removal via methylation (beet juice), the appropriate nutrients (I3C, DIM), counterbalancing progesterone cream, and fiber: The presence of plastics and other excess xenoestrogens and the problems that they cause for human biology are becoming more widely understood, including the connection to hormone disorders in humans, other mammals, reptiles, amphibians, and many other orders of life. Estrogens may be the most toxic compounds to burden the liver as we age. See Chapter 5 for more on hormones.

> **TIP** All detoxification strategies should be adopted with common sense. Too sudden a shift can "shock" the body. Everything comes as it should, in its own time. The way to create lasting change is to step outside your comfort zone, but not into your shock zone. If you want to realize greater health gains, invest your time and energy in detoxification efforts and personal development projects over a long period. The long-range projects pay off so much more because the universe rewards the virtues of discipline and perseverance.

Symptoms of Detoxification

If you're going through hell, keep going.
—WINSTON CHURCHILL

Have you ever stepped into a calm pond or lake in the early morning hours? Once you step in, the mud at the bottom is churned up. Detoxification is like this. Eating healthier, lighter foods, superfoods, and herbs, as well as taking Longevity Now recommended supplements, tends to churn up the old sludge, including past emotional residue and the buried hurt. Emotional cleansing is part of the transformation process.

Typical, Cyclical Symptoms of Detoxification

- body aches
- body odor
- bowel irregularities
- deep doubts
- emotional fluctuations
- excess mucus
- general feelings of discomfort
- halitosis
- headaches
- lack of interest in sex
- premenstrual syndrome (PMS)
- skin challenges
- soul searching
- turbid urine

These symptoms represent low-energy phenomena being flushed out by higher-energy nutrients, mental states, and emotions.

TIP If you are experiencing strong detoxification symptoms—especially through the skin—visit a reputable colon hydrotherapist. Colonics can help channel and remove the blocked-up toxicity and emotions through the bowels, instead of the skin. Again, this is like pulling the plug on a dirty bathtub. The waste must be drained out.

An important point about Longevity Now and detoxification in general is that it is usually not the organisms (such as nanobacteria, viruses, or fungi like candida) that are the cause of problematic health issues, but rather their waste products (or fecal matter—what they excrete into our system). The fastest way to immediately clean up those waste products, especially while activating the Longevity Now approach, is through colonics, which support good lymphatic drainage and help us get the blockages out of the system as quickly as possible. In addition, we want to really power up the immune system so that the white blood cells can vacuum up the rest of those waste byproducts that are generated by viruses, nanobacteria, fungi, mold, cancer cells, etc.

How to Slow Down or Speed Up Detoxification

Catabolic practices tend to speed up or accelerate detoxification symptoms. This means that a catabolic practice will move toxins through and out of the body faster. "Catabolic" means "to break down." Catabolic practices include:

- aerobic exercise
- colon hydrotherapy (also enemas)
- drinking green juices
- drinking only living spring water
- eating sweet fruit
- fasting
- herbal cleansing
- hot springs bathing
- massage (deep tissue)
- menstruation (in women)
- orgasm (ejaculation in men)
- skin brushing
- sweatlodge/sauna/infrared heat
- taking enzymes and probiotic supplements
- taking the supplements recommended in Longevity Now (zeolites, fulvic acid, MegaHydrate, Crystal Energy, shilajit, EDTA, etc.)

Anabolic practices tend to slow down detoxification. "Anabolic" means "to build up," implying that an anabolic practice will suppress the release of toxins from the body because other activities are occurring, such as muscle-building. Anabolic practices include:

- anaerobic exercise, such as heavy weight-lifting or sprints
- consuming sea salt or rock salt
- eating any kind of dairy product
- eating any type of meat, including fish

- eating cooked starches like bread, pasta, rice, or baked potato
- eating fatty foods like avocados, nuts, olives, seeds, coconuts, or durian
- eating fibrous, green-leafed vegetable salads

Neither catabolic nor anabolic practices are more important than the other. They are both valuable and useful at the correct time.

Being able to control the rate of detox is one way that this process of cleansing is a personal, unique endeavor. Self-healing through alternative healthcare, utilizing strategies for decalcification and detoxification as outlined in this book, is the wave of the future. Alternative healthcare sciences tend to view people as whole individuals in an environment with a unique history, rather than as a group of labeled symptoms and diagnoses.

> **TIP** Use your intuition and instincts to aid your own healing strategies, as well as your choice of naturopaths, physicians, or healers. If you feel that more esoteric healing regimes are appropriate, such as prayer, psychics, faith, or other methods, then by all means act upon those feelings. This is where you may have your greatest breakthroughs. The ultimate benefit of natural and spiritual healing regimes is the adventuresome, optimistic frame of mind that arises within us from using them.

Weight Loss

Enlightenment is just that—making yourself lighter. Detoxifying one's body results in heavy "gravitational" materials and energies being released.

Permanent weight loss comes through an inner transformation. This usually arises from an epiphany, a moment of clarity, a clear decision.

When the decision has been made and a new path in life is chosen, the weight is already lost.

The two primary elements to reduce and eliminate from the diet in order to lose weight are starchy carbohydrates (baked potatoes, rice, beer, bread, pasta, corn chips, potato chips, etc.) and cooked fats (high-fat meat and pasteurized dairy foods).

Overeating habits and weight gain are related to eating demineralized foods. The richer a food is in minerals, the more difficult it becomes to overeat it. When food is eaten raw, it gives a stronger signal to stop eating. This is called the "aliesthetic taste change." This taste change is stronger in more mineralized foods—and is especially strong in wild foods. It is virtually impossible to overeat wild foods. Wild foods are always higher in minerals than domesticated foods. Domesticated plants, especially those that are commercially grown, tend to be high in sugar/starch and low in minerals. These include grains (bread, pasta, rice-cakes, beer), potatoes (baked, potato chips), corn (corn chips, corn syrup products), carrots, and seedless fruits. The consumption of demineralized food often leads to addictions.

Hypothyroidism (an underactive thyroid gland) has received a lot of the blame for excessive weight gain. This can be true, though it is not always the case. If indeed thyroid challenges are the cause of excessive weight gain, then the best course of action is to get one's stress levels down, to nourish and detoxify the body, and stay grounded, while simultaneously building up androgenic hormones: progesterone (women), testosterone (women and men), vitamin D3, and DHEA. Nourishing the thyroid can include maca (superfood), coconut oil (as well as other coconut products), kelp, Brazil nuts (three to four each day), fruits rich in vitamin C (oranges, peppers), and foods high in B vitamins and enzymes (raw sauerkraut). Detoxify the body and the thyroid using the supplements recommended in Chapter 6 (Part I). Build up your healthy hormones using the suggestions in Chapter 5.

Also, it seems apparent that women with high levels of toxicity (pesticides, chemicals, solvents, petroleum byproducts, xenoestrogens, heavy metals, etc.) tend to experience more challenging PMS symptoms, as well as a more extreme menopause experience. Detoxification tools and the suggestions outlined in Chapter 5 can assist one in normalizing extremes of hormonal imbalance.

> TIP Obesity has been inversely correlated with longevity. The more obese you are, the greater the risk of leaving the planet early. Weight loss is automatic when you eat low-calorie, nutrient-rich organic foods, such as vegetables, superfoods, and superherbs, instead of high-calorie, low-nutrient foods, such as starchy carbohydrates (bread, pasta, pastries, etc.).

CHAPTER 5

Hormone Health for Women and Men

Sisyphus was a hubristic Greek king cursed with the fate of having to continuously push a boulder up a hill only to have it fall back down again upon reaching the top. He exemplifies futile effort. This is how many people feel about their nutrition, immunity, antiaging, and fitness regimes, because as we age it appears that any simple mistake or omission in our program causes the boulder to roll all the way back down the hill and we have to start over.

This chapter of *Longevity Now* focuses on hormones and addresses this frustration by aiming to increase good hormones and decrease bad estrogen and cortisol, a strategy to provide more metabolic flexibility, just as we had in our youth. The focus is on amplifying androgen hormones in your metabolism and removing bad estrogens from your system, in order to shut down hormonal signaling mechanisms that damage and inhibit health and longevity.

Leveling the hormonal playing field not only improves metabolism, it rejuvenates us, improves overall immunity, and sets the groundwork for Chapter 6.

The insights gained by research into hormones indicate that it is imperative to keep our sex hormones—our inner executives—in a system of checks and balances throughout the years of our life. This becomes particularly important as we age. Hormone health is our key to a healthy future. Answers have been found!

Recommendations in this part of *Longevity Now* utilize all-natural foods, supplements, herbs, and lifestyle/exercise strategies, representing the leading edge in "at-home" hormone health care. The strategies outlined here focus on how to:

- stop the build-up of "bad" estrogen and detoxify your body of both "bad" and "fake" estrogens
- improve the quality of your hormones in order to improve the quality of your sex life and increase your beauty—sex hormones are health hormones
- improve bone density by using *all* the dietary and supplement strategies and technologies available
- take advantage of recent scientific advances in stopping breast, prostate, and other cancers
- build up your hormones naturally and use simple, inexpensive, bio-identical hormones without doctor's bills
- simplify and have more fun with the Longevity Now approach, in order to be healthier and happier

This hormone health chapter has been put together as a research project to advance knowledge of human hormones and how longevity strategies can be implemented and improved.[1] My basic understanding and conclusion is that the correct amount of androgenic hormones improves internal levity and health within the body—meaning the correct balance of good hormones prevents and fights calcification, gravitation, and oxidation; and that estrogen dominance (estrogen toxicity) as well as low hormone levels (in general) increase calcification, gravitation, and oxidation, thus accelerating age-related degeneration.

In the Age of Information, you have access to knowledge that can improve the quality of your life. Ninety years of research and tens of thousands of studies indicate that low hormone levels, too many "bad" hormones and/or a disruption in hormone production, absorption, and detoxification are at the root of chronic health challenges, lead to calcification, and accelerate aging. Because hormone levels are critical to maintaining overall health, getting control of your hormones gives you the tools to alter your destiny and again experience the vibrancy of youth!

The Powerful Influence of Hormones

Hormones are secretions from our glands, and glandular health is a key indicator (along with levels of bad calcium and bad iron) of one's actual level of youthfulness. These all-powerful secretions known as hormones are cellular messengers that transmit information from one cell to another. They are master signaling chemicals in the body, the executives of our inner ecology. What they say to do gets done. Turn on estradiol in a thirteen-year-old girl and you have the formation of breasts and the secondary sex characteristics. Turn adrenaline on in a young mother and she is lifting a car off her pinned child. Turn on progesterone and shut down estradiol (and 16 alpha hydroxy-estrone) in a woman aged sixty and you signal her breast cancer cells to stop proliferating. Turn on testosterone in a man of sixty and keep it circulating and he regains his strength and vigor.

The new understanding emerging from extensive research is that the sex hormones are in fact our health hormones. Like face cards, aces, and wild cards in a standard deck, the main sex hormones or health hormones rule the cellular kingdom. They are the most valuable cards. These include testosterone (King), progesterone (Queen), DHEA (Jack), thryroid hormone (wild cards), vitamin D3 (Ace), and estrogens and cortisol (2's and 3's).

Let's imagine a civilization of cells that comprise a human body. Hormones rule this cellular kingdom. If the king (high testosterone) has taken control and marginalized the queen (low progesterone) and is not receiving the queen's wise counsel, and the 2's and 3's in the court are causing civil unrest (high estrogen and elevated cortisol), then health challenges or lawlessness in the empire begin to arise and develop.

Here is the crux of the hormone dilemma: due to aging, birth control pills, estrogen replacement therapy, poor nutrition, stress, xenoestrogenic pollution and/or lack of exercise, metabolic "bad" or nonmethylated

When Hormone Levels Are Off

A quick review of the scientific literature reveals that some of our most important hormones (testosterone, progesterone, DHEA, human growth hormone or HGH, insulin-like growth factor, etc.) decrease with age. This decline in hormone levels, especially sex hormones, has been scientifically correlated with age-related gains in fat, loss of lean muscle mass, decreased bone density, thinning of the skin, and other degenerations. It isn't just that decreasing hormone levels lead to menopause in women and andropause in men. Improper hormone levels are a major underlying factor related to the following health conditions:

- bone loss and osteoporosis (yes, there is a hormonal connection)
- calcification, including the development of cardiovascular disease and arthritis (yes, there is a hormone connection)
- cancer (particularly reproductive cancers)
- cellulite
- chronic acne
- chronic urinary tract infections
- diabetes
- foggy thinking
- insomnia
- low energy
- low immunity
- migraines
- ovarian cysts
- polycystic breast disease
- saggy skin
- syndrome X (pre-diabetic weight gain)
- weight gain

These are the chronic and growing problems facing the entire civilized world. High levels of stress, xenoestrogens, or fake estrogens in our environment, overall liver toxicity due to all the pollutants, sedentary indoor living, and poor nutrition are all speeding up the development of these hormone-related conditions and calcification diseases.

estrogen builds up along with the adrenal hormone cortisol and starts to swing the seesaw toward too much estrogenic metabolism and not enough androgenic metabolism. The latter is improved by building up testosterone (men), progesterone (women), DHEA, vitamin D3, and thyroid hormone while simultaneously lowering cortisol and bad estrogen levels (meaning the types of estrogen that are counterproductive to health).

The Telomerase Theory

A marked decrease in the presence of hormones in human metabolism has been associated with nearly every theory of aging, including the Telomerase Theory. This theory posits that the shortening of chromosomal tips during cell replication eventually leads, at a certain critical point, to shortening of the chromosome length, to the point where the cell no longer divides—this is also known as the Hayflick limit. This process of losing telomeres is similar to the damage one sees on the ends of shoe laces over time—eventually the tips get frayed. Telomerase is an enzyme that stops the cleaving of chromosomal genetic material during cell division and thus can lead to extended life. Research is pointing to four conclusions about the Telomerase Theory:

1. Superfood, herbal, and supplement products have been (and continue to be) developed that are targeted at protecting the telomeres. Of these product types I take and recommend both TA65, a unique and rare extract of astragalus' astragaloside IV, and Dragon Herbs' Superpill 2, containing astragaloside IV from astragalus, gypenosides from gynostemma, resveratrol, and the raw, FITT (Fingerprint Identical Transfer Technology) extracts of the following superherbs: *ho shou wu,* ginseng, Rhodiola sacra, gynostemma, and astragalus. My colleague Dr. Dave Woynarowski, author of the *The Immortality Edge,* believes that high-dose pharmaceutical-grade fish oil may be telomere-protective. I believe that the two super phenol compounds resveratrol and xanthohumol may have this property as well. Of these two, I recommend an anti-aging

Continues

Continued

product called Hops X Factor, which contains a highly bioavailable form of xanthohumol (see Resources).

2. Good, solid nutrition extends the Hayflick limit. For example, in the book *Doctors' Secrets: The Miracle of Antioxidants*, by Dr. Donald McCleod and Dr. Philip White (published by the Kelowna Health and Longevity Centre), a study is cited indicating that vitamin E is able to extend the Hayflick limit of cultured human cells from fifty duplications to one hundred duplications. This type of phenomenon has been noted with other super-nutrients.

3. My own field research indicates that Ormus minerals (and in particular Ormus gold) may be able to slow the replication of healthy cells, thus extending their lives. This was the conclusion of the chemist who I worked with on an Ormus project for eight years. Liquid Ormus Gold (total dissolved solids: 2 percent Ormus gold, 98 percent silica), used topically, was able to save him from advancing viral and bacterial infections of both feet. He is a first-class scientist, so I have every reason to believe him. I have seen the results of his case and quite a few other cases as well. For more on Ormus, see page 42.

4. HGH and bio-identical hormone replacement therapies allow the telomerase enzyme to express and therefore "turn off" aging.

Ancient Chinese Strategies for Hormone Health

With the disastrous results of estrogen replacement therapy laid bare before us, and the blind rush toward HGH supplements* and bio-identical hormones† to thwart aging, it may be prudent to review

---

*Quality HGH injections or supplementation can save a life and bring somebody back from near death, in cases of extreme fatigue and a long battle against infections or parasites.

†Bioidentical hormones are chemically identical to natural human hormones. Estrogen replacement therapies have never used bioidentical hormones.

four traditional hormone-therapy dietary technologies from China that survive into the present day and are known to stave off aging. Though in the list below only herbal therapy will appear practical or desirable for most modern readers, I think it's interesting to know about historical uses and alternative methods. We are fortunate today to have an array of more palatable and easily available natural hormone therapies, as the rest of this chapter relates.

Deer Antler

This is a natural way to do hormone replacement therapy. Deer antler is the soft antler base and/or tips harvested from these animals in the late spring before they harden. (This does not kill the deer—see the section on deer antler on page 42.) Deer antler is loaded with growth factors, hormones, and Ormus-rich nutrients that are partially digestively bioavailable and even more bio-available when dissolved in alcohol and delivered orally (sublingually). These nutrients are useful as youthening agents for all aging mammals. Even though the antlers are coming from male deer, they are still useful to both female and male humans and other mammals. Due to the prevalence of growth factors (such as insulin-like growth factors), deer antler products are not recommended for growth-factor-sensitive cancers.

Placenta

Consuming the dried or cooked placenta from newborn children has been known to provide a huge surplus of stem cells to parents and relatives. Eating one's own child's placenta, however unnerving, is a recommended practice in all traditional herbal systems I have studied. (Some of the placenta should be dried and encapsulated and/or tinctured in alcohol as a stem-cell medicine for the child as well.) Human placenta is an extraordinary source of stem cell–stimulating nutrients and growth factors, including insulin-like growth factor I (IGF-I). Stem cells are new, undifferentiated cells that are more prevalent in our youth, and that assist rejuvenation. Particularly interesting stem cell–producing substances include placenta, fresh or dried noni fruit, deer/elk antler, and phyco-cyanin (the blue pigments of spirulina and AFA blue-green algae). Dried deer or goat placenta is often used herbally when human placenta is not available. Deer, goat, and human placenta are considered primary jing herbs in Taoist tonic herbal systems and in Chinese medicine, meaning that they tonify the body—that means these substances improve the primordial longevity energy that keeps us alive and healthy.

Herbs

Generally, the Chinese tonic herb system and replenishment via core jing and adaptogenic herbs, foods, and mushrooms (such as goji ber-ries, rehmannia, cordyceps, morinda root, *ho shou wu*, eucommia, etc.) becomes more useful with age.

Urine

In China, hundreds of years ago, it was sometimes noted that elderly males in the family would consume some of the hormone-rich urine of the younger grandchildren of the same sex. If such practices are cul-turally frowned upon or impractical (as they mostly are), a more com-monly available form of urine therapy (drinking the mid-stream catch of one's own first clear urine of the day) allows one to reintroduce and conserve hormones that are normally excreted and lost. Historically, in India, this practice of drinking one's own urine is known as Shivambu (named after the Hindu god Shiva). Shivambu is associated with health and longevity, especially when done consistently. There are numerous texts written on this ancient practice in a present-day context, such as Martin Lara's *Uropathy* and Coen van der Kroon's *Golden Fountain*.

The Truth about Estrogen Replacement Therapy

Dr. Fuller Albright was a world-famous American, Harvard-trained endocrinologist. He is credited with developing the theory that low estrogen levels are associated with bone demineralization and osteoporosis. This theory has been heavily tested and proven to be incorrect.

It was Dr. John Lee of Harvard who came forth with a similar claim in the 1990s, that hormone levels are in large part responsible for osteoporosis and many other age-related degenerative conditions—except Dr. Lee theorized that low progesterone is the primary culprit (not estrogen), along with nutrition and lifestyle factors. Dr. Lee's theories have proven to be sound, based on animal studies and his own clinical experience as detailed in his books *What Your Doctor May Not Tell You about Menopause*, *What Your Doctor May Not Tell You about Pre-Menopause*, and *Dr. John Lee's Hormone Balance Made Simple*.

Since Dr. Lee's first self-published book for doctors back in 1993, hundreds of studies, including the huge and now-famous National Institutes of Health Women's Health Initiative, have confirmed his stance on progesterone's importance and the problems and challenges inherent in conventional hormone replacement therapy.[2]

Estrogen replacement therapy (ERT) may increase the risk of health problems in a small number of women. This increase in risk depends on your age, your personal risk, and when ERT is started. Using ERT may increase your risk of:

- blood clots
- breast cancer
- breast tenderness
- dementia
- fluid retention
- gallstones
- headaches
- increased growth of pre-existing uterine fibroids (rare)
- nausea
- ovarian cancer
- spotting or darkening of the skin (particularly on the face)
- stroke
- vaginal discharge
- weight gain
- worsening of endometriosis (rare)

"Bad" Estrogen and Estrogen Toxicity

The process of accumulating "bad" estrogen in the liver and in fat cells is part of aging.

What is "bad" estrogen? It's too much of the wrong types of estrogen in the wrong places: a situation that eventually starts to toxify metabolism leading to early weight gain, syndrome X, diabetes, arthritis, reproductive cancers, etc. It appears that bad estrogens are, by definition, nonmethylated estrogens (estrogens that are missing a methyl group). Estrogen toxicity builds up over time as the body loses metabolic power and begins developing methylation problems (the inability to attach methyl groups to toxins). On top of this, the body eventually loses with age the capability to control aromatization, which is the conversion of a good hormone into a bad hormone (e.g., progesterone into a bad form of estrogen).

The main categories of estrogen hormones include:

- Human Estrogens (found in the body)
- Estrone (E1): Many estrones are often considered "bad" estrogen as they can trigger reproductive cancers. Of these, the worst culprit appears to be 16 alpha-hydroxy-estrone, whereas 2 hydroxy-estrone is a good estrone that has antitumor effects.
- Estradiol (E2): When estradiol levels are elevated in late adulthood, they are often categorized as bad estrogens.
- Estriol (E3): This hormone is one of the three major estrogens produced by the human body. Although it's a weak estrogen, more and more evidence continues to indicate estriol is a good estrogen. As a topical bio-identical hormone, estriol has the following properties:[3]
  - Relieves menopausal symptoms
  - Improves bone density
  - Benefits urinary tract health
  - Protects the heart

- May be used in the treatment of multiple sclerosis
- Does not increase the risk of hormone-dependent breast and endometrium cancers.
- Decreases hot flashes and vaginal dryness with a high degree of safety.

Phytoestrogens (Found in Plants)

Some phytoestrogens (in fact, probably most) will have no direct effect on one's hormone health and can be beneficial to hormone health and metabolism (estrogen antagonists). Some phytoestrogens (e.g., soy isoflavones) are harmful (estrogen agonists) and adversely affect the hormonal health of much of the population, causing estrogen toxicity.

Xenoestrogens (Human-Made)

These are artificial, human-made chemicals that can mimic estrogen during animal metabolism (in other words, in our bodies). Xenoestrogens are suspected of causing cancer, tumors, and cysts.

Foods with Phytoestrogens

Phytoestrogen-rich foods and herbs may have beneficial, neutral, or harmful estrogenic activity (more research is needed), which can depend on the constitution of the person consuming the food. Below I discuss some foods and herbs rich in phytoestrogens that are currently controversial, giving my take on their phytoestrogen content, in particular as it relates to breast cancer.[4]

Flowers

Cannabis flower (marijuana) contains powerful antinausea agents and compounds that specifically fight certain types of cancers. THC is an extraordinary cannabinoid antioxidant. Another cannabinoid in the cannabis plant is cannabidiol (CBD). CBD is nonintoxicating, and is considered to have a wider scope of medical applications than THC, including the treatment of epilepsy, multiple sclerosis, anxiety, schizophrenia, and nausea.

Cannabis flower (bud) is specifically medicinal for certain conditions including glaucoma, multiple sclerosis, and, when extracted in oil, surface skin cancers. Nevertheless, cannabis flower contains phytoestrogens that may trigger an estrogenic response in the individual, depending on his or her metabolism.[5] *Verdict:* Neutral, because cannabis's phytoestrogens affect individuals differently depending on their hormone profile and if they have cancer and what type of cancer. Eating cannabis flowers will exert stronger phytoestrogenic metabolic effects than smoking them.

Fruits

Dates are a weakly phytoestrogenic food. *Verdict:* Positive. I feel comfortable recommending dates as a snack food, as long as the sugar content can be tolerated.

Pomegranate contains extraordinarily high levels of antioxidants, phytoestrogens of unknown estrogenicity in human metabolism, as well as ellagic acid, which draws estrogen compounds out of the body. *Verdict:* Positive. I feel comfortable recommending pomegranate.

Herbs

Black cohosh shows low/no estrogenic activity in vitro. Known to inhibit ER+ breast cancer cells in vitro. *Verdict:* This is definitely a hormonally active herb that should be assessed for use on a case-by-case basis.

Bloodroot is known to inhibit ER+ (estrogen receptor positive) and inhibits ER- (estrogen receptor negative) breast cancer cells in vitro. Bloodroot also influences PR (progesterone receptor) sites. *Verdict:* Potent, yet good anticancer medicine. Best when this plant is administered by someone with a shamanic understanding of plants.

Goldenseal may block the uptake of healthy progesterone at the progesterone receptor sites of cells. *Verdict:* This herb is inappropriate when trying to raise progesterone levels or when taking progesterone cream.

Juniper is known to inhibit ER+ and ER- breast cancer cells in vitro. *Verdict:* Overall, juniper is a solid herbal medicine for fighting breast cancer.

Licorice root, as noted in American herbalist Stephen Harrod Buhner's book *The Natural Testosterone Plan,* is too estrogenic to consume.

Although used in Taoist tonic herbalism and Chinese medicine for thousands of years, it is possible that licorice may be inappropriate now due to the enormous estrogen toxicity of our current environment. Licorice failed to inhibit ER+ or ER- breast cancer cells in vitro. Licorice may also block the uptake of healthy progesterone at the progesterone receptor sites of cells. *Verdict:* Ineffective against ER+ or ER- breast cancer and actually may block progesterone. No on licorice.

Mandrake is a shamanic plant, sacred to the druids, yet with pan-European use, as well as Biblical references. Mandrake root inhibits both ER+ and ER- breast cancer cell lines. However, mandrake may interfere with the uptake of progesterone at progesterone receptor sites. *Verdict:* This is a powerful medicine. It must be administered by someone with a shamanic understanding of plants.

Mistletoe is another wide-ranging and potentially shamanic plant that inhibits ER+ and somewhat inhibits ER- breast cancer cell lines. Mistletoe does not interfere with progesterone metabolism. *Verdict:* Potent anticancer medicine. Best when administered by someone with a shamanic understanding of plants.

Motherwort is an estrogen agonist. It does not inhibit ER- breast cancer cell growth, though it slightly slows down ER+ breast cancer cell proliferation in vitro. *Verdict:* Overall, these qualities make motherwort a poor choice to fight ER- breast cancer, although potentially useful for ER+ breast cancer.

Nutmeg is known to inhibit ER+ breast cancer cells in vitro. Nutmeg may also block the uptake of healthy progesterone at the progesterone receptor sites of cells. *Verdict:* Not recommended for those with low progesterone. Not recommended for ER- cancers.

Ocotillo is a desert plant that competes with progesterone for progesterone receptor sites. *Verdict:* This herb is inappropriate when trying to raise progesterone levels or when taking progesterone cream.

Oregano possesses relatively high progestin-binding activity and may have weak estrogenic activity in vivo. *Verdict:* Oregano is a safe and medicinal culinary herb, but is not medicinally recommended for low progesterone and/or battling hormonal cancers.

Pennyroyal may block the uptake of healthy progesterone at the progesterone receptor sites of cells. *Verdict:* This herb is inappropriate when trying to raise progesterone levels or when taking progesterone cream.

Rosemary contains weak phytoestrogens. *Verdict:* Safe to eat. Not recommended topically in oil.

Sage possesses weak phytoestrogens as well as thujones. On the positive side, sage fights Alzheimer's and contains apigenin (a natural aromatase inhibitor). *Verdict:* Safe to eat in moderation. Not recommended topically in oil.

Thyme possesses relatively high progestin and estrogen-binding activity and may create weak estrogenic activity in vivo. *Verdict:* Thyme is not recommended medicinally if someone has low progesterone or is battling a hormonal cancer.

Turmeric possesses relatively high ER-binding activity and may create weak estrogenic activity in vivo. Turmeric may interfere with progesterone metabolism, as it binds to progesterone receptor sites. *Verdict:* Although a powerful beauty food and supreme anti-inflammatory, turmeric may be an inappropriate choice for low progesterone levels and for fighting breast cancer. More research is required.

Verbena appears to be an estrogen agonist and a progesterone antagonist. *Verdict:* Overall, these qualities make verbena a poor choice to maintain hormone health.

Legumes

Peas, black-eyed peas, red beans, and **chickpeas** are very weakly estrogenic. They are rich in fiber, protein, and B vitamins. These beans should be sprouted in pure water and then cooked in order to detoxify them and make them nutritious. *Verdict:* These are safe when sprouted, then cooked.

Soy isoflavones are too estrogenic to be considered a healthy food. The research continues to indicate that soy is highly estrogenic and damaging to healthy hormonal metabolism when one consumes it more than two times a week. On top of that, soy is poisonous in its raw state and nearly all soy is now genetically modified. The harmful excitotoxin MSG is typically made of soy. *Verdict:* Thumbs down on soy and soy products.

Nuts and Seeds

Though delicious, **cashews** are, in my opinion, weakly estrogenic. *Verdict:* Ideally, one should consume no more than four handfuls of cashews in a week.

Women who consumed more than 500 milligrams of caffeine daily, the equivalent of five cups of **coffee**, had nearly 70 percent more estrogen during the early follicular phase than women consuming 100 mg or less of caffeine daily, or approximately one cup of coffee. This study indicates that coffee consumption increases estradiol levels.[6] *Verdict:* Choose chocolate over coffee. Cacao (natural chocolate) is a relatively low source of caffeine, typically containing one-twentieth the caffeine content of coffee (see the chapter "Chocolate Science" in my book *Naked Chocolate*). Some chocolate bars are high in caffeine due to the addition of guarana or kola nut.

Numerous health authorities, including William Wong, ND, PhD, and Daniel Vitalis, have popularized the concept that **flax** contains harmful estrogens. This may have been a primary reason flax was never used as a major food of any past civilization. Mineral analysis of flaxseeds indicates that they are more nutritious than chia seeds. Mineral analysis also reveals that they can contain small amounts of cadmium, which is antagonistic to zinc. Flaxseed is a complete protein and a great source of ALA omega-3 fatty acids. *Verdict:* Consuming small amounts of flaxseed and flaxseed products occasionally is reasonable. I wouldn't recommend consistently consuming large amounts of flaxseed and flaxseed oil. Consuming de-fatted flaxseed meal for estrogen detoxification purposes is still recommended.

Sunflower seeds are very mildly phytoestrogenic. *Verdict:* Safe in normal amounts.

Sesame seeds are very mildly phytoestrogenic. *Verdict:* Safe in normal amounts.

> ## Avoid These Phytoestrogenic Oils
>
> - cottonseed oil
> - lavender oil*
> - rapeseed or canola oil
> - safflower oil
> - sunflower oil
> - tea tree oil (melaleuca)†
>
> *Use only on skin irritations; not recommended for consistent topical use.
>
> †In my opinion this oil is used too often topically; it is not recommended for consistent topical use.

Roots

Cassava failed to inhibit ER+ or ER– breast cancer cells in vitro. Cassava does not interfere with progesterone. *Verdict:* Ineffective against ER+ or ER– breast cancer.

Sprouts

Alfalfa sprouts contain immunological saponins, B vitamins, and bone-building silicon. Alfalfa also contains a high level of a toxin called canavanine. It is mildly phytoestrogenic. *Verdict:* Safe if consumed no more than twice a week.

    Red clover is purported to contain powerful anticancer compounds. In Australia, around 1940, merino sheep were found to develop clover disease when they overfed on clover. This was caused by a phytoestrogen known as formononetin, so we know this plant contains strong phytoestrogens. However, humans would never eat as much clover as sheep do. Clover has a strong cancer-fighting history, and red clover is part of the Essiac Tea cancer-fighting formula. However, red clover failed to inhibit ER+ and ER– breast cancer cells in vitro (meaning it did not fight the cancer cells). Red clover also demonstrated in vitro that it may block the uptake of healthy progesterone at the progesterone receptor sites of cells. *Verdict:* Red clover is ineffective against ER+ and ER– breast cancer and probably not useful in fighting any type of reproductive cancer. Do not eat red clover if you are low in progesterone or taking progesterone cream.

White clover sprouts are known to inhibit ER+ breast cancer cell lines in vitro, yet failed to inhibit ER– breast cancer cells in vitro. *Verdict:* Recommended for ER+ breast cancer.

Hormonal Products to Avoid

Avoid the following hormonal products in order to balance and build healthy hormones:

- Birth control pills. These cause estrogen dominance.
- Cimetidine (Tagamet). Cimetide interferes with hormone metabolism and increases estrogen.
- DES
- Hormone replacement therapy (HRT)
- Premarin
- PremPro
- Progesterone creams made with paraben preservatives

Xenoestrogens: Avoid Them!

For more on xenoestrogens and excellent information about environmental factors that affect breast cancer, see The Breast Cancer Fund's 2010 State of the Evidence report, available in full at www.breastcancerfund.org/assets/pdfs/publications/state-of-the-evidence-2010.pdf.

Xenoestrogen-Rich Animal Foods

Commercial dairy products, including milk, butter, cheese, and ice cream. Avoid bovine growth hormone and the common chemical agents used on conventional farms by going organic and free-range.

🦎 Commercially raised, nonorganic meats such as beef, chicken, and pork

🦎 Farmed fish and shellfish

🦎 **Xenoestrogen-Rich Home Products**

🦎 Unfiltered tap water. Get a filter or become a filter.

🦎 Laundry detergent. According to some researchers online, avoid even the Seventh Generation and Eco brands.*

🦎 Fabric softeners. These are estrogenic and toxic.

Other known xenoestrogens include:

🦎 4-methylbenzylidene camphor (4-MBC; used in sunscreen lotions)

🦎 atrazine (an herbicide)

🦎 BHA/butylated hydroxyanisole (a food preservative)

🦎 BPA/bisphenol A (used within polycarbonate plastic and epoxy resins; present in many plastics and in Styrofoam)

🦎 DDT and DDE (insecticides)

🦎 DEHP (a plasticizer used for PVC)

🦎 dieldrin (an insecticide)

🦎 endosulfan (an insecticide)

🦎 erythrosine/FD&C Red No. 3 (food coloring)

🦎 heptachlor (an insecticide)

🦎 lindane/hexachlorocyclohexane (an insecticide that's banned in Europe)

🦎 methoxychlor (an insecticide)

🦎 nonylphenols (industrial surfactants, emulsifiers for emulsion polymerization, laboratory detergents, pesticides, etc.)

🦎 parabens and phenoxyethanol (found in cosmetics, shampoos, soaps, lotions, and toothpastes)

🦎 PCBs/polychlorinated biphenyls (industrial fluids, lubricants, adhesives, paints, etc.)

🦎 phenosulfothiazine (a red dye)

🦎 phthalates (pervasive plasticizers)

*Dr. Bronner's soap, borax powder, and (when I have it) zeolite powder is what I personally use to wash my clothes.

Osteoporosis: The Hormone Connection

The hormonal connection with osteoporosis has been developed by doctors and researchers, including Harvard-trained physician, author, international lecturer, biologist, and one of the world's foremost experts on hormones Ray Peat, PhD, who has been researching progesterone since 1968. Their conclusions are that progesterone has a protective effect against osteoporosis.

> It is very clear that progesterone can be of great benefit to women with measurable bone loss. In most such cases, progesterone will rapidly and impressively build bone, along with proper diet, weight-bearing exercise and some vitamin and mineral supplements.
> —Dr. John Lee*

The leading edge of improving bone density is innovative, yet simple to understand. The following are contributing factors to maintaining healthy bone density and avoiding osteoporosis:

- Adequate hormone levels, especially progesterone levels in women and testosterone levels in men.
- Adequate vitamin D3 levels, or sunlight. Note that even if you get enough sunlight, you may not be absorbing enough D3. This is because vitamin D3 can be washed off the skin by harsh soaps. It takes thirty-six to forty-eight hours to absorb the D3 once it's produced in the skin.
- Appropriate minerals and the amino acid lysine work to increase bone density. The minerals required for creating healthy bone and marrow include hydrogen, boron, carbon, magnesium, phosphorus, potassium, silicon, and sulfur.
- Grounding to the earth and using the appropriate technologies. Grounding or "Earthing" simply means touching the earth or a body

*Dr. John Lee is a Harvard-trained physician, author, and international lecturer and is one of the world's foremost experts on hormones. Learn from him at www .johnleemd.com/store/truth_osteoporosis.html or by reading *Dr. John Lee's Hormone Balance Made Simple* and *What Your Doctor May Not Tell You about Menopause.*

Continues

Continued

of water in the Earth with your skin (e.g., walking barefoot, swimming in the ocean, lying in the grass). The technologies referenced include grounding or "Earthing" devices and vibration plate machines.

- Weight-bearing exercise. It's alarmingly clear that the incidence of osteoporosis is on the rise. The following statistics, provided by the International Osteoporosis Foundation, are indicative of current and future trends:[8]

  - In women over forty-five years of age, osteoporosis accounts for more days spent in hospitals than many other diseases, including diabetes, heart attack, and breast cancer.
  - One in three women over fifty will experience osteoporotic fractures, as will one in five men.
  - Osteoporosis affects an estimated seventy-five million people in Europe, the United States, and Japan.
  - In the year 2000, there were an estimated nine million new osteoporotic fractures, of which 1.6 million were at the hip, 1.7 million were at the forearm, and 1.4 million were clinical vertebral fractures. Europe and the Americas accounted for 51 percent of all these fractures, while most of the remainder occurred in the Western Pacific region and Southeast Asia.
  - Nearly 75 percent of hip, spine, and distal forearm fractures occur among patients sixty-five or older.
  - Between 1990 and 2000, there was a nearly 25 percent increase in hip fractures worldwide. The peak number of hip fractures occurred at 75–79 years of age for both sexes; for all other fractures, the peak number occurred at 50–59 years and decreased with age.
  - By 2050, the worldwide incidence of hip fracture in men is projected to increase by 310 percent and by 240 percent in women.
  - The combined lifetime risk for hip, forearm, and vertebral fractures coming to clinical attention is around 40 percent, equivalent to the risk for cardiovascular disease.
  - In white women, the lifetime risk of hip fracture is one in six, compared with a one in nine risk of a diagnosis of breast cancer.
  - Osteoporosis takes a huge personal and economic toll. In Europe,

the disability due to osteoporosis is greater than that caused by cancers (with the exception of lung cancer) and is comparable or greater than that lost to a variety of chronic noncommunicable diseases, such as rheumatoid arthritis, asthma, and high blood pressure-related heart disease.

- Most fractures occur in postmenopausal women and elderly men at moderate risk.

The research and data are in. The technology is here. The strategies have been identified. Because of the explosion of osteoporosis worldwide, it is time to address the leading edge in bone-density improvement research.

Hormone Health the Natural Way

Longevity nutrition is an art form designed to help the body build androgenic sex hormones, keep them available for signaling one's metabolism to remain young, and keep hormone cell receptor sites open. Our first step in building up healthy hormones is understanding methylation, methyl donors, and methylators.

Methylators

The liver is the first place to focus as we begin the process of building up healthy hormones. The accumulation of bad estrogens in the liver has been associated with a deficiency in methyl groups, aging, estrogen dominance, and a decrease in the body's ability to detoxify carcinogens.

A methylator is a substance that is able to donate methyl groups. The liver uses methyl groups (CH3) by attaching them to toxins as part of its phase-one detoxification mechanisms. Once a methyl group attaches to a toxin, such as a bad estrogen molecule, the liver can deal with the toxin and move it down the pathway to elimination.

Methyl groups consist of one carbon and three hydrogen atoms, and they are more abundant in fresh food and deficient in cooked food. Certain foods and supplements are considered good methylators as they are able to donate significantly more methyl groups. These foods and supplements are listed below.

Choline is a "tetra-methylator" (donates four methyl groups) and is found most abundantly in egg yolks. I recommend you consume eggs that are sunny-side up (yolk is raw, white part is cooked). The yolk not only contains choline, but also lecithin; vitamin D3; vitamins B5, B6, B9, and B12; protein; numerous trace minerals; and (in some cases) DHA (docosohexaenoic omega 3 fatty acid).

Beet roots, beet root juices, and **goji berries** are the best natural sources of betaine (tri-methyl-glycine or TMG), a gentle liver detoxifier that works by adding methyl groups (CH3) to the liver's arsenal of metabolic detoxifiers. Methyl groups aid the liver in detoxifying bad estrogens. Dr. Norman Walker, who lived to be 109, wrote of the liver-supportive and longevity power of beets in his classic book *Fresh Vegetable and Fruit Juices.* Next to beet roots, goji berries are the second highest of any food in betaine concentration. This may explain part of the goji berry's action in keeping the body young and rejuvenated.

TMG and **DMG** are also available as independent supplements. TMG has three methyl groups; DMG (di-methyl-glycine) has only two. Sometimes people metabolically agree with DMG more than TMG, perhaps due to its slightly different and simpler structure. When isolated, TMG betaine is a sticky, sweet substance that hints of the beginning of carbohydrate formation found in sweet spring water. In fact, when small amounts of betaine are added to water, it makes the water taste like fresh spring water.

Methyl-cobalamin B12 is a methyl-donating form of protective B12 that builds blood, detoxifies homocysteine, and helps the liver lower bad estrogen levels.

MSM (methyl-sulfonyl-methane) is a methylated form of sulfur. Each molecule of MSM is able to donate one methyl group to liver metabolism.

SAMe (S-adenosyl methionine) is also a methyl group donor. This molecule has been used as an antidepressant and as a treatment for osteoarthritis.

Vitamins B6 and **B9** are methyl group donors that detoxify the liver of bad forms of estrogens.

"Bad" Estrogen Removers

Even though some of the recommended items below are phytoestrogens, that does not necessarily mean that they increase bad estrogens. Phytoestrogens in soy (isoflavones) may metabolize in certain people into bad estrogens, whereas lignans in kale may actually block bad estrogens from the hormone receptor sites on cells. Therefore, based on our current understanding, some phytoestrogens may damage hormone health, some may be neutral, and others may improve hormone health. However, if you are already experiencing an estrogen dominance, you may want to avoid certain phytoestrogenic plants, such as soy isoflavones, that could make the problem worse.

- **Berries:** Not only are they delicious, but berries are also an excellent natural source of lignans, calcium d-glucarate, quercetin, and ellagic acid, all of which help to lower bad estrogen in the body.[9]
- **Button mushrooms:** Also known as *Agaricus bisporus,* this mushroom is maligned by Dr. Robert Young and Dr. Gabriel Cousens and is blamed for causing poor blood quality based on live-blood microscopy. Nevertheless, the jury is still out on the hidden powers of this mushroom. What *is* known is that it breaks down bad estrogen better than any other mushroom studied.
- **Calcium D-glucarate:** Found in berries, apples, and cruciferous vegetables, C-D-G is a fiber that draws bad estrogen out of the body via the intestines. It also inhibits beta-glucuronidase, high levels of which are associated with increased bad estrogen receptors. Because of its ability to enhance intestinal detoxification, it may also be used to treat autism.
- **Citrus essential oil:** Citrus essential oils have been associated with dissolving bad estrogen accumulation in fatty tissue, especially in areas affected by cellulite. Usually the oils are massaged directly into the cellulite topically.

- **Citrus peel:** Lemon, lime, and kumquat peels dissolve bad estrogens and may be eaten raw. Other citrus peels must be prepared (e.g., cooking, drying, etc.) due to high levels of toxins. "Prepared citrus peel" is a common additive to youthening formulas and dishes in Chinese and Persian herbal medicine and food systems.

- **Cruciferous vegetables:** An excellent natural source of lignans, calcium d-glucarate, and quercetin, cruciferous vegetables also metabolize into I3C and DIM (see below). All these elements help to lower bad estrogen in the body.

- **Defatted flax:** If you purchase this product in stores, it must be in the refrigerated section and vacuum-packed for maximum freshness and effectiveness. The lignan fibers in defatted flax draw bad estrogens into the intestines for removal. This is a critical action. Bad estrogens may be detoxified all the way to the intestines, only to be reabsorbed again; defatted flax prevents this.

- **DIM:** Also known as diindolylmethane, DIM should be taken with I3C (see below). This important supplement is a metabolic breakdown product of I3C, which itself is a breakdown product of glucosinolate glucobrassicin, found in cruciferous vegetables. DIM works indirectly and uniquely by helping the cells understand how to create proteins that detoxify bad estrogens. DIM possesses antiviral, antibacterial, antiangiogenesis, and cancer-fighting qualities. It is also known to inhibit nuclear factor kappa beta.

- **Ellagic acid:** This compound is a natural selective estrogen receptor modulator (SERM) believed (based on the science) to be an important component of a breast-cancer-fighting protocol.[10]

- **I3C:** Also known as indole-3-carbinol, I3C should be taken with DIM (see above). I consider I3C to be one of the most important supplements of the twenty-first century. I3C is a breakdown product of the compound glucosinolate glucobrassicin, found in cruciferous vegetables. Research continues to indicate that I3C has anticarcinogenic, antioxidant, antiviral, and antiatherogenic effects.[11] I3C along with DIM are integral nutrients to assist in lowering bad estrogen levels.

- **Iodine:** This is the "Queen of the Halogens." Iodine gradually displaces toxic halogens including fluoride, chlorine, bromine, and radioactive iodine—all of which could be damaging to the endocrine system. Iodine stops and may even reverse polycystic breast disease. It is typically an adjunct to the natural treatment of any reproductive cyst formations. Iodine is one of the most important supplements to protect yourself from the toxicity of the fluoridated-chlorinated water, chemtrails (ethylene dibromide or bromine), and nuclear age that we all live in.

- **Lignan-rich foods and herbs:** These encompass a wide range from flaxseeds, sesame seeds, berries, and vegetables (broccoli and kale) to green tea. These appear to be moderately effective in lowering breast cancer risk in post-menopausal women by approximately 14 percent.[12] My feeling from reviewing the literature on the subject is that lignans from berries, vegetables, and green tea are likely more protective than lignans from flaxseeds. The weak estrogenic effects of protective lignans may allow them to affix themselves to estrogen receptor sites, thus blocking the growth signals of stronger estrogens such as estradiol that could trigger breast cancers.

- **Melatonin:** This tryptamine, which is a close chemical relation to I3C, inhibits some forms of estrogen and the estrogen response pathways of certain cancers.[13] Living in an environment saturated with electromagnetic pollution (EMF) may inhibit melatonin's protective properties against cancer.[14]

- **Raw carrots:** Raymond Peat reports in his pro-progesterone book *From PMS to Menopause* that carrot fiber helps draw bad estrogens out of the body.

Natural Aromatase Inhibitors

Natural aromatase inhibitors prevent the conversion of androgens to bad estrogens.

- **Chamomile:** Chamomile contains apigenin and, according to some accounts, also chrysin. Both of these compounds are natural aromatase inhibitors. For this reason, chamomile tea may have longevity properties.

- **Damiana:** Though known to inhibit ER+ breast cancer cell lines in vitro, damiana failed to inhibit ER– breast cancer cells in vitro. Damiana does not interfere with progesterone metabolism. Because damiana is an aromatase inhibitor, this may account for its aphrodisiac properties.[15]

- **Hops extracts** (prenylated chalcones from hops): Hops is most well-known for its use as a preservative and flavoring agent in beer. The prenylflavonoids extracts from hops—xanthohumol, isoxanthohumol, and 8-prenylnaringenin—exhibit aromatase-inhibition properties.[16] However, isoxanthohumol and 8-prenylnaringenin exhibit mild estrogenic properties, yet xanthohumol is a "pure estrogen antagonist."[17] A patented highly bioavailable form of xanthohumol is now found in two products: the Longevity Bliss chocolate bar and the supplement Hops X Factor (see the Sacred Chocolate section on page 377 and Hops X Factor section on page 379). Hops X Factor is the most promising anti-aging longevity product I know of. It works by itself and also in conjunction with other longevity compounds such as resveratrol and astragaloside IV (TA 65, Superpill 2) as well as high-dose omega 3 fatty acids. I drink a dropper-full every day and use Hops X Factor topically as well.

- **Nettle root** (for men): Aromatase inhibitors have been studied closely and have shown promise in generating hair growth (Dr. Sheffield). In addition to inhibiting the binding of sex hormone binding globulin (SHBG), at least six constituents of the methanolic extract of nettle root inhibit aromatase, reducing the conversion of androgens to estrogens.[18]

- **Oleuropein:** This antifungal, antiviral compound is found in all parts of the olive tree. Oleuropein may be responsible for some of the longevity and health-promoting properties of olive oil.

- **Passionflower:** Chrysin, a chemical compound found in passionflower, is a natural aromatase inhibitor. It is best delivered

Dark grapes are an excellent source of anti-aging resveratrol.

in a stronger-than-normal, 35 to 40 percent (or more) alcohol tincture of passionflower herb.

- **Quercetin:** This longevity-inducing aromatase inhibitor is found in many raw fruits and vegetables including onions, apple skins, berries, and cruciferous vegetables.

- **Resveratrol:** Resveratrol must reach your cells within three and a half hours after ingestion. That explains why the traditional methods of consuming this compound are in high-phenolic and/or port wine alcohols. Alcohol is a driver and drives the poorly soluble resveratrol into the body. Because of its short "half life," most resveratrol products are for the most part ineffective. Resveratrol is found in dark grapes, blueberries, Saskatoon berries, Japanese knotweed root *(Polygonum cuspidatum),* and in other sources.

- **Soy extract genistein:** The soy isoflavone phytoestrogen genistein suppresses estradiol synthesis by direct genistein inhibition of aromatase and the 17B steroid oxidoreductase enzymes necessary for the conversion of androgens to estrone and estrone to estradiol. But it, its partner daidzein, and/or their metabolites in digestion—in my opinion—are too estrogenic to be useful in creating healthy hormones.

Natural Hormone Builders

Following is a list of foods, food extracts (fats/ oils), and/or herbal substances that promote the natural production of healthy hormones.

- **Bee pollen:** This is arguably the most nutritious, complete-protein food on Earth. Fresh bee pollen contains enough fat and protein to help the body produce hormones. Always obtain fresh bee pollen if possible; failing that, obtain freeze-dried bee pollen. Store your bee pollen in the freezer. For more, see the chapter on bee pollen in my book *Superfoods: The Food and Medicine of the Future.*

- **Cacao:** An excellent source of fat-soluble minerals, cacao is able to influence the endocrine system glands to produce natural hormones.

- **Chaste or vitex berry (for women):** This contains bioidentical progesterone. To obtain the full benefits, it is best if the alcohol tincture is consumed sublingually, as digestion will break down the bioidentical progesterone.

- **Cistanche:** This obscure Chinese herb is gaining greater and greater prominence as an aphrodisiac. It increases the production of testosterone and DHT (di-hydro-testosterone). In one study, cistanche doubled the level of testosterone in mice as compared to the control group.

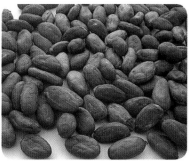

Raw cacao beans

- **Coconut cream and oil:** Coconuts are one of Nature's great superfoods. Coconut fat can fairly easily be converted to pregnenolone, a fantastic androgenic hormone precursor.

- **Deer antler:** See the "Adaptogen Herbs" section in Chapter 6 on deer antler.

- **DHA:** Docosahexaenoic acid is a long-chain omega-3 fatty acid usually of marine origin (e.g., fish, krill, algae). DHA is a nutrient precursor that leads to the formation of the androgenic memory hormone DHEA.

- **Fennel:** This group of plants is known to increase the flow of breast milk and to fight estrogen-induced migraine headaches.

- **Maca:** This adaptogenic super-root influences the hypothalamus and, subsequently, the rest of the endocrine system. Maca provides hormone precursors that help the glands produce more and better-quality hormones and neurotransmitters. Maca is often recommended for hypothyroidism and for low progesterone and testosterone. For more, see the Maca chapter in my book *Superfoods: The Food and Medicine of the Future.*

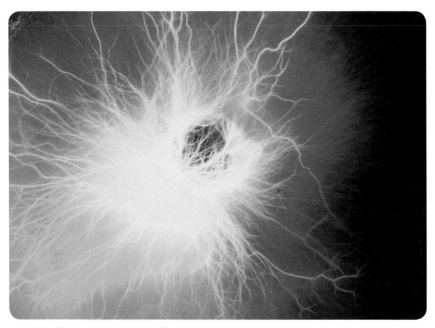

A Kirlian image of maca

- **Oats:** Oats (seed and blade) are known to contain avenacosides A and B as well as a saponin (sulfated in products) that is purported to raise free (unbound) testosterone and lower the stress hormone cortisol.
- **Pregnenolone:** This androgen precursor helps build progesterone and testosterone. It is available in supplemental powders and capsules. This is a very safe androgen-building supplement.
- **Progesterone cream from wild yam root:** This is perhaps the most important protective bio-identical hormone for healthy adult female metabolism. Progesterone deficiency appears to be at the root of nearly all age-related degenerative conditions. In general, hormones taken orally are 80 to 90 percent metabolized and broken down by the liver on the first pass. However, when progesterone is applied to the skin, it is directly absorbed by the body without being damaged. Thus, any skin dose is ten times stronger than an oral dose. In addition, progesterone is toxic to

the liver when taken orally, yet perfectly safe when consumed through the skin. I consider progesterone cream an essential health tool, to be used when needed. Can men use progesterone cream? The answer appears to be yes, but in a limited fashion (three to five days per month). Men will typically convert the progesterone immediately into testosterone. Apply a designated quantity of the cream (differs per brand) to one of the following areas each day you use it: thin-skinned areas behind the knees, around the genitals, in the inner crook of the elbows, under the breasts, along the breastbone, on the neck, and on the belly. The idea is to change up the location and even the time of application each day. Menstruating women: Begin twelve days after your cycle starts and continue for two weeks. Nonmenstruating women should take more progesterone cream—select a random day and use the cream three weeks straight followed by a weeklong break. Choose chemical-free progesterone cream products.

- **Raw, organic butter:** Perhaps the best dairy product, raw organic butter contains a large fraction of saturated fat, a great hormone-building material. Always choose the purest form of butter available, as butters may concentrate xenoestrogens, AGEs, nuclear fallout, fire retardants, and probably a number of other different chemicals.

- **Reishi mushroom spore products:** The book *Ling Zhi: From Mystery to Science* (about the reishi mushroom, published by the Peking University Medical Press) cites research indicating that reishi mushroom spore oil increases testosterone.

- **Pine pollen:** This contains bioidentical testosterone. To obtain the full hormonal benefits of pine pollen, it is best to use pine pollen alcohol tincture sublingually, because digestion will break down the bio-identical testosterone.

- **Saturated fat:** Saturated fat is required to produce cholesterol, which is the mother molecule needed to form the health hormones. Some people have shunned saturated fat. Based on my experience, these folks may end up with serious hormone deficiencies.

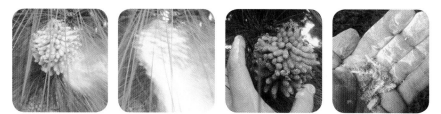

Pine pollen contains plant steroids that act as antiviral compounds in humans and mammals.

- **Tongkat Ali (for men):** An extraordinary root from Indonesia, *tongkat Ali* means "Ali's walking stick." This superherb and its extracts are known to significantly increase testosterone.
- **Tribulus (for men):** This is one of the key herbs recommended to increase testosterone levels in men.
- **Yam/sweet potato:** Anecdotal evidence continues to pile up in support of the androgenic qualities of yams and sweet potatoes. However, no conclusive scientific evidence exists that yam or sweet potato varieties increase progesterone.[19] Overall, this is a great food, either raw or cooked. If you eat yam or sweet potato raw, be aware that they contain trypsin inhibitors that prevent excessive consumption. These trypsin inhibitors are destroyed by cooking.

Hormone-Building Exercise and Fitness

From my review of the research, I believe anaerobic exercise is better for building hormones and making you young than aerobic exercise. I also believe that when one balances yin aerobic exercise practices (most yoga asanas, yoga classes, walking, gardening, etc.) with yang anaerobic exercises such as sprinting, cross-fitness workouts, heavy weights, sports, mixed martial arts workouts, etc., something unique is felt: perhaps this fusion of exercise styles is in fact the fitness balance required to thrive in our everchanging, multifaceted world of limitless adventure.

Grounding as a Hormone-Regulating Technology

Multiple clinical studies on "grounding technology" presented to this author by research scientist and inventor Clint Ober (and written about in his book *Earthing*) indicate that hormonal fluctuations within metabolism are "referenced" to innate rhythms that electromagnetically emanate from the Earth itself.

For example, in one unpublished study, in eight weeks of using grounding technology, the cortisol levels of the study group were reduced (normalized) and also synchronized, suggesting a higher organizational power—the Earth itself.

This type of research indicates that rubber-soled shoes and living on carpets and dead, dry wood have had profound impacts on the erratic fluctuations within our hormonal system. Essentially, this research demonstrates that a lack of direct "skin-to-skin" electromagnetic connection with the Earth can throw our hormone cycles out of balance.

Of course, in our original state within Nature's wild lands we would be without shoes, grounded twenty-four hours a day, which is the best situation according to Clint Ober. However, living within civilization precludes consistent grounding. Sleeping using grounding technology (making an electrical Earth-to-metal-to-skin connection, thus bridging the insulation gap) appears to be the easiest way to solve this challenge, as it gives us five to eight solid hours of being grounded per day, and a chance for the hormone rhythms to be reset and normalized. See the pages 307–317 for more on grounding technologies.

Herbal Hormone Helpers

- **Ashwagandha** (for men): See the "Adaptogen Herbs" section on ashwagandha (page 268).

- **Catuaba:** This is the most famous of the aphrodisiac Amazonian plants. It stimulates the nervous system, improves memory, and modulates immunity (antiviral and antibacterial). It also demonstrates dopamine-mediated antidepressant effects. Catuaba improves erections and normalizes prostate function.

- **Dong quai** (for women): See the "Adaptogen Herbs" section on dong quai (page 267).

- **Epimedium** (horny goat weed): This Chinese herb has been used traditionally to treat fatigue, arthritic and nerve pain, and low sex drive. In-vitro studies suggest that epimedium exhibits neuroprotective, immunomodulatory, and anticancer effects. The flavonoids present in epimedium were shown in a randomized trial to prevent bone loss in postmenopausal women.[20] Epimedium contains phytoestrogens that may negatively influence hormone-sensitive cancers. Taoist tonic herbalist Ron Teeguarden has indicated that based on his research, combining epimedium with eucommia may activate antiaging telomerase enzymes in metabolism.

- **Eucommia** (jing herb): See the "Adaptogen Herbs" section on eucommia (page 275).

- **Ginseng:** See the "Adaptogen Herbs" section on ginseng (page 276).

- **Goji berry:** An excellent source of betaine, which is a basic "sticky" carbohydrate that helps nutrients to nourish the cells by maintaining good cellular hydration. Betaine helps the liver detoxify bad estrogens.

- **Gynostemma:** This super adaptogenic leaf lowers cortisol and helps build a stress-defense shield. See the "Adaptogen Herbs" section on gynostemma (page 277).

- ***Ho shou wu*** (jing herb): See the "Adaptogen Herbs" section on *ho shou wu* (page 278).

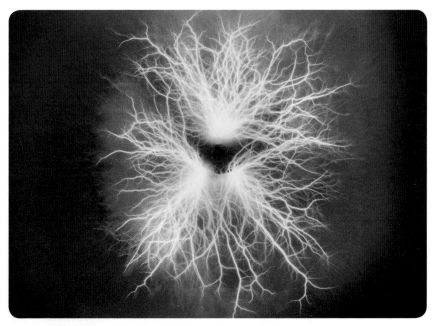

A Kirlian image of a single goji berry

- **Kelp:** "The queen of the sea." Consuming kelp is believed to lower bad estrogen levels. Kelp is a superfood and an estrogen antagonist that prevents bad estrogen from binding to estrogen receptors. For more, see the Kelp chapter of my book *Superfoods: The Food and Medicine of the Future.*

- **Muira puama:** Purported to increase testosterone, this Amazonian herb is used by men as an aphrodisiac to increase erections. Women can use this herb as well and report better-quality orgasms.

- **Poria** (mushroom): An excellent spleen-nourishing yin tonic medicinal mushroom, poria is cooling and drying; it expels excess heat and dampness. This mushroom calms and tonifies the heart. Poria is often mixed in yin jing formulas with rehmannia, and this combination has a particularly balancing effect on those who follow a raw-food diet.

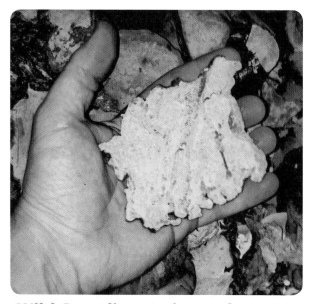

Wild Canadian poria mushroom

- **Rehmannia root:** "The kidney's own food." This extraordinary root nourishes yin jing and blood; it also supports a healthy heart. It is generally considered cooling and helps expel heat. Rehmannia has slight aphrodisiac effects. Rehmannia is often mixed in formulas with poria, and this combination has a particularly balancing effect on those who follow a raw-food diet.

- **Red raspberry leaf** (for women): This herb is a uterus tonic that is particularly useful in pregnancy to prepare the uterus for birth. Raspberry leaf works by directly interacting with the uterus and not through the use of plant estrogens.

- **Sarsaparilla** *(Smilax officinalis):* Sarsaparilla root contains the steroid saponin, also known as diosgenin. This is the same compound found in Mexican wild yam. Diosgenin is the key laboratory building block of estrogens, testosterone, and progesterone; although in human metabolism (outside the laboratory), the conversion of diosgenin into hormones has never been proven. Nevertheless, reports of the aphrodisiac effects of sarsaparilla continue.

- **Saw palmetto** (for men): Unlike finasteride (Proscar/Propecia), saw palmetto does not function as a 5 alpha reductase inhibitor that results in lower serum DHT (at least according to Merck). It works instead by reducing the uptake of DHT at the receptor sites by a factor of 40 percent.[21]

- **Suma:** Known as "Brazilian ginseng," this root *(Pfaffia paniculata)* is actually unrelated to ginseng. It is an adaptogen with immunological properties, considered a testosterone booster, although there is no clear in-vivo scientific proof of this. Its extensive historical use speaks to its efficacy and safety.

- **Tulsi** (for women): See the "Adaptogen Herbs" section on tulsi (page 281).

- **Yohimbe** (for men): Yohimbe and its derivative substance yohimbine have been used as male aphrodisiacs to treat impotence and erectile dysfunction. Its action as an alpha 2-adrenergic antagonist raises adrenaline and norepinephrine. Yohimbe and yohimbine vary dramatically in their effectiveness.

Healthy Hormone-Promoting Supplements

- **Beta-carotene:** According to Raymond Peat, beta-carotene has antiestrogenic properties.

- **Sea salt:** I reviewed a dozen major websites for what they prescribe for pregnancy-related morning sickness. The top recommendation among those websites was, not surprisingly, salty crackers. Salt is antiestrogenic, and high estrogen levels are considered the primary cause of morning sickness. Because of the toxicity of synthetic salts sold as food preservatives and used as "table salt," I recommend using one type of salt above all others: sea salt.

- **Vitamin D3:** This vitamin turns on more healing genes than any substance yet known. D3 is antiestrogenic, anticortisol, and it promotes an androgenic metabolism of healthy hormones. Vitamin D3 works best when one gets adequate sleep and rest.

- **Vitamin E:** Raymond Peat recommends 100 units per day of vitamin E in his book *From PMS to Menopause*. Vitamin E is known to normalize the ratio of estradiol to progesterone in a woman's body.

Remember, conquering estrogen dominance and improving androgenic metabolism:

- accelerates wound healing
- improves athletic performance
- improves arthritic conditions
- improves lean muscle mass
- improves mental facility and acuity
- increases anti-inflammatory actions in the body
- increases healthy libido and improves sexual performance
- increases production of red blood cells
- increases sense of well-being
- slows the deteriorating effects of aging
- supports the cardiovascular system
- supports the entire endocrine system

Frequently Asked Hormone Questions

After learning about how many everyday foods and common products negatively influence hormone balance, some folks have questions about how to avoid them. Here are some simple answers.

- Q: What do I do about sunscreen?
- A: Many sunscreens are toxic and estrogenic. Use a hat and long-sleeved shirt and long pants.
- Q: What kind of cosmetics should I use?
- A: Only use cosmetics you would be willing to eat. Cosmetics should use vitamins, minerals, and/or grapefruit seed extract as a preservative.
- Q: What should I use as a weed killer?
- A: Avoid all Monsanto products, including RoundUp. Use a quarter-liter of salt in four liters of vinegar instead. Or decide to either pull the weeds by hand or love and eat weeds instead.
- Q: What should I eat?
- A: Go organic and eat lower on the food chain. Avoid animal products whenever possible due to potential contamination.
- Q: What should I use for birth control?
- A: Use natural latex condoms without spermicide (or, if you are going to use coconut oil and/or olive oil with spermicidal neem oil, use oil-resistant polyurethane condoms). Avoid birth control pills and other prescription forms of chemical birth control such as Depo-Provera.

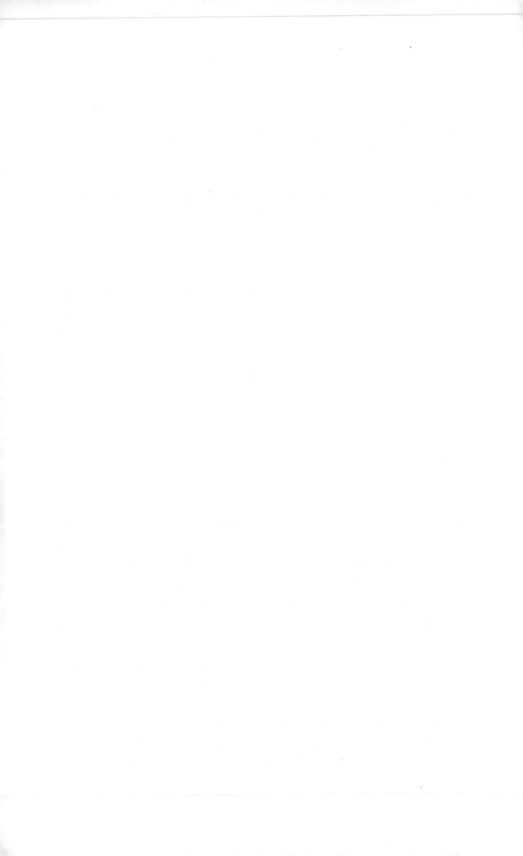

CHAPTER 6

Calcification, the Great Undertaker

Who has calcification? If you have taken inorganic calcium supplements or have acute aches in your muscles and/or arthritic pains in your joints; if you've ever suffered from a sports- or accident-related injury that has never completely gone away; if you have scar tissue, wrinkles, or stiff joints; if you have experienced a loss of hearing, cataracts in your eyes, or you are just getting older, there is a good chance that you have elevated levels of calcification, especially in the painful areas.

Nanobacteria: A Primary Cause of Calcification

Longevity Now presents cutting-edge insights in science and nutrition. I have spent twenty years investigating why we age, why our body breaks down prematurely, and why we suffer. What I found during the course of my twenty years of research was a number of culprits behind aging—common denominators that cause aging and premature death and destroy our potential to experience vibrant, incredible health. Calcification is one of the biggest of these threats.

I discovered research indicating that shell-forming, coral-like micro-organisms (similar to coral, barnacles, and clams) appear to be causative agents in calcification. These organisms have been given one name thus far (more will come) and are known in medical journal science as "nanobacteria." Calcification and calcium-forming organisms are part of Mother Nature's recycling system; it appears to me that they are found in the earth (in layered, calcium-rich strata), in many of the waters of the Earth as a natural effect of contact with calcium-rich strata, and perhaps some may also pleomorph from bacteria or cells in a chronically stressed unhealthy growing environment. In order to avoid aging we have to avoid becoming silted up with calcium, as well as calcium-forming organisms and/or their residues (shells). We also have to avoid consuming dead calcium supplements that are either mineral residues from the earth, coral residues, or oyster shell residues, all of which make the calcification problem even worse.*

Nanobacteria, or *Nanobacterium sanguineum,* were discovered in the 1980s by Finnish scientist E. Olavi Kajander and Turkish researcher Neva Ciftcioglu at the University of Kuopio in Finland. Nanobacteria

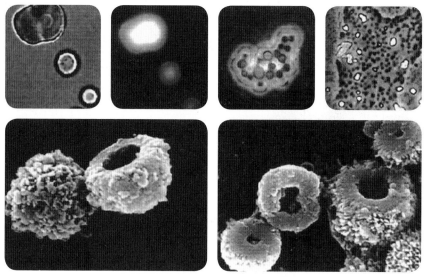

Calcium-forming nanobacteria

Source: NASA website; www.nasa.gov, study from NASA and Nanobac Pharmaceuticals

*Just as we should avoid calcium supplements, more and more research indicates that we should also avoid iron supplements. Elevated iron levels in hair samples have been conclusively correlated with aging and disease. The presence of elevated iron levels in the tissues increases oxidation. The higher the iron levels in the body, the greater the danger of dying prematurely from numerous causes; hence the logic of the ancient idea of bleeding patients via leeches and the Chinese idea of giving blood to increase longevity.

are microscopic living organisms that are roughly the same size as most viruses (approximately one hundredth the size of normal bacteria).

Nanobacterium sanguineum appear to be only one of what may be numerous types of nano-size shell-forming organisms. Theoretically, these shell-forming organisms appear to be the basic unit of recycling organisms, and as such they silt up (or calcify) the great families of reptiles, birds, amphibians, and mammals in order to make room for the next generation of creatures to inhabit the planet.

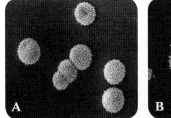 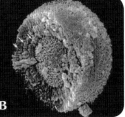 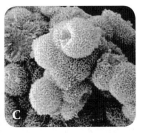

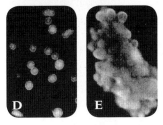

(a) Scanning electron microscopic (SEM) observation of calcified nanobacteria cultured in serum-free condition. (b) Detail from fractured nanobacteria showing mineral formation as layers shown by arrows. (c) SEM image of human apatite kidney stone showing apatite units. (d) Immunofluorescent (IF) staining of the nanobacteria similar to those shown in (a), and (e) the kidney stone shown in (c) with an anti-nanobacteria monoclonal antibody. Bars: a and c, 10 micrometers; b, 1 micrometer.

Source: Neva Ciftcioglu, Mikael Björklund, Kai Kuorikoski, Kim Bergström and E Olavi Kajander; Department of Biochemistry and Biotechnology, University of Kuopio; Kuopio University Hospital, Clinical Physiology, Kuopio; Central Hospital of the Central Finland, Jyväskylä, Finland

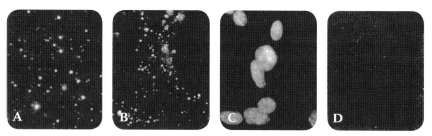

(a) Immunofluorescent (IF) staining of demineralized nanobacteria. (b) Double staining of 3T6 cells infected with nanobacteria cultured from a kidney stone. (c) DNA staining. (d) Control IF staining of noninfected cells.

Source: Neva Ciftcioglu, Mikael Björklund, Kai Kuorikoski, Kim Bergström and E Olavi Kajander; Department of Biochemistry and Biotechnology, University of Kuopio; Kuopio University Hospital, Clinical Physiology, Kuopio; Central Hospital of the Central Finland, Jyväskylä, Finland

A growing body of scientific evidence indicates that shell-forming nano-organisms are found in vaccines, urine, and even autoclaved medical and dental tools. These discoveries alert us to potential dangers we should all be aware of. Conventional vaccines are of dubious quality and are coming into more and more disfavor amongst doctors worldwide—the presence of bad calcium (as well as mercury and viruses) in vaccines furthers our awareness. Advances in urine therapies indicate that centrifuging one's own urine (dropping the calcium and fat to the bottom of the test tube and only using the lighter fraction of the urine as an injection into fatty tissue) is vastly more beneficial as a vaccine. There is a risk that medical and dental tools may not be completely sterilized by current autoclaving (heating) techniques. Virkon, a sterilization agent, should be used to completely eradicate calcium-forming organisms from used equipment.

Nanobacteria form shells made of calcium phosphate and other stone-like mineral compounds (otherwise known as apatite). Research indicates that the secreted shell first appears as a biofilm around the nanobacteria and then hardens around the organism, forming a defensive "outer armor" that helps shield it from the body's immune system. During the formation of the biofilm (before the shell hardens), it appears that toxins such as mercury, pesticides, and plastics are attracted, trapped, and stored there. When the shell hardens, these compounds are incorporated into the "bad calcium" they create, helping to further disarm our immune system against their removal.

Remarkable Facts about Nanobacteria

According to research found in the book *The Calcium Bomb,* by D. Mulhall, nanobacteria:

- are found in human blood
- replicate much more slowly than most viruses or bacteria
- require special methods to observe and culture them
- uniquely form a hard calcium phosphate shell in blood-like conditions
- resist radiation and heat that kill most bacteria and viruses
- trigger the same type of swelling and clotting found in heart disease and injuries
- cause kidney stones in lab animals injected with them
- contaminate vaccines and slip through conventional filters
- lead researchers to mislabel them by emitting a "false positive" for other infections
- have been found in arterial plaque, heart valves, ovarian cancer, dental stones, and kidney stones
- have been found in every heart disease patient who participated in a clinical trial
- are a reliable indicator of coronary artery calcification
- are treatable with a novel combination of well-known chemicals and drugs

---

Nanobacteria can reproduce themselves, forming aggregate, "budding-like" clusters (similar to coral), or they can remain in a state of "relative calcified dormancy" and hide inside our bodies, clogging up our system for years (such as what we find in scar tissue).

These hardened shells shield the nanobacteria in the same way a clam's shell shields a clam. Because the immune system has trouble breaking down these hardened shells to get at the "bad guys" inside, this protective layer forms an excellent living space, not only for the calcium-forming organisms, but also for opportunistic viruses, bacteria, and fungi.

Why Is Calcification Harmful?

Theoretically, once a calcium-forming organism infection has become manifest in the body, and the continually multiplying mass of shelled organisms has been established, the nanobacteria will continue to geo-metrically colonize the body over one's lifetime until one dies of a calci-fication disease. This indicates that an aggressive course of action must be taken against calcification.

Over the years of our life, the body will attempt to sequester and wall in harmful forms of bad calcium using fibrin, which causes the body's tissues to harden around the shells. Hence we have the terms *hard of hearing, hardening of the arteries, hard-headed,* etc. This is the reason we have the hardening of scar tissue and damaged skin, as well as the hard tissue of cysts.

Over our lifetime calcification or calcium phosphate crystallization (basically, "coral reefs" in our internal ocean) eventually build up in size, creating inflammation and sclerosis, and laying the foundation for what will eventually become any one of a number of painful chronic conditions, some of which have been previously listed.

Calcium-forming organisms such as nanobacteria take many years, sometimes decades, to grow to a population number with calcifica-tion debris significant enough to cause harm. Longevity Now was cre-ated in order to alert you to the dangers of calcification and how to avoid them. By incorporating Longevity Now we can rid our body of bad calcium and reverse the degeneration and inflammation that has occurred—in other words, we can reverse aging. When our system is no longer clogged with all the calcium-forming organisms (nanobacteria), viruses, harmful bacteria, candida, mutated cells, and other unwanted guests, as well as toxic waste from unhealthy foods, iron, pollutants from the environment, and harmful chemicals such as fire retardants and pesticides, we will be able to achieve our highest potential for longevity in the material realm.

Calcification has many disguises that undermine our health, age us, and cause our untimely death. The following terms are all used to describe conditions associated with calcification:

- apatite formation
- biomineralization
- brain sand (calcium deposits in the brain)
- calcified deposits
- calcified scar tissue
- calcium build-up
- calcium phosphate crystals
- calcium salts
- cataracts
- cellulite
- crystallization
- cysts
- dystrophic calcification
- gallstones
- hardening of body systems: arteries, hearing, eyes, etc.
- hard plaque (which is often found in the arteries and gums)
- kidney stones (calcium phosphate, calcium oxalate, magnesium ammonium phosphate, uric acid stones, cystine stones)
- metastatic calcification
- microcalcification
- ossification
- scars (internal and external)
- spurs (bone)
- stones (kidney stones, gallstones)

Calcification plagues all areas of the body, commonly including the brain and nervous system, the eyes, the heart and circulatory system, digestive system, reproductive system, endocrine system, urinary system, breasts, teeth and gums, skin, and bones.

The Shocking Truth about Calcium Supplements

> The fact that an opinion has been widely held is no evidence whatsoever that it is not utterly absurd.
>
> —BERTRAND RUSSELL

Bad calcium, as we are discovering, has been linked to inflammation and the production of more bad calcium in the human body. Nearly every troublesome condition known to humans, mammals, reptiles, and birds involves calcification.

Should you stop taking calcium supplements? Yes. Stop taking them immediately, including and especially coral calcium, oyster shell calcium, and any calcium in any form that was originally mined out of the Earth (e.g., calcium citrate, calcium carbonate). Calcium supplements of nearly every sort and description actually cause calcification. They act like sand in the gears of our tissues. They are deposited in the body as sediment. The use of calcium supplements must be stopped in order for us to decalcify and remineralize our bones. Calcium supplements cause aging and prematurely drag us into an early, permanent retirement six feet under the ground. On top of that, they do not do what they are stated to do: increase bone density and strength.

According to the great philosopher Rudolf Steiner (the developer of Waldorf education and creator of biodynamic farming), most calcium is "gravitational," meaning that it channels or conducts forces that accelerate gravity. The more calcium supplements one takes, the quicker one is dragged back into the earth for recycling.

Not all calcium is bad. Longevity Now identifies both good and bad forms of calcium. Basically, the two types differ in electrostatic charge: bad calcium compounds lack electrons (they are positively charged); good calcium contains surplus electrons (they are negatively charged).

The calcium naturally found in plants (vegetables, the pith of citrus fruits, carob, mesquite, wheatgrass, etc.) has a surplus of electrons and is perfectly safe for consumption. In particular, good calcium from green-leafed vegetable sources is essential for detoxification, muscle relaxation, lowering tension, and creating alkalinity. Raw dairy products from free-range animals are another source of good calcium (if you have the enzymes to digest them).

Pearl calcium is safe to consume if you feel you require a calcium supplement. Pearl carries the proper negative charge, is time-proven to be safe, and carries signal proteins that increase mineralization. Pearl also assists in calcium's natural function of detoxification and relaxation.

The "calcium theory"—which holds that we have to eat calcium to produce calcium for our bones—has led to more suffering than just about any theory ever developed by humanity. It is based on Lavoisier's Law, which states that a mineral is a mineral and cannot be changed (nothing is lost, nothing is gained, everything is transformed). Lavoisier's Law gave us the idea that a lack of calcium in the bones indicates that we need to eat more calcium. Calcium = calcium. The European alchemists never bought into Lavoisier's Law and always opposed it. Subsequent discoveries by Ernst Rutherford in 1919 indicated that Lavoisier was incorrect, because Rutherford found that radiation could change one mineral into another.

Later, in the 1950s, the French scientist Professor C. L. Kervran discovered that multiple types of low-energy transmutations of one mineral into another were occurring inside living organisms and also were naturally happening in the biosphere and geosphere. Kervran's work led to the rediscovery that supplemental silicon (horsetail herb extract, bamboo sap, hemp leaf, etc.) as well as magnesium (cacao/chocolate, chlorella, green vegetables) could remineralize porous or damaged bone with calcium. (These facts were always well known to herbalists from many traditions.) This rediscovery indicates that silicon and magnesium are being biologically transmuted into calcium in the bones; therefore, in order to increase our bone density we need to consume the minerals silicon and magnesium (as well as other minerals and nutrients)—but not more calcium.

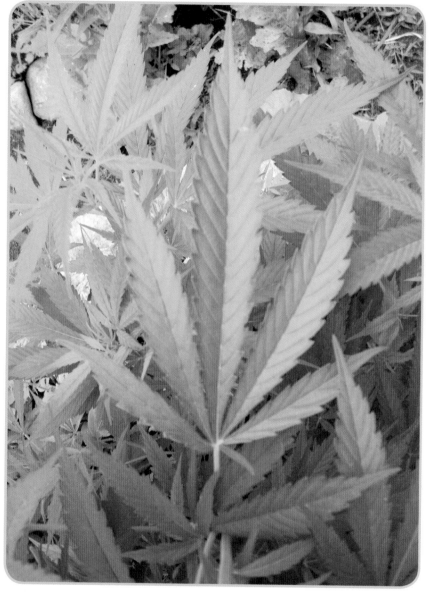

Hemp leaf is rich in bone-building silica and medicinal CBD compounds. Due to the influence of Dr. Courtney, patients are now fighting cancer by drinking hemp leaf juice.

> # TIP
> To remineralize bones and reduce calcification, consume silicon-rich herbs (horsetail, nettle, hemp leaf, oatstraw), silicon-rich supplements, and silicon-rich waters, as well as magnesium-rich superfoods (cacao or raw chocolate, chlorella, etc.) and magnesium-rich supplements.*
>
> *For more information on the subject of bone remineralization and biological transmutations, see my books *Eating for Beauty* and *Naked Chocolate*, as well as C. L. Kervran's *Biological Transmutations*. Also, key information about grounding and its important effects on mineralization is provided on pages 307–309.

The distinctions of good and bad calcium should not be applied to soil science, only to the healing sciences of animal biology; many forms of bad calcium that are toxic in animal biology are required for useful, productive, healthy soil.

Reversing Calcification with the Longevity Now Approach

This section consists of five specific strategies designed to break down and evacuate bad calcium from the body; to modulate the immune system; to ward off calcium-forming organisms and other parasites from multiplying in our bodies; and to create an overall superior level of health and well-being so that disease symptoms, illness, bacteria, virus and/or fungi cannot proliferate. These five specific strategies are more effective once the suggestions in Chapter 5 have been heeded, so that androgenic hormones are up and bad estrogen and cortisol hormones are down.

Decalcification System, at a Glance

Below is an at-a-glance breakdown of the decalcification system detailed in the following pages. I recommend incorporating all five parts, as well as implementing as many steps as possible within each part. If you feel this is too much for your body to take on, then incorporate at least one thing in each of the five parts, as well as anything you understand from this book. Add in as many powerful healing tools as you can, but please keep in mind that incorporating any single idea in this book will deliver at least some positive results!

- **Part 1. Bad calcium dissolvers:** Dissolve bad calcium detritus found in the body. Strip down the hard shells that surround infections and calcium-forming microorganisms.
  - **Step 1.** zeolites, MSM, and fulvic acid
  - **Step 2.** MegaHydrate, Crystal Energy, and DMSO
  - **Step 3. (optional)** shilajit and EDTA
- **Part 2. Herbal immune boosters:** Develop super immunity. Destroy and evacuate any opportunistic unwanted guests, calcium-forming microorganisms, viruses, bacteria, and fungi.
  - **Step 1.** aged garlic extracts, Triple Herbal Treasures (cloves, wormwood, black walnut)
  - **Step 2.** medicinal mushroom extracts, noni fruit-seed powder
  - **Step 3.** mangosteen, cat's claw (extract, powder and/or tea), citric acid (citrate)
- **Part 3. Cell-rejuvenating supplements and foods:** Modify the internal terrain using the best superherbs, superfoods, and supplements. Accelerate and support Parts 1 and 2 by acting as a "clean-up crew," repairing damaged, aged tissue and removing any debris lingering in the body.
  - **Step 1.** enzymes, adaptogen herbs (superherbs)
  - **Step 2.** probiotics (friendly bacteria), vitamin C plant powders (camu camu, amla, and/or acerola)
  - **Step 3.** krill oil, marine phytoplankton, additional cell-rejuvenating supplements, stone-breaking herbs, and Wulzen factor foods

> · **Part 4. Longevity technologies:** Destroy and evacuate bad bacteria and other unwanted guests through cutting-edge electronic technologies while normalizing all your circadian rhythms.
>   · **Step 1.** Zapper
>   · **Step 2.** grounding technologies
> · **Part 5. Deep tissue bodywork and yoga:** Break up and massage calcification on the bones and in the tissues and muscles by utilizing the power of deep-tissue bodywork, yoga techniques, and other discoveries.
>   · **Step 1.** yoga, rebounding, Bongers
>   · **Step 2.** deep-tissue massage, Rolfing, Body Electronics
>   · **Step 3.** David Wolfe's Neckwork Protocol, Chinese *gua sha*, Maori romi romi bodywork

Determining Your Intensity Level

There are three levels of intensity of the Longevity Now decalcification approach—low, medium, and high. In order to determine the level at which you should begin, please consider the following guidelines. **Note:** These are general guidelines. When in doubt, *always* start with a milder approach. Remember, you know your body better than anyone. Please proceed with caution. If you continue to have questions or concerns, please seek the advice of a qualified health practitioner.

Go with a **low-intensity approach** if you:

- eat processed foods regularly (3–7 times per week)
- drink tap water
- drink alcohol regularly (3–7 times per week)
- consume coffee regularly (5–7 times per week)
- have a history of abusing sugar and carbohydrates
- have neurological imbalances
- have a history of taking prescription drugs
- have a history of taking over-the-counter medication

- consume animal products (meat, fish, pasteurized dairy) regularly (3–7 times per week)
- have *never* taken herbal supplementation before
- take recreational drugs (I advise you to completely avoid recreational drugs when using the Longevity Now approach)
- do not floss regularly
- do not exercise regularly (at least 3 times per week)
- are overweight
- do not get a good night's sleep regularly (at least 3–4 times per week)

You may consider trying **medium-intensity** approach if you:

- eat mostly vegetarian and organic (5–7 times per week)
- drink from a pure water source regularly (spring water or purified water)
- rarely eat processed foods
- rarely drink alcohol
- rarely consume coffee
- do not have a history of taking prescription drugs and over-the-counter medication
- have taken herbal supplementation before
- rarely take recreational drugs
- floss regularly (5–7 times per week)
- exercise regularly (3–5 times a week)
- are at a reasonably healthy weight
- get a good night's sleep regularly (up to 5 times a week)

You may consider trying **high-intensity** approach if you:

- are eating raw, organic fruits and vegetables as part of your daily diet
- drink from a pure water source (low in calcium and iron) regularly
- are abstaining from all meat and fish products
- are abstaining from pasteurized dairy products
- are abstaining from alcohol
- are abstaining from daily coffee intake

- do not have a history of prescription drugs or over-the-counter medications
- already have familiarity with superfoods and supplements and take them regularly (5–7 times per week)
- abstain from recreational drugs
- floss your teeth regularly (5–7 times per week)
- exercise regularly (3–5 times per week)
- are at a reasonably healthy weight
- get a good night's sleep (at least 5 times a week)

Part 1. Bad Calcium Dissolvers

If you have ever scrubbed scale (calcium residues) off a sink, bathtub, or toilet surface, then you are aware of how calcification needs to be dissolved and scrubbed with an appropriate solvent. The "bad calcium dissolvers" are designed to go into your body and safely dissolve, detoxify, and facilitate the excretion of bad calcium.

Step 1: Zeolites, MSM, and Fulvic Acid

Zeolite

Zeolite is a natural volcanic type of rock that possesses a uniquely complex crystalline structure and is similar to clay. It is one of the most powerful negatively charged minerals in Nature, acting as a magnet, drawing toxins to it, capturing them in its cage-like molecular structure, and then permanently removing the toxins from our bodies. I have included zeolite in Longevity Now for its extraordinary abilities to detoxify the body.

Humans have been exposed to more toxins through water and air pollution, household cleaning supplies, pesticides, chemtrails, disinfectants, furniture finishings, construction materials, and food additives than ever before in history. The toxicity in our environment has a direct effect on our health, reduces our quality of life, and causes us to age prematurely, to get sick, and to lose our vitality. In order to combat the toxicity and pollution that is harming our bodies, many

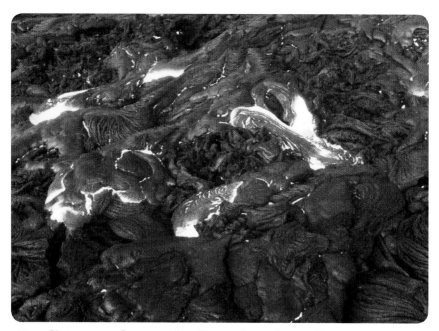

Zeolites are formed where hot lava flows into the ocean.

health-seekers have turned to the time-tested healing power of raw earth compounds such as fulvic acid, humic acid, humates, shilajit, salts, clays, and other unique natural mineral compounds.

Like salt, clay is an edible form of earth that is highly absorptive. This means that clay can draw into itself and trap toxic gases, liquids, and solids. Clay (like other raw earth compounds) is negatively charged (has extra electrons) and therefore has the ability to attract highly positively charged (electron-deficient) substances like bad calcium, plastics, petrochemicals, heavy metals, food toxins, etc. These toxins are then "locked up" in the clay and safely eliminated from the body. Clay eating and clay bathing are traditional solutions to help free ourselves from environmental and food toxins.

For centuries, the powdered forms of specific zeolites have been used as traditional remedies throughout Asia to promote overall health and well-being. Although zeolites are not technically forms of clay, they produce a similar effect. Like clay, zeolites have a strong detoxification ability, yet they are dramatically more powerful than clay. Because of this, I like to think of zeolites as a form of "superclay."

Today zeolites are available in an extremely finely ground, micronized liquid form. This method of preparation significantly increases the bio-availability of the zeolites, so that they are more easily assimilated into the body. In comparison to clays, which are bulky, heavy, and unpalatable, zeolites in liquid form are extraordinarily potent, simple, and convenient to use.

Zeolite appears to have an especially powerful chelating effect, removing heavy metals such as mercury, cadmium, arsenic, lead, and aluminum. These heavy metals are considered highly toxic and are often carcinogenic, neurotoxic, and mutagenic.

Zeolite has also been found to help remove pesticides, herbicides, and other positively charged toxins from the system. It seems to do this in a hierarchical manner. It first acts strongly to remove lead, mercury, cadmium, and arsenic. It then acts to remove the pesticides, herbicides, furans, and other toxic chemicals called volatile organic compounds.

Zeolite has a strong antioxidant component. In fact, zeolite is the only scientifically known substance to remove harmful oxidants such as mercury, lead, arsenic, and volatile organic compounds such as formaldehyde, dichlorobenzene, toluene, methylene chloride, etc. These are all *highly* toxic, free radical–causing substances that we definitely want out of our bodies.

Volatile organic compounds (VOCs) are carbon compounds that turn into gases at room temperature, especially when they come into contact with sunlight. VOCs can cause skin and eye irritation, nausea, respiratory problems, headaches, and weakness. Some VOCs can lead to serious illnesses, including the mutation of cells. VOCs are found in paint, mattresses, carpets, and other common items. One example of a VOC is formaldehyde, which has been shown to cause cancer in animals.

Because these toxins and VOCs lead to an increasingly weakened immune system, by removing these substances, zeolites support a healthy immune system.

VOCs Removed by Liquid Zeolite

According to research, liquid zeolite product Natural Cellular Defense removes the following volatile organic compounds (VOCs):[1]

- formaldehyde
- o-dichlorobenzene
- toluene
- methylene chloride
- benzene
- tetrachlorodibenzodioxin
- p-dichlorobenzene
- tetrachlorodibenzofuran
- xylene hexachlorobiphenyl

Zeolite also seems to increase the rate of glucuronidation in the liver. This is a process whereby toxins are made water-soluble so that they can be eliminated more easily from the body. When we take zeolite, the amount of pesticides, herbicides, and xenoestrogens released through the urine has been shown to increase as a result of the liver letting go of all its stored-up toxins. As we take zeolites over time, the burden on our organs significantly decreases.

Along the same lines, zeolite is the only scientifically known compound to remove uranium-238 and may be capable of removing radioactive plutonium and cesium as well. Uranium-238 is a type of radioactive uranium regularly used by the United States and NATO military forces in depleted uranium weapons. It is also found as a byproduct of nuclear power plants. It is radioactive, neurotoxic, an immunotoxin, and is linked to genetic abnormalities and "Gulf War Syndrome." When substances like uranium-238 or plutonium begin to decay, they cause a massive oxidation reaction, or free-radical attack, in the human body. Zeolite is scientifically shown to stop these oxidation reactions.

In the context of Longevity Now, zeolite also acts as a clathrating compound, which is defined as having the ability to remove calcified substances (bad calcium) from the body as well as heavy metals and volatile organic compounds (see below).

Once the zeolite has done its job, it is then excreted from the body in a process that from start to finish takes about 5–7 hours. What is very important to note in this process is that once trapped by the zeolite, the bad calcium, heavy metals, and other toxic compounds cannot be redeposited elsewhere in the body. Because of the way the zeolite molecule is shaped, it is impossible for any of the waste to escape; it stays tightly bound up inside the zeolite "cage" structure.

Due to its powerful role of cleaning up the debris inside our bodies, it is essential that we consistently take zeolite throughout the entire duration of Longevity Now. This ensures that we remove all the "leftover" byproducts that arise from deep cleansing.

Other than mild dehydration (which occurs as a result of not drinking enough water) and too-rapid detoxification among beginners who take too much of the zeolite at once, no negative side effects should be expected from ingesting zeolites. If you increase the amount you take, make sure to increase the amount of water consumed, in order to stay properly hydrated.

Edible zeolites are 100 percent natural, nontoxic, and regarded as safe for long-term use.

Recommended Use: Zeolite in liquid form or powdered forms are both recommended. Ingest with at least 1 ounce of drinking water per drop of liquid zeolite or 1,000 mg capsule of powdered zeolite. Liquid zeolite is not homeopathic, so it is not necessary to hold it under the tongue. Add the powder into your favorite beverage, elixir, tea, or drinking water.

MSM (Methyl Sulfonyl Methane)

MSM is a crystallized, oxidized form of DMSO, otherwise known as $DMSO_2$, that can be taken daily. MSM helps to maintain lubrication of the joints, flexibility of the tissues, and rejuvenation of the skin, hair, and nails. MSM is a strong antioxidant and anti-inflammatory, and assists the immune system in breaking down bad calcium. MSM is also a "methyl donor," which means that it donates a methyl group to the liver to help detoxify nonmethylated bad estrogens.

It is known from scientific evidence that the more MSM and biologically available sulfur we take, the more difficult it is for calcium-forming organisms to "get a hold of us." These organisms are like barnacles or oysters, and they are always looking for a stagnant part of our body that is easy to hook on to. When we take in enough sulfur, the areas where calcium-forming organisms like to grow—for example, our joints—become so "slippery" that the nanobacteria can no longer hold on and continue to grow. MSM has a long history of helping improve conditions known to be connected to the production of bad calcium, including all arthritic conditions, bursitis, damaged joints, and inflammation.

Rheumatoid and psoriatic arthritis are autoimmune disorders whereby the immune system attacks the tissues of the joints. Calcium-forming organisms (nanobacteria) appear to be responsible for the build-up of calcium crystals in the joints, and appear to be implicated along with viruses in these conditions.

In the geosphere, sulfur converts the excessive calcium that Earth organisms produce and deposit in layered strata into calcium sulfate (gypsum). Gypsum, when added to your garden, creates sweetness. MSM does something similar to this when we take it in—it converts bad insoluble calcium into bio-available calcium.

If we take significant amounts of MSM, over a period of time we are going to see a powerful shift in the way our hair and nails grow, in our skin, in our digestive abilities, and in our flexibility. The calcification and hardening of the joints will also change. We may find relief from pain and inflammation in both the short term and the long term. In addition, as we have seen, MSM is a methyl group donor and therefore is highly bioavailable and detoxifies the liver of bad estrogens. Because of all these factors, I believe that MSM is one of the great discoveries, or rather rediscoveries, of the twentieth century.

MSM comes in powders and capsules. Pine resin MSM is the best type and most highly regarded; however, all forms of MSM will do the job. The innovation of capsule technology protects the substance inside from oxidation—a level of oxygen protection greater than the bottle itself.

MSM can also be applied topically. MSM lotions/creams do more than just soften and moisturize the skin; they help restore and rejuvenate dry, rough skin, leaving it smooth and silky. These pure creams deliver all the value of MSM directly to the skin surface. Because a past or present MSM deficiency may have allowed for the creation of scar tissue and wrinkles, MSM cream should be applied daily, directly to areas of skin damage. Applying MSM to the joints, to sunburns, mosquito bites, and skin irritations is also highly beneficial.

Warning: Some people who are allergic to sulfur-containing drugs may have reactions to MSM and therefore cannot take it. It is rare, but it does happen. If you are one of these people, you can instead use liquid zeolite (orally and topically), fulvic acid (orally and topically), shilajit (orally), and/or liquid Ormus gold (topically). EDTA (suppository or intravenous) may be used as well. You will still obtain the desired results.

Recommended Use: Because MSM is such a powerful compound, we always recommend starting light. Take two doses per day, one in the morning and one in the evening. You can add MSM to water, juice, or smoothies.

Fulvic Acid

Fulvic acid (not to be confused with folic acid) is a nutritious and detoxifying compound created in extremely small amounts by millions of beneficial microbes working on decaying plant matter in sediment and soil. The fulvic acid is layered in humic acid and other compounds in sediments set down over tens of thousands of years. These are sediments that were never stripped to the bedrock and washed into the ocean. Some beds containing fulvic acid are estimated to be millions of years old.

Fulvic acid has always occurred naturally in soils. The more fulvic acid in the soil, the more powerful the growth of plants in that soil. The agricultural benefits of adding fulvic acid to soils have enormous potential to heal damaged soils all over the world.

Scientists have found that fulvic acid is an elemental compound that when consumed by humans makes nutrients more absorbable. Because of fulvic acid's low molecular weight and small molecular size, it has the ability to readily dissolve bad calcium, to bond minerals, and to draw nutritional elements into its molecular structure. Once chelated by fulvic acid these substances are in an ideal and healthy form to be either detoxified and removed from the body or absorbed by living cells. One single fulvic acid molecule is capable of carrying sixty or more minerals and trace elements into the cells. Fulvic acid is also one of the most efficient transporters of vitamins into the cells.

Fulvic acid is a provider of powerful natural electrolytes. It is also one of the most powerful antioxidants ever. Fulvic acid detoxifies and helps eliminate from the body bad calcium, bad iron, other toxic metals, and pollutants. This process is called "chelation." Research shows that fulvic acid improves enzymatic reactions in cells. Many years of observation of the effects of human consumption of plant-derived mineral fulvic complexes show that they do not build up in body tissues the way metallic minerals do.

Fulvic acid is concentrated out of natural sediments and is available in powdered or liquid forms at various concentrations.

Recommended Use: Consume fulvic acid with detoxifying lemonades, spring water, elixirs, or smoothies.

Step 2: MegaHydrate, Crystal Energy, and DMSO

MegaHydrate

Dr. Patrick Flanagan was considered one of the top ten scientists in the United States when he was only seventeen years old. That was more than fifty years ago.

Dr. Flanagan's research on the fabled longevity water from the Hunza Valley in Pakistan, sometimes called "glacial milk," led him to the development of his famous longevity products: MegaHydrate and Crystal Energy. He found that this water contained unique silica compounds as well as massive levels of embryonic negatively charged hydrogen ions or "reactive hydrogen." From these discoveries he was able to develop his famous "Flanagan microclusters," which are tiny silica-rich mineral clusters loaded with negatively charged hydrogen—also known as silica hydride. These microclusters are perhaps the strongest antioxidants known; they deactivate free radicals and convert dangerous reactive oxygen to pure water. These microclusters are the key ingredients in MegaHydrate and Crystal Energy.

When oxygen in the body loses one or more electrons it becomes a free radical, which can roam throughout the body, damaging DNA and cell membranes while stealing electrons, thus creating more free radicals and aging. This cycle continues until the oxygen molecules are quenched with spare negatively charged hydrogen ions found in fresh spring water, raw plant foods, colored plant pigments, raw fats/oils, and in vitamins (such as A, C, E), mineral/nutrient complexes, and the supplements MegaHydrate and Crystal Energy.

Dr. Flanagan is an advocate of raw-food nutrition and believes that the presence of reactive hydrogen in raw food is the main scientific difference between raw and cooked food. Dr. Flanagan believes that we should give our bodies as much reactive negatively charged hydrogen as possible.

MegaHydrate is encapsulated, powdered, reactive hydrogen on a silica carrier—which is the most powerful type of antioxidant and hydrating substance known. MegaHydrate has an ORAC value of 6,271 (umoleTE/g). That's more than ten times higher than chocolate, more than thirty times higher than açaí, and more than one hundred times higher than blueberries.

MegaHydrate is the only scientifically proven supplement known to increase hydration in double-blind placebo studies. MegaHydrate decreases the surface tension of water and allows the cells of the body to absorb much more water. Water molecules are the sailors, and Mega-Hydrate is the captain. One uses the other for maximum success.

MegaHydrate's microclustered "silica hydride" compounds are known to positively influence the "zeta potential" of blood cells. Zeta potential is an electrical charge that describes the distance between cells. Greater zeta potential helps each cell to expel toxins, viruses, and other unwanted guests from their dehydrated and/or calcified hiding places.

MegaHydrate is also known to make bad calcium soluble. Once calcium is dissolved in water, the human metabolism has a much easier time detoxifying the bad calcium. This research may be viewed pictorially on page 47 in Lim Cheu Song's e-book entitled *Stay Younger, Healthier Naturally: Long Life with Negative Hydrogen and Biological Water.*

Recommended Use: MegaHydrate capsules are great to take supplementally with water or food (on an empty or full stomach—most people prefer to have a little bit of food in their stomach when taking Mega-Hydrate). Due to its powerful antioxidant properties, MegaHydrate powder is great to add to smoothies and juices that one desires to keep fresh for several days. Simply open up a couple of capsules and add the powder to your beverages, stir, then refrigerate. But be careful, MegaHydrate releases hydrogen and fizzes upon contact with vitamin C compounds in foods.

Crystal Energy

Crystal Energy is a hydrogen-rich zeolite supplement. Like other forms of zeolite, it has detoxification and clathrating (bad calcium-removing) properties. It is a similar product to MegaHydrate; the two products are designed to be used together. Crystal Energy differs from MegaHydrate in that it is a liquid. One can add it directly to drinking water or other beverages, thus making them "wetter" by lowering their surface tension (to a lower dynes number).

Crystal Energy acts as a catalyst, reducing the surface tension of water, thus making it a more efficient solvent and wetting agent. Adding Crystal Energy to water and beverages has been shown to increase hydration and nutrient absorption, and to improve digestion and eliminate toxins. Crystal Energy contains the powerful Flanagan "microclusters."

Crystal Energy may be added to herbal alcohol tinctures to increase their efficacy and upgrade their potency. One bottle contains 94 forty-drop servings.

Crystal Energy is highly recommended by Dr. Gabriel Cousens, MD.

Recommended Use: Add 10–50 drops of Crystal Energy for every 32 fluid ounces of drinking water. Also, Crystal Energy drops can be added to smoothies, juices, coffee, and teas.

DMSO (Dimethyl Sulfoxide)

DMSO is a particularly popular substance in the Longevity Now approach, one that we like to call "alchemical sulfur." It is strongly believed that the ancient alchemists figured out how to create this substance many hundreds of years ago. It was then rediscovered in 1866 by the Russian scientist Alexander Saytzeff, who reported his findings in a German chemistry journal in 1867. DMSO has been with us ever since. It is included in the first step of Longevity Now because it is a time-proven healing sulfur compound, an extraordinary topical and intravenous delivery system for healing substances, and a known catalyst in the breakdown of bad calcium. DMSO-type compounds are naturally found in tree bark, aloe vera, noni fruit, marine phytoplanktons, grasses, several different types of sulfur-bearing amino acids, and in animal organs and muscle tissues as well.

Most of what is happening as we age does not involve needing more calcium; in fact, we are accumulating too much of the wrong kind of calcium. Using DMSO in conjunction with MSM is a very powerful way to dissolve the calcified waste materials within the body.

A long-standing nutritional deficiency of sulfur (as well as silica, Ormus minerals, and polysaccharides) appears to be directly related to the ability of viruses, fungi, and calcium-forming microorganisms to grasp, adhere, and penetrate into the negative pressure bladders that protect each joint.

Warning: DMSO is a chemical solvent and is for external use only. *Do not ingest DMSO internally.* Because our mouths are so often full of heavy metals (as in amalgam fillings), bacteria, and their debris, the DMSO will drive all these things into the bloodstream and body without filter. We do not want this happening.

Recommended Use: Apply DMSO topically to troublesome areas. First transfer the DMSO from the "mother" bottle into a spray or dropper bottle. Use "straight" DMSO—70 percent to 99.9 percent liquid DMSO products are both fine because they have no additives except distilled water. Before applying, wash the area with water and a very small

TIP If we do not have enough sulfur (e.g., DMSO MSM), silica, Omega-3 fatty acids (DHA, ALA, EPA), hydrogen, Ormus minerals, and polysaccharides (from aloe, noni, medicinal mushrooms, etc.) to seal and give flexibility to the negative pressure bladders that surround each joint, then we may be subject to an infection breaching the shielding of our joints. Sulfur compounds not only prevent infection of the joints and related infections (psoriasis and eczema),* they can help fight existing infections of this sort. If our joints are damaged by infections (e.g., arthritis), then instead of operating on the joint, which can oxidize the joint and permanently damage it beyond repair, I recommend seeking out prolotherapy (preferably using injections of aloe vera extracts into the joints) and autologous mesenchymal stem cell treatments.

*Psoriasis and eczema notably occur on the skin around joints. And they appear to be "rooted" in the joints near to where psoriasis and eczema repeatedly occur.

amount of natural soap, and then spray with food-grade hydrogen peroxide. This process ensures that any chemicals, bacteria, or other undesirable things are not absorbed into the skin. Finally, spray the DMSO on the areas where needed. Apply just enough DMSO until a slight heating reaction is felt—not too little where nothing is noticed, but not so much as to cause a burn.

TIP Keep DMSO in a tightly closed bottle. This liquid has a high affinity for water molecules. If we open up a bottle in a humid climate we will see the DMSO come out of the bottle (like steam) and move right into the water molecules that are in the atmosphere.

DMSO must be applied on the skin when it is free and unencumbered by clothing, as the dyes in clothing can be carried directly into your skin by DMSO. Your skin must be completely dry, or the DMSO wiped off after ten minutes by a clean undyed rag, before putting your clothes back on.

Start with small amounts of DMSO. If you apply too much, wash and then rub it off with water as quickly as possible.

Please be careful and educate yourself on this product *before* using it. Excellent resources on DMSO include *DMSO: Nature's Healer,* by Dr. Morton Walker, and *The DMSO Handbook,* by Bruce Halstead.

> **TIP** DMSO is a localized delivery vehicle of healing compounds. For example, DMSO can be topically combined with some of the other bad calcium dissolvers where calcification skin conditions (psoriasis) repeatedly occur. Simply wash the area so it is completely clean with no soap residue, put liquid fulvic acid on top of the skin, and then spray the area with DMSO. The DMSO will act as a potentiator and drive the fulvic acid into that particular area under the skin. DMSO can deliver multiple alcohol-based herbal tinctures such as pau d'arco and neem through specific areas of the skin. DMSO can also deliver colloidal silver through the skin. This insight can be enormously valuable as a technique in healing.

Step 3. (Optional) Shilajit and EDTA

Shilajit

The highest-concentration, natural-source, readily edible form of fulvic acid is shilajit. Shilajit is a blackish-brown mineral pitch, resin, or tar that exudes from layers of rocks in several mountain ranges of the world, especially the Himalayan and Hindu Kush ranges of the Indian subcontinent. It was noted by ancient healers in the regions where shilajit arises from rock strata that all the animals who consumed it (especially white monkeys) were particularly healthy and happy. Soon shilajit was incorporated into the medicinal repertoire of those regions. Eventually, through thousands of years of time-proven benefits, shilajit came to be considered the primary adaptogen in Ayurvedic medicine, the traditional herbal system of India.

> Like other black tonics, superherbs, and foods (including chaga mushroom, eucommia bark, prepared rehmannia root, black ant, dried schizandra, black wild rice, black maca, black sesame seeds, black walnut hull, naturally ripened olives, black honey, black-bean prepared *ho shou wu*, mucuna (ripe black pod), etc.) shilajit possesses jing-building super longevity and tonic properties associated with its black color. Shilajit can be ingested nearly every day.

Because of its source in the high Himalayas and the science behind the substance, I have concluded that shilajit confers additional adaptogenic properties including more resistance to cold weather and greater ability to handle lower-oxygen environments.

Shilajit can be purchased in powdered form and as a tar substance.

Recommended Use: Shilajit possesses strong, smoked, earthy, slightly bitter flavor notes that offer hints of chocolate. Shilajit is best incorporated into one's diet using cacao or chocolate, which naturally disguises shilajit's strong flavors. The two are a natural marriage.

EDTA

EDTA is absorbed directly into the bloodstream. It then begins to "chelate" or remove bad calcium, toxic metals, and other excessive mineral deposits. When metals and minerals remain in the bloodstream, they accumulate and harden, causing poor circulation. By removing debris from the body's arteries and veins, the blood flow is increased. This increased blood flow is better able to supply the body's organs, muscles, tissues, and nerves with ample nutrients and oxygen, thus allowing them to recuperate, regenerate, and function normally.

EDTA has a recent history of human use, having been utilized for more than sixty years to clean up food substances that have heavy metal contamination.

EDTA is a false amino acid that, when properly administered, the human body recognizes and uses effectively to remove heavy metals and excessive calcium. EDTA has also been extensively studied for its potential to heal cardiovascular problems. This makes sense, as EDTA is an antiplaquing agent in the bloodstream. EDTA has traditionally been used intravenously to help chelate and pull out the bad calcium particles and heavy metals from the bloodstream. EDTA suppositories have also been found to be effective against cardiovascular calcification.

EDTA may be even more effective when used in conjunction with sulfur-bearing N-acetylcysteine (NAC) and/or MSM (usually taken orally). To clarify, the EDTA would be taken as a suppository or via IV and the NAC or MSM would be taken orally.

Warning: EDTA (ethylene diamine tetra-acetic acid) is a very powerful compound that is not necessarily beneficial for everyone. Please use extreme caution if you choose to include EDTA as a part of your research. EDTA should be administered as a suppository or by intravenous chelation (see a qualified professional). Even then there may be adverse reactions from the use of this product. Oral EDTA is not recommended; it has been shown to be harsh on the digestive tract and potentially dangerous in depleting our bodies of essential zinc, copper, and other trace minerals. Oral EDTA may produce no positive results at all.

Recommended Use: EDTA can be taken as a suppository or in the form of IV chelation therapy with a certified naturopathic or other type of physician who can determine the appropriate number and frequency of treatments. Generally, it takes twenty treatments of chelation therapy to clean out the circulatory system and get back to a state of health where one's life would no longer be threatened (for example, by a heart attack).

If your teeth begin to become translucent due to taking EDTA, back off to lighter usage and/or treatments, as the EDTA may be pulling too many minerals from your body. Remember to take EDTA with MSM and/or NAC (N-acetylcysteine).

Part 2. Herbal Immune Boosters

The immune system includes the organs, tissues, chemistry, and processes by which an organism maintains its resiliency against destructive decay and parasite attack. The immune system's primary role is to recognize and eradicate pathogenic bacteria, calcium-forming microorganisms, viruses, fungi, parasites, and cancer cells. This is done through use of the body's macrophages, interferon secretions, T cells, and natural killer cells. These vital mechanisms can be greatly enhanced by consuming specific herbs, superfoods, and other natural "medicines" containing compounds that support the production of immune system elements.

The immune system is also responsible for "clean up"—the location, removal, and/or recycling of waste products, toxic particles, and dead tissue. In order to activate our highest longevity potential, it is critical to maintain a highly functioning immune system. This helps our bodies cope with and remove the deeply rooted nanobacteria, parasites, bad calcium, and toxic wastes that can build up over the years.

Step 1. Aged Garlic Extracts and Triple Herbal Treasures

Aged Garlic Extracts

Garlic (*Allium sativum*) is one of the most powerful and aggressive medicinal herbs in the world. It has been used as both food and medicine in many cultures for thousands of years, dating as far back as the ancient Egyptian civilization and before.

Garlic is a scientifically proven, broad-spectrum immune-boosting antibiotic that combats and helps flush out harmful bacteria, parasites, viruses, and nanobacteria. There is no more powerful antiviral and anti-infective food/herb on the Earth than garlic. Garlic contains multiple compounds and antioxidants including organo-sulfur compounds (diallyl sulfides), which are believed to be responsible for most of its pharmacological and antimicrobial actions. Garlic also contains minute amounts of the neurotransmitter-like EPA, an essential long-chain omega-3 fatty acid. These antioxidants protect the body's tissues from free-radical damage, help stop cell mutations, and enhance the nervous system.

In addition, garlic contains at least thirty-nine different known antibiotics, including its main constituent, allicin, which has been found to be a more effective antibiotic than penicillin or tetracycline. Garlic is known to contain many sulfur compounds, including the sulfur-bearing amino acid cystine, as well as various enzymatically active sulfur oils. It is believed that the sulfur compounds in garlic facilitate the breakdown of bad calcium. The multiple other antibiotic compounds in garlic are known to kill whatever harmful organisms are left.

During detoxification processes, blood pressure may temporarily increase as thick, soupy materials pass out of the lymph into the blood. When you implement Longevity Now in combination with a healthy diet, the lymph and blood systems will naturally unburden themselves and normalize. An elevated blood pressure is caused by obstructions in the blood vessels (cooked fat, cooked protein, oxidized food particles, toxins, bad salt, and bad calcium), an increased thickness of the blood, and/or a constriction of the arteries due to stress, all of which cause the heart to work harder to push blood through the vessels. By using garlic and aged garlic extracts (see below), we can easily and quickly unclog our arteries and decrease our blood pressure to safe levels, as the sulfur compounds in garlic have been scientifically proven to help the blood normalize.

Because garlic has a noteworthy history as a preventative for heart disease (which is usually caused by a coronary calcium occlusion resulting from an infection), it is highly beneficial to the health of the cardiovascular system. Garlic is also very useful in clearing up sinus and lung congestion, temporary symptoms that one may intermittently experience while getting rid of toxins in the body.

Recommended Use: Fresh raw garlic is a very aggressive herbal food with powerful medicinal properties and is reasonable to eat when required, but it can overwhelm the nervous system if consumed in excess daily for more than three weeks in a row. This is why aged garlic extracts are recommended—an alchemical product created by aging the garlic in various ways and for various amounts of time in order to obtain a more tonic, odorless herb. Aged garlic extracts contain powerful medicinal substances, including various antioxidant properties that you can ingest nearly every day without overstimulating yourself. Aged garlic extracts have been made for thousands of years by the Persians and Chinese. They are available in liquid and capsule form—both are great choices.

Triple Herbal Treasures

The Triple Herbal Treasures comprise a critical component of Longevity Now. This three-herb combination of cloves, wormwood, and black walnut is well tested, well known, and proven to help remove certain parasites from our bodies. These "unwanted guests" are a burden to the immune system and undermine our health and vitality. We need to get them out as quickly and safely as possible. The Triple Herbal Treasures provide a powerful way to do this.

The Triple Herbal Treasures act against unwanted guests taking up residence in the digestive tract. Bacteria and parasites may be continually producing viruses and creating conditions for nanobacteria and other calcifiers to flourish. These undesirable elements keep the immune system chronically suppressed and in a constant state of overdrive, unable to function effectively or keep the body running at an optimal state.

Parasites usually increase with increasing calcification. Viruses love bad calcium. Usually bad bacteria are found on top of viruses and bad calcium, which attract fungi. These fungi then create an environment friendly to parasites that have entered the body through contaminated water sources, foods, people, and/or animals. These unwanted, opportunistic guests and their friends are part of a chain reaction of decay and destruction. It is imperative to strategically and regularly flush them out.

We add the Triple Herbal Treasures to the Longevity Now approach for 100 days to kill both parasites and their second-generation eggs. Generally their life cycle is ninety days; therefore, by continuing to take these herbs for 100 days, the unwanted guests will be inhibited in their ability to reproduce and survive. As long as these freeloaders are in our system, our immunity will remain compromised, and it will be easier to become sick and suffer from colds and flus. This is a truth that must be told—from my personal experience after having evacuated these unwanted guests from my system, I feel it is imperative to inform you of the transformation in my immune system. This transformation is so significant that it seems impossible for me to get sick—that means no flus, coughs, colds, etc., under any stresses or circumstances.

The fact that most people have parasites in their body is not something that is widely heard or recognized in the mainstream health "news." When, for example, a dog gets sick, there is no hesitation to diagnose it with parasites; however, when a human's health is compromised, parasites are usually the last thing suspected. As unpleasant as it is to imagine, the vast majority of us have unwanted guests in our system. It is a reality that we must address now in order to move forward with having the best health ever.

According to Dr. Hulda Clark's book *The Cure for All Diseases,* almost every variety of commercial meat available is loaded with parasites of numerous types. Cooking may not always destroy calcium-forming and other harmful extremophile organisms present in the meat. Parasites are also present in tainted water sources (e.g., giardia), in our pets, our family, and friends. Remember, parasites are always looking for a warm home. They thrive in an unhealthy body because they feed and live most happily in an environment of excessive toxicity. They particularly enjoy foods you are allergic to: cooked starchy foods, sugar, and decaying cooked animal byproducts. When the body becomes so weakened from a toxic lifestyle, the unwanted guests will breach the digestive tract and enter the internal organs. This is when major health problems arise.

An effective strategy to stop any more parasites from coming into your body is to avoid all factory-farmed meat, fish, and fowl products, as well as potentially contaminated water sources. Avoid raw fish (sushi), which is known to be contaminated with tapeworms. Avoid kissing your pets or putting your hand to your mouth after being licked by your pet. Be aware that you can pick up parasites from people as well.

I believe that the highest concentrations of bad calcium and perhaps even calcium-forming microorganisms are found in some well or hard tap water (this will leave a white film called "scale"). Any water filter system must remove calcium and iron for starters. Any factory-farmed animals that consume hard well or tap water become, like us, contaminated with bad calcium and calcium-forming organisms. If we eat these animals their internal organisms are transferred to us (even if cooked), since calcium-forming microorganisms are extremophiles and may withstand high heat. In general, free-range animals usually consume higher-quality water and therefore are safer for us to consume.

It is critical to adopt a well-balanced, mineral-rich, plant-based diet in conjunction with the Longevity Now tools. We can also take special care to send "spicy" foods through the digestive tract regularly—such as garlic, onions, hot peppers (e.g., cayenne), ginger, and radishes—in order to help eliminate these critters. These foods may be mixed into juices, salads, blended foods, or eaten whole with raw plant fats such as avocados. Colonics will also help flush parasites out of the system.

Let's take a closer look at each component of the Triple Herbal Treasures.

Cloves

Cloves *(Eugenia caryophyllata)* are one of the most antibacterial of all spices. These popular and delicious aromatic flowers come from a tree indigenous to Asia. They help remove parasites in the intestines by killing their eggs. Cloves can be easily crushed and added to all sorts of drinks and smoothies to enhance the flavor. Clove extracts or alcohol tinctures do not produce the same results as the powdered form of the whole herb because cloves appear to work mechanically on intestinal parasites.

Cloves have also been known to:

- eliminate nausea
- expel gas from the stomach or bowel
- act as a powerful antiseptic
- soothe toothaches and gum pain
- provide nutrients to the body, including manganese, omega-3 fatty acids, and vitamin K
- reduce inflammation
- increase sexual function

- aid in digestion
- fight acne
- destroy candida
- treat cuts and bites in the form of a poultice

Warning: Cloves should not be taken if you are on anticoagulant or antiplatelet drugs, nor should they be used by pregnant women.

Recommended Use: Clove powder possesses bright yet deep antiseptic flavor notes. As long as one is conscious enough to avoid using too much, clove powder may be added to fruit smoothies, elixirs, homemade toothpastes, parasite cleanses, or simply added to other herb powders (e.g., black walnut hull, wormwood).

Wormwood

Wormwood *(Artemisia absinthium)* is a common species in the genus *Artemisia.* This powerful herb contains very strong medicinal compounds that are extraordinarily effective at removing unwanted organisms within the body—hence the name "wormwood." Because its effects are so profound, the FDA has regulated this herb as toxic in concentrated forms. However, these claims have yet to be proven and the fact still stands that wormwood has been safely used medicinally for at least two thousand years.

Wormwood has the following medicinal and health effects:

- treats liver, gallbladder, and stomach ailments
- expels parasites from the intestines
- stimulates the digestive process
- increases digestive enzymes
- has antiseptic, antispasmodic, and mild anti-infective properties
- promotes the discharge of bile from the liver
- helps to expel gas from the stomach and bowel
- improves blood circulation
- relieves symptoms related to menstruation
- treats candida
- helps alleviate arthritis, bruises, and sprains
- repels insects, moths, and fleas

Warning: Wormwood essential oil is toxic when ingested internally. Also, people with stomach problems, liver challenges, or intestinal ulcers should not use wormwood, nor should pregnant women.

Recommended Use: I recommend taking wormwood in a powder form, because mechanical cleansing properties remain active in the powder that directly alter the living environment of intestinal parasites. Also, parasites consume the wormwood powder as it passes through and are poisoned by it. A wormwood alcohol extract does not produce that same effect because the extract never makes it into the lower intestine. Start with a lesser dosage if you feel you are sensitive to strong-acting, bitter herbs.

Black Walnut

Black walnut *(Julgans nigra)* is actually a fruit. The nut itself is the seed of the fruit, and the flesh of the fruit is called the walnut hull. The walnut hull turns from green to black as the walnut ripens. Black walnut hull kills the adult and developmental stages of at least a hundred different types of parasites.

When taken internally, black walnut hull (and walnut leaf) remove toxins and parasites from the blood, lymph, liver, kidneys, brain, heart, and intestinal tract. Black walnut is also helpful in treating fungal infections. When extracted and applied topically, black walnut has been known to speed the healing of eczema, herpes, psoriasis, and other skin conditions.

Black walnut's range of action includes the following:

- reduces constipation
- heals acne and canker sores
- alleviates jock itch, ringworm, athlete's foot, and other fungi that attack the body
- lowers levels of harmful cholesterol and lowers risk of heart attack
- lowers high blood pressure
- cleanses and detoxifies the body
- assists the immune system in fighting cancerous tumors

Black walnut trees planted in your yard will help control your weeds—the same properties that make it antifungal and antiparasitic also act as a natural herbicide.

Recommended Use: Both the hull and the leaf taste reasonably good. When the black walnut hull and/or leaf powders move through our lower bowels, they act as toxic compounds that directly poison parasites. It is critical that the black walnut reach deep inside our gut—alcohol extracts lack the ability to accomplish this.

Step 2. Medicinal Mushroom Extracts and Noni Fruit-Seed Powder

Medicinal Mushroom Extracts

A big part of Longevity Now involves the cleansing and detoxification that comes from what I call "inner terrain modification." This is what results when we transform our tissues in a way that eliminates stagnation and restores intelligence. This modification drives all manner of decay organisms out of our bodies and removes the debris that they have left behind.

Medicinal mushrooms enhance the intelligence of the human immune system. They help it create all the weapons possible, such as the T-fighter cells, NK cells, Helper T cells, and lymphocytes. Mushrooms also help the immune system produce more weaponry that white blood cells use to conquer viruses, bad bacteria, and other harmful microorganisms.

Medicinal mushrooms are more than 80 percent genetically identical to the human body (closer than plants). What does this mean? It may mean that the mushrooms are utilized by our immune system, nervous system, cardiovascular system, heart, liver, and kidneys more efficiently than most other botanical compounds.

Medicinal mushrooms are dual-directional and work in whichever way is needed. This means that medicinal mushrooms have the ability to stimulate an immune response as well as to subdue overly reactive immune effects. Another way of saying this is that they are intelligent. They create more intelligence at the interface of our immune system's

> ### Mushroom Safety
>
> Be careful regarding the quality of mushrooms found at certain Asian markets. Also, be extremely careful about misidentifying mushrooms in the wild—do not take chances. Medicinal mushrooms mostly grow on trees as opposed to the forest floor, and nearly all tree mushrooms are safe to consume; therefore tree mushrooms are the easiest ones to identify and utilize. If you do not know exactly what you are doing, avoid picking mushrooms yourself and find an expert. To stay on the safe side, I recommend taking the easily available, pre-prepared medicinal mushroom extracts available online and in health food stores until one becomes a mushroom-picking expert.

armada and pathogens (whether those pathogens are nanobacteria, viruses, fungi, molds, yeasts, and/or parasites).

Medicinal mushrooms are some of the most healing and powerful anticandida substances in the world because they give the immune system the ability to fight back against bacteria and fungi, using the same chemical weaponry they themselves must produce in their own natural forest environment. In fact, the very first thing we recommend to someone with candida is to start taking medicinal mushrooms, especially reishi.

Quality medicinal mushrooms may come from different sources: some are grown in controlled conditions (e.g., mycelium biomass, planned log-growing environments); some are found growing on trees in the forest or are extracts therefrom. If you pick wild tree mushrooms you can leave them outside, upside down, in the sun to dry (for 24–48 hours) and they will actually develop vitamin D2 upon the under surface. It is possible to then make a tea out of dried wild tree mushrooms and get more vitamin D2 into one's diet during the cold, dark months of winter in the northern hemisphere.

The generally recommended technique for extracting medicinal compounds from tree mushrooms is to steep the mushrooms over time (preferably at least one hour) in hot (not boiling) water (ideally spring water), and then drink the tea/broth. To extract properly the water temperature should be 150–170°F (65–75°C). Whole mushrooms do not need to be cut up into little pieces or mechanically ground down. Instead, when putting the medicinal mushrooms in water, take the entire mushroom and break it up by hand (cutting with a metal knife increases oxidation, damages polysaccharides, and decreases the medicinal value). The general rule is that wild tree mushrooms (which are for the most part medicinal mushrooms) are too woody to consume and therefore should be used for tea. Chaga mushroom is a slight exception to this rule. In addition to being consumed as a tea, chaga can be ground down with a mortar and pestle and eaten directly or added in to any recipe.

With mushroom tinctures or mycelium biomass there is no preparation necessary by the consumer. Mycelium biomass comes as a powder

For Those Sensitive to Alcohol

Medicinal mushrooms may be obtained in alcohol tincture, similar to many other herbs. This is the process by which an herb's fluids are extracted into a solution of alcohol. This process maintains the vital ethers of a plant without temperature adulteration. In this way, the alcohol-soluble (often anti-viral) compounds found in the fresh-picked super-herbs are extracted, and are then able to act medicinally within the body.

If one does not wish to consume alcohol yet still wants to use alcohol tinctures, pour or dropper the desired amount of tincture into an open glass of water and let the alcohol evaporate over several hours (heating the water will rapidly speed up this process, as alcohol boils before water). What happens is that the alcohol-soluble fraction of the substance will be left behind, but the alcohol will have evaporated. This is a very good way to use tinctures without ingesting any alcohol. If you do not mind the alcohol (it is only a small amount), you can simply take the tincture under the tongue, or mix the tincture into water and drink everything together.

and may also be encapsulated. The powders can be added directly into beverages, superfood-superherb drinks, elixirs, smoothies, and food.

Let's take a look at some of the most powerful mushrooms on the planet.

Recommended Use: Medicinal mushrooms are useful in all kinds of forms: mycelium biomass powder may be added to smoothies, elixirs, sauces, and dips; wild mushrooms make great bases for teas and broths; alcohol tinctures of medicinal mushrooms may be consumed directly, in elixirs, and evaporated off (leaving the medicine behind) in hot teas; encapsulated extracts of mushrooms are easy to travel with and consume; and they are less oxidized, thus slightly more potent.

Reishi

Reishi is indeed the supreme protector, protecting us on every level—physically, immunologically, mentally, and spiritually. It helps us adapt to the world and provides additional power for us to achieve a superior level of life. When we are so protected and so provided for, we can achieve things that would otherwise be impossible. That is why Reishi has been called the Herb of Good Fortune.

—RON TEEGUARDEN, *THE ANCIENT WISDOM OF THE CHINESE TONIC HERBS*

Reishi *(Ganoderma lucidum)* has been the most revered herbal mushroom in Asia for at least two thousand years. The Taoists consider it an "elixir of immortality" that increases the spiritual heart or *shen* energy. Its reputation for causing radiant health and extreme longevity and its superior antiaging properties make it an essential addition to Longevity Now.

Reishi is celebrated for its ability to significantly improve the functioning of the immune system, regulating and fine-tuning it so that we are protected from the onslaught of viruses, bacteria, parasites, pollution, chemicals, molds, and the toxicity we are often subjected to in the current configuration of our world. Using sufficient doses of reishi to boost and modulate our immune system helps prevent pathogens from invading the body, gaining a foothold, and causing disease, aging, calcification of joints, and other chronic and acute conditions.

Reishi has been proven effective in aiding in the treatment of arthritis, and it possesses antiallergic, anti-inflammatory, antiviral, antibacterial, and antioxidant properties.

Reishi is also an excellent anti-stress and antistimulant herb. It is known in Taoism as a "shen stabilizer"—it is antianxiety and normalizes our heart energy along with our aura. Herbally, reishi counterbalances stimulants such as coffee, chocolate, yerba mate, green tea, etc. Overall, reishi is an excellent choice to aid in reducing anxiety. When we are holding stress and tension physically, emotionally, and mentally, we are compromising our immune system. Our body's ability to fight illness and calcification, as well as maintain detoxification mechanisms, is significantly weakened by stress. Reishi is known to ease tension, elevate the spirit, and promote peace of mind by transforming negative energy in the body in the same way that the mushroom transforms decayed material in the tree into life-giving nourishment.

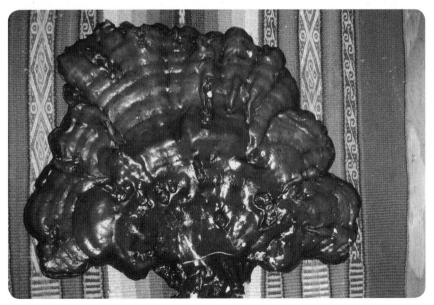

Reishi often appears bone-smooth and shiny red.

Reishi is one of the safest herbs and is nontoxic. It is the most well studied herb in the history of the world. You can take reishi continuously and it does not produce any side effects. Reishi is a powerful aspect of Longevity Now and I highly recommend it to those who are just starting on the path to create the best health ever.

Reishi mushrooms are available as dried mushrooms (either cultivated or wild); in powders, concentrated tablets, and capsules (these are usually derived from reishi mycelium grown on rice); or as a liquid tincture (preferably a dual extract of reishi tea mixed with the alcohol-soluble fraction of reishi).

Extraordinary reishi spore and reishi spore oil products are also available and recommended.

Reishi has also been known to provide the following benefits:

- acts as a neuroprotective
- improves and nourishes the immune system
- lowers high blood pressure
- alleviates anxiety
- acts as an antiviral (the alcohol-soluble fraction fights the common cold, herpes, hepatitis, HIV)
- acts as an antifungal
- fights candida
- helps prevent cancer
- protects the heart, kidneys, liver, and lungs
- fights radiation
- alleviates nausea

Cordyceps

Cordyceps *(Cordyceps sinensis)* has been one of the most highly revered longevity herbs for thousands of years in Taoist tonic herbalism and Traditional Chinese Medicine. At one time the procurement of this caterpillar-eating mushroom that thrives just underneath the glacier sheets of the Himalayas was punishable by death unless it was for the emperor and his family. It has long been celebrated as one of the most effective immune-modulating, life-enhancing herbs on this planet. Its potent antiaging, rejuvenation, jing-building properties make cordyceps a rare and highly treasured herb and an excellent addition to the Longevity Now approach.

Cordyceps, like reishi, helps the body resist a wide range of viruses, pathogens, fungi, and nanobacteria. The polysaccharides present in cordyceps help strengthen the immune system, thereby helping slow down the aging process and causing us to experience extraordinary levels of vibrant health and well-being.

Cordyceps is known for its ability to help increase stamina, energy, and endurance levels. In the 1990s, cordyceps was brought to public attention by a Chinese Olympic team whose members attributed their record-breaking runs to the use of this mushroom.

Cordyceps has also been known to provide the following benefits:

- restores energy
- relieves stress
- reverses aging
- strengthens the lungs
- improves sexual function and appetite
- improves stamina and endurance
- increases brain power and protects the brain
- accelerates healing, detoxification, and immunity
- relieves fatigue from excessive exercise and mental work
- strengthens jing energy, as well as one's adrenals, kidneys, hearing, eyesight, lower back, knees, and ankles

Note: Common powdered cordyceps products are techno-grown on rice; these products are called cordyceps mycelium and are not grown on caterpillars. These are good products, but there are better. The second tier up would be cordyceps grown on silkworms. The highest and most powerful cordyceps product is actual dried worms containing the cordyceps fungi or products made from it.

Agaricus blazei

Backed by more than twenty-five years of research studies, *Agaricus blazei* is a widely recognized medicinal mushroom from Brazil, known for its ability to significantly enhance immune system function. In addition, agaricus promotes natural responses within the body that seemingly decrease and control mutated cell creation, multiplication, and proliferation.

Agaricus contains a special class of polysaccharides called beta glucans, which are found to play an important role in preventing normal cells from turning carcinogenic by triggering the body's own natural antitumor response. *Agaricus blazei* contains more beta glucans than any other medicinal mushroom known. Agaricus also seems to effectively reduce blood sugar and control high blood pressure.

Agaricus blazei has been known to have the following benefits:

- fights and prevents certain cancers, including breast, colon, lung, and prostate
- enhances the effectiveness of alternative and mainstream cancer therapies, including chemotherapy
- activates helper-T lymphocyte cells and macrophage white blood cells
- promotes antiallergy effects without causing the drowsiness of antihistamines
- increases the number of "natural killer" or NK white blood cells, making them more powerfully effective in defending against infection
- improves liver function
- prevents diabetes-related complications
- treats hepatitis B

Ronald Reagan took this mushroom to treat his skin cancer!

Lion's Mane

Lion's mane mushroom *(Hericium erinaceus)* may have the ability to stimulate the production of a substance known as nerve growth factor, or NGF. This specialized protein is necessary for the growth of sensory neurons, and studies have shown that extracts of this mushroom promote myelin sheath growth on nerve cells. Since the myelin sheath is the component of nerve cells most closely associated with the transmission of nerve messages, research suggests that lion's mane mushroom may help to slow the progression of degenerative neurological conditions such as Parkinson's disease. In the absence of a health challenge of this nature, lion's mane may provide an additional cognitive boost to help us through times of high demand on our concentration and intellect.

In addition to the possible benefits it offers to the nervous system, lion's mane has also been used in Taoist tonic herbalism to address ailments of the digestive tract. The glyconutrients (polysaccharides) found in lion's mane, like those found in other medicinal mushrooms, have been shown to have significant immune-enhancing properties.

Lion's mane has been used to:

- regulate blood sugar and cholesterol levels
- combat underlying causes of Alzheimer's and dementia by stimulating nerve growth factor (NGF)
- alleviate pain symptoms associated with HIV-AIDS
- speed the healing of ulcers
- promote digestive health
- reduce inflammation
- boost memory and overall nervous system function
- relieve indigestion and constipation

Maitake

The medicinal mushroom maitake *(Grifola frondosa)* is best known for its ability to detoxify carcinogens, due to its high content of beta glucan polysaccharides, which have been found to promote natural cell growth and energize the cellular immune system to an astounding degree. However, the health benefits of maitake are not limited to these two traits. Maitake supports the healing of a broad spectrum of conditions including helping protect the liver as it processes chemical toxins; fighting hepatitis B; battling blood, stomach, and bone cell mutation; lowering high blood pressure and blood lipid levels (two key risk factors in cardiovascular disease); aiding digestion in the stomach and intestines; and providing nutritional support by enhancing the colon's ability to absorb micronutrients, especially copper and zinc.

Maitake has also been known to:

- support cardiovascular health by regulating blood pressure and normalizing cholesterol and blood lipids
- support the appropriate production of insulin
- stimulate the immune system
- activate macrophages, which consume mutated cells
- help block the growth of tumors
- treat leukemia, stomach, and bone cancers
- relieve side effects of chemotherapy
- aid digestion by eliminating food stagnation
- support liver health, especially as related to hepatitis
- fight bacterial and viral infections

Shiitake

Another powerful immune-supporting medicinal mushroom, shiitake *(Lentinula edodes)* contains a free-radical-fighting polysaccharide compound called lentinan, which appears to stimulate immune-system cells to specifically clear the body of tumor cells.

Shiitake mushroom has been extensively studied and proven efficient in lowering cholesterol. In addition, shiitake appears to be effective against some of the more serious viruses we face today, including HIV and hepatitis B. Not only can shiitake relieve symptoms of these conditions, but complete inactivation of these viruses has also been documented.

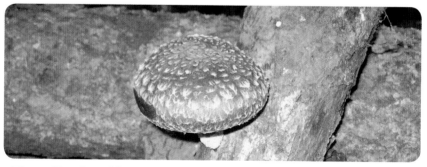

First flush of log-grown shiitake

On top of being an excellent source of iron, shiitake is known to:

- boost the immune system, including the immune system of HIV-AIDS patients
- combat HIV-infected cells more effectively than the AIDS drug AZT
- stop cell damage from herpes simplex I and II
- relieve hepatitis-B symptoms
- fight flu and other viruses
- promote the creation of reticular fibers, which fight mutated cells
- lower cholesterol
- function as an antioxidant
- fight nanobacteria in the form of gout and kidney stones
- inhibit platelet aggregation, therefore possibly preventing thrombosis
- increase survival rates for patients with gastric cancers

Chaga

The chaga mushroom *(Inonotus obliquus)* grows in birch forests of Russia, Korea, Europe, Canada, northern regions of the United States, and in the forests of the Appalachian mountains. Chaga resembles a large piece of burnt charcoal and was/is used by the primitive-skills community as a coal extender, hence it is sometimes referred to as "tinder mushroom." Chaga contains one of the highest amounts of cancer-fighting compounds of any of the medicinal mushrooms known, especially in the form of betulinic acid, which is a powerful antimutagen naturally present in the white part of the birch bark. Chaga mushroom essentially concentrates birch bark and therefore concentrates betulinic acid in large amounts.

Chaga is unique in the medicinal mushroom family because its beneficial compounds can be directly absorbed by simply eating it. Chaga does not harden into a wooden consistency as most of the other tree mushrooms do when they mature.

Chaga is extremely high in vital phytochemicals, nutrients, and free-radical-scavenging antioxidants, especially melanin. Melanin is the same compound and pigment found in human skin, the retina of

The legendary chaga mushroom

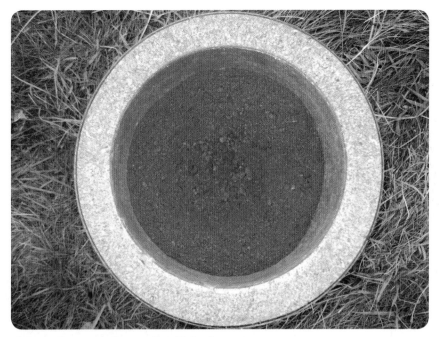

Hand-powdered wild chaga

the eye, the inner ear, the pigment-bearing neurons within the brain stem, etc. Chaga is second only to cacao in antioxidant content. Please refer to my book *Chaga: King of the Medicinal Mushrooms* for more on this fascinating superherb.

Chaga can be used to:

- enhance the immune system
- fight nearly all cancers and tumors
- fight candida
- protect cell components against free radicals (it is a powerful antioxidant)
- protect cells against DNA degradation
- increase longevity by slowing the aging process (it is a black food-herb, known to possess a high zinc content and jing nourishing qualities)

- treat chronic fatigue syndrome, flu, stomach problems, HIV, and cancer
- inhibit the cell mutations associated with cancer
- fight hepatitis and herpes (using the alcohol soluble fraction or chaga tincture)
- nourish skin, eyes, glands, and hair with its melanin compounds
- improve digestion
- treat ulcers, diabetes, gastritis, and inflammatory diseases
- provide good nutrition to connective tissue
- be a great source of vitamin D2 (wild chaga)
- deactivate radiation, perhaps more powerfully than any food-herb in the world

Trametes versicolor

Popularly (though no longer correctly) known as *Coriolus versicolor,* or turkey tail mushroom, *Trametes versicolor* is a medicinal mushroom that has been recognized for centuries as a powerful healing tool in traditional Asian medicine. It helps maintain excellent immune function, especially during times when the immune system would be otherwise compromised.

The *Trametes versicolor* mushroom has also demonstrated strong antiviral, antimicrobial, and antitumor properties, which have been attributed to a protein-bound polysaccharide called Polysaccharide K (PSK), also known as krestin. In the 1980s, the Japanese government approved the use of PSK for treating several types of cancers, and it is currently used to combat the disease alongside surgery, chemotherapy, and radiation.

Polysaccharide P (PSP), another compound from trametes, was discovered more recently, and it has been studied mainly in China. Initial research suggests that PSP may slow the growth of certain tumors and help protect the immune system, especially from the effects of cancer treatment.

Trametes versicolor can be taken in capsules, as mycelium, as an extract, or as a tea. Certain additional extracts of the herb, including VPS, are also sold.

Trametes's primary benefits include fighting and preventing certain cancers, especially liver cancer, and nourishing the immune system.

Noni Fruit and Noni Seed Powder

Noni is the common name for *Morinda citrifolia,* a tropical tree native to Polynesia, especially popular in Tahiti and Hawaii. The fruit, seeds, leaves, stems, and roots have all been used in foods and beverages by Polynesian *kahuna,* or traditional healers, for at least two thousand years. The plant produces an irregular, lumpy, egg-shaped fruit reaching a dozen or more centimeters in length. Ripe noni fruit and noni powder have a strong, pungent odor that is particularly synergistic with citrus fruits. Citrus fruits wonderfully mask the odd noni flavor, hence the noni species name: *citrifolia.*

Scientific research has identified numerous important and beneficial nutritional compounds in noni. Studies have suggested an exciting finding: that noni increases the efficacy of the immune system by feeding white blood cells. Polysaccharide compounds (6-D-glucopyranose pentaacetate) found in the fruit are generally believed to increase the overall killing power of white blood cells. Noni fruit is full of many powerful antioxidants and compounds that are believed to promote wellness, such as selenium (skin elasticity, skin health), xeronine (cell structure health and regeneration), glycosides (defense against free radicals), scopoletin (anti-inflammatory properties), terpine (helps the body detoxify), limonene (a biological solvent with citrus odors), and anthraquinones (antiseptic, pain-killing properties).

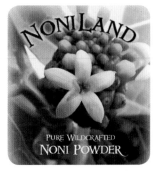

"Noni juice" is a potent antimicrobial and antifungal beverage created during the fermentation of the noni fruit and seeds, yet it is not as powerful as the fresh fruit or dried fruit powder. Noni juice is not really a juice, but a noni vinegar.

Noni fruit is a premier longevity superfood and immune system enhancer with a

NoniLand Noni powder

special concentration of Ormus elements in the polysaccharide fraction of its sugars. At least some of these Ormus elements (e.g., Ormus gold) are known to fight bad calcium. Noni seeds contain omega-3 fatty acids.

Step 3. Mangosteen, Cat's Claw, and Citric Acid

Mangosteen

Mangosteen *(Garcinia mangostana)* is used as an herbal product in the form of the alkaloid compounds in the mangosteen fruit rind. This rind contains forty antioxidant nutraceutical xanthone alkaloids, each with a different array of healing properties. Antioxidants are found in Nature and they are also produced within the body. These hydrogen-rich and electron-rich compounds are usually visible to our eye as pigments of color in plants (such as the reds and blues of berries). It is the availability of the excess electrons that allows antioxidants to deactivate free radicals. (Free radicals are molecules that are missing electrons and can cause oxidation and tissue damage, resulting in aging conditions ranging from wrinkles to cancer.)

Richly pigmented plants prove to be the easiest way to identify where high-density antioxidants can be found. Superfoods and superherbs including cacao, açaí, goji berries, spirulina, blue-green algae, mangosteen, marine phytoplankton, and chaga all have extraordinarily high pigment/antioxidant content. Consuming these types of superfoods and superherbs is recommended as part of the Longevity Now approach.

Antioxidants can be water and/or fat-soluble. All raw, pure fats and oils are antioxidants as they contain excess electrons. This means that not only are richly colored foods loaded with antioxidants, but so are all raw organic olives, avocados, nuts, seeds, and coconuts.

The three most well-studied xanthone antioxidants in mangosteen at this time are alpha-mangostin, gamma-mangostin, and garcinone E. These alkaloids assist the immune system in fighting nanobacteria as well as whatever viruses, fungi, yeasts, and infections have been lying dormant in the body. The xanthone antioxidants in the rind of the

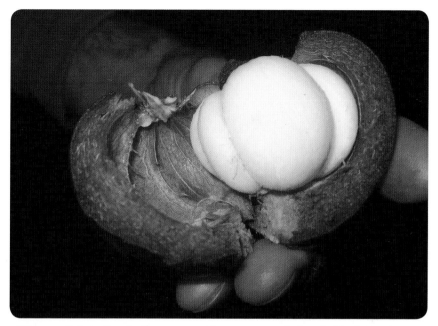

The white fruit is eaten because it's delicious. The surrounding rind is consumed because it's medicinal.

mangosteen fruit are also known to fight the organisms that cause rheumatism and arthritis better than any other known botanical substance.

Mangosteen is also a powerful anti-inflammatory. Inflammation is the response of the body to intrusions to the tissue such as a wound, infection, or toxins. It is the result of bringing focused circulation to the area so that the immune system can allow healing to occur. In cases where toxins are backed up and there is chronic inflammation, the root cause is often a deeply sequestered calcification or infection of some type. When this occurs, the body gets into a chronic state of what would normally be considered a temporary biological inflammatory response.

Overall, mangosteen has been found to:

- protect the health of the joints
- reduce inflammation

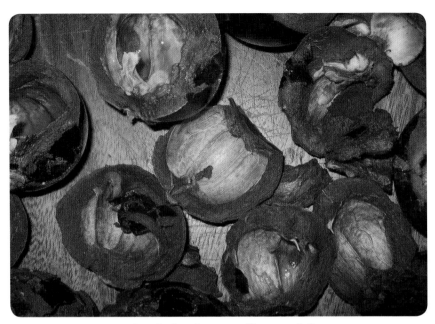

Mangosteen rinds being collected for tea

- prevent free-radical damage
- increase mental energy, focus, and attention span
- enhance the immune system
- increase longevity

Recommended Use: With fresh mangosteens, the rind can be peeled and then thrown directly into tea, or it can be dried and powdered and made into tea or added to smoothies at a later time. Concentrated mangosteen powders are also available and are best when blended into smoothies or elixirs.

Cat's Claw

Cat's claw *(Uncaria tomentosa)* grows as a vine in the Amazon. Native people strip the root bark to make herbal teas. It is among the most revered medicinal herb in all of South American herbalism. The alkaloids found in cat's claw have been documented to nutritionally support the immune system in a variety of powerful ways. Used in Longevity

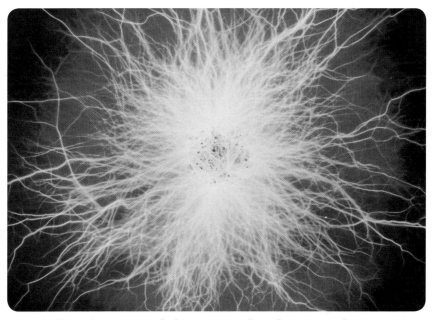

A Kirlian image of the superherb cat's claw

Now primarily for its antiviral effects, cat's claw also improves our emotional disposition due to its monoamine oxidase inhibitor (MAOI) content. This herb can be easily used in either tea or extract form.

Cat's claw has tremendous antiviral properties, in addition to being one of the most delicious and incredible-tasting Amazonian teas. A highly medicinal herb, cat's claw is now regularly used as a natural remedy for many conditions, ranging from the common cold to hepatitis to herpes to Lyme's disease.

Cat's claw appears to be effective at combatting numerous calcium conditions that may appear throughout the body, including calcification of the coronary artery (heart disease), calcification of the circulatory system (atherosclerosis), calcification of the ear (hard of hearing), and calcification of the eye (cataracts).

Recommended Use: Use in tea, extract, powder, or capsule form.

Citric Acid

Citric acid is used within Longevity Now to quickly dissolve both the harmful calcium phosphate shells and the exposed nanobacteria organisms underneath the shells. The medical history and peer-reviewed medical journals on nanobacteria have conclusively demonstrated that citric acid dissolves bad calcium and kills nanobacteria.

Citric acid is the acid we taste in citrus fruit. It was first extracted from lemons. In fact, if one does not like taking a concentrated supplement of citric acid, fresh lemon juice and white lemon pith can be substituted instead (at least one lemon a day). Both lemon and lime have extensive beneficial properties beyond simply making our drinks taste good. It has been found that these citrus fruits help increase hydration, cleanse the body, dissolve bad calcium, dissolve bad estrogens, and support longevity with their citric acid component. There is a demonstrated correlation in herbal literature between the breakdown of calcium deposits and the consumption of lemon juice. For example, citric acid has the proven benefit of helping to prevent and break up kidney stone formations.

Warning: Higher dosages of citric acid are not recommended. Citric acid does not necessarily agree with everyone, so we recommend that you test your own metabolism and see what works for you. If citric acid supplements do not work for you, please consider consuming at least one lemon or lime each day for a similar effect.

Recommended Use: Citric acid is available in tablet, capsule, and powder form. Because citric acid is so potent, it is recommended that one ingest it in small amounts (as recommended below) along with water.

Super Electrolyte Lemonade Superhero Cleanser

To easily add a balanced portion of the great substances discussed in the first two parts of the decalcification system into your daily routine while retaining metabolic balance during cleansing, try the following beverage.

- 1.5 liters spring water
- 1–2 pinches sea salt, Miracle salt, Himalayan salt, or some other super salt
- Juice of an entire lemon (with white pith blended in if possible)
- 1000–2000 mg MSM
- 1–2 tbsp of local wild honey or the best organic honey you can find*
- 5–15 drops of liquid zeolite
- 5–15 drops fulvic acid (or 1 tsp shilajit)
- 1000–2000 mg noni powder

Next thing you know, you have activated a whole piece of the Longevity Now approach, simply by drinking your daily lemon water! Stacking the different tools provided in Longevity Now will help you get more goodies into your body quickly, easily, and effectively. I encourage you to create your own recipe formulas like the Super Electrolyte Lemonade Superhero Cleanser. Come up with your own recipes, and enjoy the process of becoming younger.

*In my opinion, honeys (especially dark honeys) are superior to other sweeteners (e.g., maple syrup, molasses, etc.) due to their extraordinary enzyme and Ormus mineral content.

TIP The Super Electrolyte Lemonade Superhero Cleanser is best consumed primarily in the morning. To balance this cleanse formula and maintain alkalinity while detoxifying, I recommend drinking at least one liter of fresh vegetable juice each afternoon or evening (consisting of at least 60 to 95 percent celery and cucumber, with the other 5 to 40 percent of ingredients made up of carrots, beets, and parsley).

Part 3: Cell-Rejuvenating Supplements and Foods

It appears from my review of the research evidence relating to nano-bacteria (the catch-all term for calcium-forming microorganisms) that the process of bad calcium formation in the body concentrates and incorporates into itself all kinds of toxic materials (e.g., mercury, pesticides, plastics, etc.) from the internal environment of the human body. Theoretically, it is possible that these calcium-forming microorganisms use these toxic substances as part of their protective biofilm, which then solidifies into calcium phosphate armor (calcification). Basically, the idea is that calcification is laden with built-in toxic debris as shielding.

As our bodies start breaking toxic, bad calcium down, the heavy metals, pesticides, etc., can be excreted, and the toxins are all of a sudden back out again, coursing through our blood. This is one of the reasons we have to be very careful with cleansing.

Because we have brought in substances that break down the bad calcium, and due to the biological impact of using the tools in Parts 1 and 2, we need to have a great "clean-up crew" to come in next and support the immune system and detoxification mechanisms, making sure that we clean out all the toxins being released.

The tools provided in this third part of the decalcification section are designed to ensure that you do not retoxify yourself by releasing toxic substances back into your system. This portion is about cleaning up the debris left over on the "battlefield." We use cell-rejuvenating supplements to help our healthy tissues and immune system take out all the toxins and waste products that have been stirred up during Parts 1 and 2, as well as through lifestyle changes. This third part is focused primarily on modifying our inner terrain by taking enzymes, adaptogens, probiotics, vitamin C botanicals, microalgae/animal superfoods, as well as other cell-rejuvenating supplements and foods. This is how we empower our biology with the best of the best. Cell-rejuvenating supplements assist our bodies in eating up all the garbage and making everything inside of us brand-new.

⬛ Step 1: Enzymes and Adaptogen Herbs

Enzymes

> Enzymes are substances that make life possible. They are needed
> for every chemical reaction that takes place in the human body.
> No mineral, vitamin, or hormone can do any work without
> enzymes. Our bodies, all our organs, tissues, and cells are run by
> metabolic enzymes. Enzymes have many important functions in
> the body.
>
> —Dr. Edward Howell, *Enzyme Nutrition* and *Food Enzymes*
> *for Health and Longevity*

The discovery of enzymes is one of the greatest breakthroughs ever achieved in nutrition. Enzymes are the foundation of extraordinary health—catalysts and transformative elements of positive change that scrub and cleanse organs and the circulatory system by helping cells assimilate nutrients. By transforming amino acids, fats, starches, and minerals into a form that our bodies can use, enzymes aid healthy weight loss, accelerate detoxification and cleansing, rejuvenate aged skin and internal organs, and greatly assist the digestive process.

For the most part (not always), enzymes are destroyed by the cooking process. They can only be found in raw foods (or foods and herbs that have been dehydrated at low temperatures), enzyme supplements, and living cells. Enzymes that come from raw plant foods are particularly beneficial for human health because plant enzymes provide the most action throughout various pH (acid/alkaline) conditions in the body. In other words, the enzymes remain potent and effective catalysts despite the body's chemistry. Typically, plant enzymes are recommended. However, enzymes from animal sources such as pancreatin and chymotrypsin are also important enzymes recommended against pancreatic cancer.

Enzymes are especially known for their ability to reduce what is called C-reactive protein, a marker of inflammation. When blood work shows a high level of C-reactive protein, it means that there is a bad-calcium problem somewhere in the body. If the inflammation continues to increase—month after month—you know that a time bomb is ticking; and underneath the inflammation, the bad-calcium-forming action is starting to significantly hinder normal metabolism. Because calcification precedes inflammation, both are often found together in the cardiovascular system, in the joints, in the lymphatic system, the liver, the kidneys—anywhere in the body. By consuming enzymes we can get our C-reactive protein levels down, reduce inflammation, and get at the calcification.

In addition, enzymes facilitate the breakdown of scar tissue. Calcium-forming microorganisms (nanobacteria) are suspected of having an affinity for growing and reproducing where we have been injured (scarred).

There are two different categories of enzymes: digestive enzymes and metabolic enzymes. **Digestive enzymes** are the essential enzymes that primarily help us digest food and overcome digestive lethargy. Digestive enzymes are present in raw, living foods, herbs, and superfoods. Digestive enzymes can also act metabolically when taken between meals (see below). **Metabolic enzymes** help with our daily bodily functions, and thus their benefits are limitless. When we move our body, when we breathe, when we walk and do all the different things we do in a day, even if we are just sitting, we are using enzymes. Metabolic enzymes support the liver in its clean-up function; they support the movement of our muscles, our thinking, breathing, cellular reproduction, the cleansing of the cardiovascular system, and the purification of the nervous system. Taking significant doses of metabolic enzymes can increase the speed of healing by a factor of two or three. Metabolic enzymes function specifically to help break down excess waste and allow the body to excrete it naturally through the bowels, kidneys, urine, skin, sweat, and through the lungs when we breathe out toxins.

Digestive and metabolic enzymes both have a tremendous history of research and benefit that are worthy of your investigation. I recommend reading *Food Enzymes for Health and Longevity,* by Dr. Edward Howell.

Recommended Use: Enzyme supplements are usually sold as encapsulated powders and tablets. They travel well and can be a lifesaver at social dinners. Look for digestive enzymes with some or all of the following ingredients:

- alpha galactosidase
- amylase
- beta glucanase
- bromelain
- cellulase
- glucoamylase
- hemicellulase
- invertase
- lactase
- lipase (I, II, and/or III)
- maltase
- papain
- pectinase
- protease (I, II, III, and/or IV)
- xylanase

Adaptogen Herbs

Traditionally, adaptogen herbs are considered to be rejuvenative, tonic, and restorative. In present-day scientific literature, they are considered to counteract the impact of stress upon the body caused by physical exertion, chemical or pathogenic exposure, emotional trauma, and electromagnetic stress. They have been shown to improve the physical health of different organ systems by as much as 10–15 percent.

The following recommendations are based on traditional Chinese and Ayurvedic medicinal wisdom that is thousands of years old. I include the top adaptogenic herbs on the planet because of their time-proven ability to remove the causes of aging and to create incredible, abundant health.

Angelica Root *(Dong Quai)*

Commonly known as a primary yin jing "female" herb in Chinese medicine, angelica root *(Angelica sinensis)* carries analgesic, anti-inflammatory, antispasmodic, aphrodisiac, blood tonifying, and sedative effects. As a hormone regulator, angelica root is a valuable botanical for keeping the immune system operating optimally and providing the body with the energy it needs to carry out detoxification. *Dong quai* inhibits estradiol synthesis (lowers age-related bad estrogen). It is also known to inhibit ER+ (estrogen receptor positive) breast cancer cells in vitro.

Angelica root is known to:

- prevent the growth of various bacteria
- fight colds, bronchitis, and respiratory infections
- improve anemia
- aid circulation and digestion
- treat rheumatism and arthritis
- treat sore throat and mouth when used to gargle
- prevent acne (when used as a face wash)
- treat fungal conditions (candida, etc.)
- weaken symptoms of PMS by dilating blood vessels and relaxing uterine muscles (angelica root is a popular Chinese remedy for PMS)
- regulate the menstrual cycle
- treat symptoms of menopause
- relieve allergies by boosting the immune system

Warning: Angelica root is fairly toxic when fresh; it must be dried thoroughly before use. When using angelica root, you may be more susceptible to sunburn. Angelica root should not be used by people with diabetes, nor should it be used in large doses by pregnant or breastfeeding women.

Ashwagandha

Ashwagandha root *(Withania somnifera)* is a powerful immune tonic with a strong tradition of use in Northern Africa, India, Pakistan, and other parts of Asia. It acts partly as a mild sedative, relieving the body of stress, and boosts the immune system to operate at optimum active levels. Depending on the part of the plant used (root, leaves, seeds), ashwagandha contains antibacterial, antimicrobial, and adaptogenic properties.

Ashwagandha root contains nerve growth factors and is known to:

- repel insects
- regulate the body's ability to withstand stress

- increase the body's general performance
- increase stamina and relieve fatigue
- boost the immune system
- speed recovery from chronic illness
- soothe and calm without producing drowsiness
- improve memory
- slow the aging process
- be an effective treatment for anemia, arthritis, asthma, bronchitis, cancer, chronic fatigue syndrome, common colds, and many other ailments

Recommended Use: Ashwagandha is available in pills, capsules, powders, tinctures, and just about every form that an herb can be in. I prefer ashwagandha powder mixed in cacao elixirs.

Asparagus Root

Asparagus root *(Asparagus officinalis)* has long been one of the most highly prized tonic herbs in China and Korea. It has been used for thousands of years in the Chinese medicinal system to support and uplift both the spirit and physical body.

Asparagus root is considered an important lung tonic. It moistens and purifies the lungs, assists our breathing, and dispels toxins from the respiratory tract. When taking asparagus root all respiratory functions tend to continuously improve. Asparagus root is particularly useful for those living in cities where they are exposed to environmental pollution, smoke, and smog.

Because of its excellent ability to aid in lung function, asparagus root has tremendous benefits for the skin. This is because beautiful skin results from healthy lungs and pure blood. By consuming asparagus root regularly, we will achieve the radiant health we desire, as exemplified by our smooth, soft, and supple skin.

Asparagus root is known to:

- increase vitality
- beautify the skin
- build the immune system

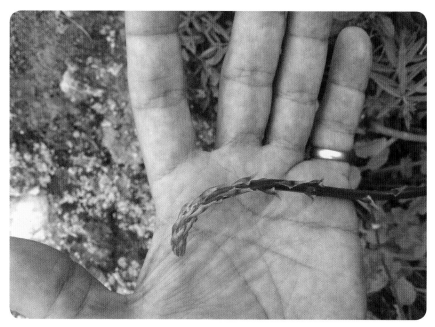

An asparagus shoot. The roots of this common plant are medicinal.

- calm the mind
- enhance sexual function
- enhance yin chi
- improve homeostasis
- act as an overall restorative

Good-quality asparagus root is mildly sweet, chewy, and soft. Most wild asparagus root is yellow in color. The red variety of wild asparagus root is rare and considered a treasure, dubbed "the flying herb" by Taoists. If you ever have the good fortune to come across best-ever-quality wild red asparagus root, get as much as you can!

Recommended Use: You can simply chew raw wild asparagus root, allowing it to melt in your mouth. It offers a well-rounded, metabolically balancing flavor and may even be considered delicious! You can also make a tea out of it along with your favorite tonic herbs.

Astragalus

Astragalus *(Astragalus propinquus or Astragalus membranaceus)* is an adaptogenic root, time-proven by Taoist tonic herbalism as an immune enhancer, mild stimulant, tonic, and antiviral. Astragalus has a strong action upon the marrow and lymph, stimulating the production and maturation of stem cells into active immune cells, while also raising the level of production of the hormones that signal for virus destruction. Astragalus makes a great addition to teas and can be consumed as a broth to strengthen and improve digestion.

Astragalus's primary medicinal components have been identified as 24 astragaloside saponins. Of these, a fraction of astragaloside IV is used to make the anti-aging, telomere enzyme activating product known as TA65. Astragaloside IV is also utilized in Dragon Herbs' longevity-enhancing product Superpill 2.

Recommended Use: Astragalus is available in pills, capsules, powders, tinctures, tea-cut, and just about every form that an herb can be in. My favorite ways of consuming astragalus include: tea-cut version made into tea; concentrated, encapsulated material either by itself or mixed with other superherbs (which travels well); tincture form (which also travels well).

Brahmi (Bacopa)

Brahmi *(Bacopa monniera)* is an Ayurvedic adaptogenic herb rich in antioxidants that has gained popularity as a brain tonic that helps to promote memory and mental alertness. It is unique in that it is able to increase intellectual and cognitive functioning without over-stimulating the body. In fact, brahmi has been found to have a calming and stress-relieving effect, which makes it an ideal tonic herb to use when under pressure or within unnatural environments.

Brahmi helps the body maintain a balanced state, especially while cleansing, detoxifying, and experiencing physical, mental, and emotional upheavals or transformation. In addition to its antiasthmatic, anti-inflammatory, and calming properties, brahmi is known to:

- assist in controlling neurosis
- help prevent cancer
- improve memory recall and learning ability
- lower anxiety and tension
- provide healing nutrition for those with head/brain injury

Recommended Use: Brahmi is available in pills, capsules, powders, tinctures, and just about every form that an herb can take. Brahmi powder is very intense and nearly impossible to make taste good. The encapsulated forms seem to be the only way to deal with any high-quality brahmi product.

Deer Antler Velvet *(Cervus nippon)*

In the springtime each year, male deer regrow their antlers in a very swift explosion of energy that lasts ninety days. During that growth spurt the young male deer antler velvet grows from a soft spongy material into hard antlers. During the young spongy stage, wild male deer may be herded and have their young velvet antlers removed (in a way that avoids permanently harming the animal; they regrow their antlers, are not killed, do not kill each other, and the process is sustainable). The removed antler material is then extracted and used herbally to improve kidney, bone, marrow, and liver strength, and to amplify hormone levels in humans.

Deer antler has been used for thousands of years in the Taoist tonic herbal system as a primary jing herb. Today New Zealand leads the world in antler removal specifications and quality. Only the white deer antler tips contain the stem cells, so purchase deer antler products that exclusively use the tips. You can determine this by the color of any deer antler tincture product. If the tincture is white, then it is made from tips; if it is pink or red, then it contains blood and is inferior in quality.

Deer antler velvet contains at least twenty-four growth factors including IGF-1 (insulin-like growth factor). It is a glycine-rich, complete-protein source that also contains twenty amino acids. Deer antler is known to:

- increase yang jing energy and tonify yin jing, chi, blood, and shen*
- increase longevity
- improve immunity
- fight inflammation
- increase strength, endurance, and lean muscle mass
- improve sexual appetite and performance
- improve reflexes and endurance
- strengthen the skeleton
- improve mental acuity
- strengthen the nervous system
- improve the health of the heart and cardiovascular system

Deer antler is Nature's natural answer to athletic steroids. Because of its powerful androgenic effect, it is banned in some sports.

Deer antler possesses numerous nutrients that support the joints. One interesting nutrient is chondroitin sulfate A; another is hyaluronic acid, a natural substance produced in the human body that maintains juicy elasticity of the skin, joints, and connective tissue. Deer antler is rich in mucopolysaccharides, pantocrine, and ectosaponin, which all promote the regeneration of tissue.

Who should take deer antler products? They are recommended for individuals looking to protect their joints, energize their body, increase will power, improve feelings of well-being, grow younger, and stimulate the immune system. Deer antler may be used by both men and women and possesses aphrodisiac qualities. In addition, deer antler has historically been recommended in Asia for slow-growing preteen and teenage children.

Internet and book research indicates that deer antler contains the following unique compounds:

- beneficial collagen (types I, II, III, IV, VI, X)
- choline (for neurotransmitter support and liver detoxification)
- chondrocytes (cells that build cartilage)

*In Chinese medicinal traditions, deer antler is said to fortify the yang jing essence (the kidney/adrenal/reproductive meridians).

- chondroitin sulfate (known to protect the joints and fight arthritis)
- glucosamine (a nutrient that supports healthy cartilage while protecting the joints and fighting arthritis)
- interleukins (types 1, 2, 6, 12)
- linolenic acid (omega-3 fatty acids)
- minerals: good calcium, copper, iron, magnesium, manganese, phosphorus, potassium, selenium, sodium, sulfur, zinc
- phospholipids (assist with the uptake of omega-3 fatty acids)
- polysaccharides (these long-chain, often high-molecular weight sugars are known to carry Ormus minerals)
- prostaglandins (potentially anti-inflammatory lipid compounds)
- protein (deer antler is a complete protein source and contains twenty amino acids)
- the following growth factors:

    bone morphogenetic proteins (BMPs)

    insulin-like growth factors I and II (IGF-I and IGF-II)

    epidermal growth factor (EGF)

    fibroblast growth factor (FGF)

    nerve growth factors (NGF), which stimulate nerve regrowth, and which are also found in ashwagandha, lion's mane, and chaga mushrooms

    transforming growth factors alpha (TGF-A) and beta (TGF-B)

Recommended Use: Select cruelty-free deer antler products from reputable sources. Deer antler is most effective when taken in an alcohol extract (tincture) sublingually. Tonifying herbs, such as the goji berry or *ho shou wu* (fo-ti), are often added to the deer antler velvet in order to balance its effects. Yin jing herbs such as morinda root are also used to balance the intense yang energy of the deer antler. Using a natural aromatase inhibitor (such as: olive oil, olive leaf extract, resveratrol-rich wine, xanthohumol (Hops X Factor), passionflower alcohol tincture, or nettle root alcohol tincture) is also a good idea when one is using deer antler products. This is particularly recommended for individuals over forty, in order to preserve the build-up of progesterone and testosterone without them becoming bad estrogens. Essentially, these superfoods, foods, herbs, and supplements are an important herbal adjunct to assisting the hormone-building power of deer antler products.

Eucommia Bark

Eucommia bark *(Eucommia ulmoides)* is the last surviving member of temperate-climate rubber trees that once dominated the northern hemisphere. Eucommia adds elasticity to collagen, tissues, muscles, and skin. It is a premier jing-restoring herb. Jing herbs such as eucommia, cordyceps, and *ho shou wu* strengthen our adrenal/kidney/reproductive/hearing/lower back/knee energies. Eucommia is especially good for alleviating back pain. Its overall effect is to help keep us flexible and limber as we age, by keeping calcification out of our bodies.

Eucommia is the number-one recommended herb for pregnancy. In addition, it is known to:

- improve joint health and relieve joint pain
- treat lower back pain
- increase ligament flexibility
- improve reproductive health and sexual function
- help heal tissues that are normally slow to mend, especially due to stress or aging
- reduce inflammation
- nourish the liver and kidneys
- enhance immune function

Studies show that eucommia bark is an effective treatment against hypertension and its related stress disorders.

Taoist herbalist Ron Teeguarden mentions Chinese research indicating that eucommia in combination with epimedium (horny goat weed) may have telomerase-activation properties.

Recommended Use: The collagen-creating compound found in eucommia bark is largely destroyed during the drying process. For this reason, alcohol tinctures made from the fresh bark of eucommia work best.

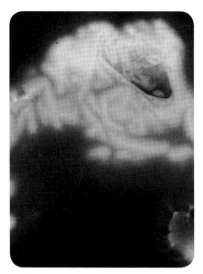

The astonishing Kirlian field of ginseng

Ginseng

Ginseng *(Panax ginseng)* is the king of herbs, considered one of the most powerful adaptogens, with a long and prominent history in Chinese Taoist tonic herbalism dating back some six thousand years. Ginseng contains saponins, which are phytochemicals that have been found to specifically stimulate the immune system and thereby aid the body in protecting against disease.

Generally, Asian ginsengs are heating and American ginsengs are cooling. Taoist tonic herbalists recommend using ginseng roots that are a minimum of seven years old, so that the plant gains its tonic, dual-directional activity. Ginseng is gonadotropic, meaning that it signals the body to produce more androgen hormones. However, I recommend consuming ginseng that is at least thirteen years old, because somewhere between twelve and thirteen years of age ginseng activates a gene or a set of genes that essentially allow it to live indefinitely. Nobody knows how long a ginseng may live. Ginsengs have been picked that have been dated at more than two hundred years old, and rumors of ginseng finds range to much older ages.

Ginseng is known to:

- improve concentration
- increase alertness (though unlike caffeine, ginseng does not provoke overstimulation or disrupt sleep)
- improve physical energy
- regulate blood sugar levels
- help balance hormone levels in both men and women
- increase stamina

- speed up recovery time from surgery, illness, exercise, and other activities that might cause stress in the body
- lower pain in cancer patients and protect against radiation/chemotherapy treatments

Recommended Use: Do the research and select reputable brands or sources when it comes to ginseng. Most of the ginseng on the market is younger than four years and possesses unbalanced stimulating properties. Remember one principle beyond reputable brand or source: the older the ginseng, the better.

Gynostemma

Gynostemma *(Gynostemma pentaphyllum)* is a major adaptogenic herb that is considered in Asia to be one of the top anti-aging longevity herbs. Many Chinese octogenarians drink gynostemma tea daily. It is used as a virtual "cure-all" because it has so many benefits. Even though it is an entirely different plant, gynostemma is considered the "female" counterpart to the "male" ginseng because they share many characteristics. Gynostemma is often referred to as "southern ginseng."

Gynostemma contains amino acids, vitamins, and important major and trace minerals, including selenium, magnesium, zinc, calcium, iron, potassium, manganese, and phosphorus, making it an excellent source of nutrients for the body.

According to Ron Teeguarden's book *The Ancient Wisdom of the Chinese Tonic Herbs:* "Gynostemma acts as a scavenger in the stomach and intestines, ridding the body of toxins, microbes, and waste that otherwise may become lodged in the intestines."

Gynostemma strengthens the immune system and has been reported in both China and Japan to be clinically effective in the treatment of a wide range of health problems, including coronary heart disease, arthritis, rheumatism, high blood pressure, and dozens more conditions. In China, gynostemma is also used to treat acute and chronic inflammation.

Gynostemma is likely the richest herbal source of healing, immune-system-stimulating saponins. Gynostemma contains over 100 different medicinal saponins called gypenosides. Of these, gypenoside 49 is believed to have longevity-enhancing, telomere-protective properties. Dragon Herbs' anti-aging product Superpill 2 contains a concentrate of gynostemma saponins amongst other herbal compounds.

For those who seek quick results, I highly recommend drinking gynostemma tea daily. It tastes delicious and has so many extraordinary health benefits for your body, including the following:

- slows down the aging process
- reduces fatigue and increases vigor
- improves digestion
- calms the nerves
- eases pain
- de-stresses the body and brings it into balance
- increases longevity

Recommended Use: Gynostemma exists in powder, tincture, and in encapsulated forms, yet is most pleasant and desirable as a tea.

Ho Shou Wu

Ho shou wu (Polygonum multiflorum) is one of the most important adaptogenic root herbs in Chinese Taoist tonic herbalism. Its extraordinary ability to strengthen the kidneys and adrenals, as well as to modulate the hormonal system, results in its classification as a "jing tonic"—a substance that boosts sexual energy, fertility, mental clarity, and the development of tissues and fluids like hair, tendons, and blood. Most of all, *ho shou wu* is considered to be the number-one antiaging Taoist tonic superherb. It is also known as *"he shou wu"* and has been misnamed "fo-ti" (but is so well known by that name that it stuck). The herb is known to:

- relieve itching, eczema, and dry skin
- reduce symptoms of alopecia—*shou-wu* means "head full of black hair" in Chinese
- slow the degradation of glands
- reduce the accumulation of lipid peroxidation
- reduce the risk of cancer
- improve cardiovascular health by reducing cholesterol
- enhance immune function

- cleanse the liver and kidneys
- protect and maintain blood vessel health
- protect against free-radical damage from ultraviolet light
- feed the bone marrow
- improve and build yin jing longevity energies

Recommended Use: To prepare *ho shou wu*, the fresh material is cooked in water with black beans. This is to tonify (take the edge off) the strong laxative effect of the raw material. Prepared *ho shou wu* is one of the world's great superherbs and is available in pills, capsules, powders, tinctures, tea-cut, and just about every form that an herb can be in. My favorite ways of consuming *ho shou wu* include: tea-cut version made into tea; concentrated, encapsulated material either by itself or mixed with other superherbs (which travels well); tincture form (which also travels well); and especially the FITT (Fingerprint Identical Transfer Technology) extract powder put out by Dragon Herbs.

Rhodiola

Rhodiola varieties *(Rhodiola rosea, Rhodiola sacra)* are adaptogenic herbs that survive in the harshest and most unforgiving climates of the high-altitude regions of Asia, Europe, and other parts of the northern hemisphere. They are widely used to help the body defend against the debilitating effects of stress, which suppresses our immunity and ability to cope with the various forms of bacteria and viruses that we encounter every day.

Rhodiola is known to:

- improve nervous system function
- enhance cognitive function, memory, and mental productivity
- increase endurance, strength, stamina, and resistance to stress
- aid in the oxygenation and blood supply to the body's cells (excellent for high-altitude environments)
- treat nervous-system conditions, altitude sickness, headaches, anemia, gastrointestinal problems, infections, colds/flus, depression, and chronic fatigue
- catalyze the breakdown of stored fat

🍃 increase endorphin levels of the brain by helping it to retain quantities of "feel good" neurotransmitters such as serotonin and norepinephrine

Recommended Use: Rhodiola is available in pills, capsules, powders, tinctures, tea-cut, and just about every form that an herb can be in. My favorite ways of consuming rhodiola include: tea-cut, made into tea; concentrated, encapsulated material, either by itself or mixed with other superherbs (which travels well); tincture form (which also travels well).

Schizandra Fruit

Schizandra *(Schisandra chinensis)* has been used for thousands of years in Chinese medicine as a major tonic herb. It is one of the most popular herbs in Asia because of its ability to prolong life, increase youth and vitality, and enhance beauty. In fact, the schizandra fruit is depicted in art as a symbol of longevity and represents the ability to attain immortality.

Its Chinese name is *wu wei zi,* which means "the five-flavor fruit." Schizandra has an unusually sour, sweet, bitter, warm, and salty taste, hence the name. The herb is considered balanced by virtue of this distribution of flavors.

Schizandra is renowned as a beauty tonic and youth-preserving herb. It has been used for centuries to make the skin soft, supple, and radiant. Its number-one attribute is its ability to cleanse and purify the liver.

Schizandra is known to:

🍃 purify the blood
🍃 improve memory function
🍃 rejuvenate the kidneys
🍃 increase sexual function
🍃 protect the skin from sun damage
🍃 sharpen concentration and alertness
🍃 cleanse the liver and treat hepatitis
🍃 remove toxicity from the body

Recommended Use: Schizandra is one of the world's great superherbs and is available in pills, capsules, powders, tinctures, a whole dried state, and just about every form that an herb can be in. My favorite ways of consuming schizandra include: a few whole dried schizandra berries made into tea with other herbs; concentrated, encapsulated material, either by itself or mixed with other superherbs (which travels well); tincture form with goji berries; and especially the FITT (Fingerprint Identical Transfer Technology) extract powder put out by Dragon Herbs.

Tulsi (Holy Basil)

> If you don't have a tulsi plant in the front of your home, you don't have a home.
>
> —ANCIENT VEDIC PHRASE

Revered as the most sacred herb in India for more than five thousand years, tulsi *(Ocimum tenuiflorum)* is traditionally used as an Ayurvedic adaptogenic supertonic to protect the brain, nervous, and respiratory systems. Tulsi is an especially excellent herb to use during a cleanse.

All basils are very active medicinally, and tulsi is no exception. It is rich in free-radical-fighting antioxidants and restorative phytochemical compounds. Tulsi is known to:

- boost immunity
- reduce stress
- relieve inflammation
- balance cholesterol
- improve stamina
- promote a healthy metabolism
- eliminate toxins
- protect against radiation
- purify the body of wastes and excess phlegm
- reduce fevers
- support a healthy liver
- prevent gastric ulcers
- support the heart
- enhance the nervous system
- regulate blood pressure
- control blood sugar levels

- aid in the elimination of colds
- aid in the elimination of lung and sinus infections
- calm stomach and digestive upset

Recommended Use: Tulsi is one of the world's great superherbs and is available in pills, capsules, powders, tinctures, dried leaves, and just about every form that an herb can be in. My favorite ways of consuming include: dried leaves made into tea; fresh off the plant; and the freshening encapsulated supercritical (carbon dioxide) extract.

Advice on Buying Herbs

When choosing and purchasing herbs, I recommend keeping the following five critical points in mind.

- Use certified organic or ethically wildcrafted herbs.
- Look for low-temperature drying. This is critical. We want to keep the enzymes in our herbs intact. We do not want to overheat or boil the substances to the point where the life force is destroyed.
- Herbs should be as freshly processed as possible. There are volatile elements in all foods; over a period of time foods, even dried herbs, do break down.
- Listen to your body. Some herbs will agree with you more than others. Tune into what is going on in your body and you will find the right adaptogen formula for you.
- Pick two or three herbs that work in combination with each other. The basic idea of herbalism is that you have the primary herb, the secondary supporting herb, and then the third herb that helps with the synergy and brings it all together. Three herbs working together form a specific adaptogen result. On top of this, other herbs may be added, but it is always important to have a strong base.

Step 2. Probiotics and Vitamin C Plant Powders

Probiotics

According to the World Health Organization and the Food and Agriculture Organization of the United Nations, probiotics can be defined as "live microorganisms, which, when administered in adequate amounts, confer a health benefit on the host." Microorganisms are tiny living organisms such as bacteria, viruses, and yeasts that can be seen only under a microscope. Probiotics are "friendly microorganisms."

Most often, the friendly bacteria primarily (though not exclusively) come from two groups, Lactobacillus and Bifidobacterium. Within each group there are different species (for example, *Lactobacillus acidophilus* and *Bifidobacterium bifidus*), and within each species there are different strains or varieties. A few common probiotics such as *Saccharomyces boulardii* are yeasts, which are different from bacteria.

A healthy adult can have more than four hundred species of good bacteria in the digestive tract. In total, the microorganisms may collectively weigh anywhere from two to four kilograms. Because bacteria may be a hundred or more times smaller than human cells, the total number of bacteria in the digestive tract may greatly exceed the number of all the cells in the human body.

Probiotics modify our internal terrain and create a healthy digestive environment. We cannot live without them. These friendly microorganisms help us digest food in both the small and large intestines. They secrete compounds that normalize and heal the digestive environment, along with compounds that are absorbed into our blood, providing us with vitamins B, C, K, and E, as well as amino acids, butyric acid, and dozens of other healthy substances. Probiotics play a critical role in our immunity as they directly drive out pathogenic organisms and secrete substances that are used by the immune system.

Different probiotics have different effects. Probiotic organisms include:

- *B. bifidum* (effective in normalizing the intestinal pH while driving out fungus and mold)
- *B. breve* (improves immune response)
- *Bifidobacterium infantis* (the first probiotic we receive from our mother; lives mostly in the lower intestinal tract)
- *B. longum* (prevents cancer; stimulates immune system; effective in normalizing the intestinal pH while driving out fungus and mold)
- *Enterococcus faecialis* (knowledge on the benefits of this bacteria was pioneered by Dr. Ohhira; this bacteria is found in the products bearing his name)
- *Lactobacillus acidophilus* (the natural enemy of candida; lives mostly in the upper gastrointestinal tract)
- *L. brevis* (improves the immune system)
- *L. bulgaricus* (fights herpes)
- *L. casei* (many strains are anti-inflammatory)
- *L. helveticus*
- *L. plantarum* (anti-inflammatory probiotic that assists *L. salivarius*)
- *L. salivarius* (eats away at intestinal plaque and mucus)
- *Streptococcus thermophilus* or *Lactococcus thermophilus* (improves immune response)

Probiotics have been found to:

- prevent growth of harmful bacteria, yeast, and fungi
- maintain the chemical and hormonal balance within the body
- produce and regulate vitamins (especially B vitamins, including vitamin B12)
- assist the digestive system
- aid the proper function of the immune system and correct nutritional deficiencies
- lower calcification levels and severity of calcium-related illnesses
- decrease body odor (because probiotic bacteria digest putrefaction—a friend of mine feeds probiotics to her dogs, and as a result they have no body or breath odor)

Recommended Use: Probiotics are available in foods and dietary supplements that come in the form of capsules, tablets, and powders. Examples of foods containing probiotics are kombucha, sauerkraut, coconut kefir, and other fermented foods. These food sources and supplements can be purchased in any health-food store and online.

The Causes of Dysbiosis

Many people who are suffering from poor health have a disturbance in their inner probiotic "garden." A **dysbiosis** is a disturbance in the natural balance of friendly bacteria as compared to unfriendly bacteria. The following circumstances can disturb our internal probiotic environment, creating a dysbiosis:

- excessive antibiotic use
- consumption of factory-farmed meat and dairy products (indirect antibiotics use)
- high-stress environments
- high-sugar diets and excessive carbohydrate intake
- heavy-metal toxicity
- chronically disturbed lifestyle patterns (e.g., excessive traveling, lack of sleep, inability to find a quiet toilet, etc.)
- exposure to radioactivity (depleted uranium) and X-rays
- "unwanted guest" exposure (too many parasites)
- artificial-chemical exposure
- hormone replacement therapy and oral contraceptives

A dysbiosis occurs when natural friendly bacteria are unable to proliferate due to heavy antibiotic or garlic use, or because unfriendly bacteria, yeast, mold, viruses, calcium-forming organisms, and/or other parasites have gained the upper hand in one's digestive tract. Supplementing the diet with friendly bacteria (probiotics) helps heal dysbiosis. Even if we do not suffer from digestive disturbances, an understanding of the overall importance of probiotics is a key ingredient in our recipe for vibrant health and longevity.

Probiotics can be taken in capsule form, or one can use capsules or other probiotic "starters" to culture one's own foods and beverages in order to flood the body with friendly bacteria. Culturing is an entire art in itself; for more information on culturing, please read Sandor Katz's book *Wild Fermentation* and Donna Gates's *Body Ecology Diet.* Getting probiotics into the lower gastrointestinal tract may require larger dosages and/or enteric-coated probiotic capsules that survive the stomach and upper gastrointestinal environment to implant in the lower regions.

Vitamin C–Containing Plant Powders

It is known that ascorbic acid is required for the synthesis of connective tissue. This fact provides an explanation for the reported value of large quantities in the treatment of rheumatoid arthritis and other connective-tissue diseases.

—LINUS PAULING, *VITAMIN C AND THE COMMON COLD* (1970)

There is no doubt that ascorbic acid [vitamin C] is required for the synthesis of collagen in the bodies of human beings and other animals. One of the important functions of collagen is its service in strengthening the intercellular cement that holds the cells of the body together in various tissues. It is not unlikely that part of the effectiveness of vitamin C against the common cold, influenza, and other viral diseases can be attributed to this strengthening effect, and in this way preventing or hindering the motion of the virus particles through the tissues and into the cells.

—LINUS PAULING, *VITAMIN C, THE COMMON COLD, AND THE FLU* (1971)

The vitamin C complex has a tremendous research history to suggest that it is effective in supporting the immune system, healing connective tissue, and building collagen, as well as detoxifying the liver, brain, and kidneys.

The best kind of vitamin C is found naturally in plants. Whole-food vitamin C sources include camu camu, kakadu plum, acerola, amla, and rosehips. (Below I detail camu camu berries, but I could detail out each of these berries, or even write a short book on berries.) Dry these at low temperatures to make powders that can easily be added to your smoothies, water, and food.

Vitamin C helps to rejuvenate and repair tissue quickly. If you are injured or have had a surgery, taking large quantities of vitamin C–containing plant powders can help speed up the healing process. Vitamin C is also critical in improving the effectiveness of both MSM and medicinal mushrooms. If one is taking sulfur (MSM) and medicinal mushrooms, taking vitamin C plant powders on top of that can actually triple the effectiveness of these substances.

Vitamin C plant powders come in vegetarian capsules as well as powder form. The powder can be added to anything, or even taken straight—just put it on the tongue! Vitamin C has a slightly tangy yet great taste and flavor. It can even be added to desserts! One can encapsulate these powders or purchase them pre-encapsulated. However you choose to take it, vitamin C is a super-critical part of Longevity Now.

Camu Camu

Consider the words of Dr. James Duke, USDA scientist and author of *The Green Pharmacy*: "I take vitamin C for colds . . . I prefer to get mine from camu camu, the amazing Amazonian fruit that has the world's highest vitamin C content."

Camu camu *(Myrciaria dubia)* is a native bush of the South American rainforest that produces a fruit containing more vitamin C than any other known botanical source. For comparison: a fresh camu camu berry may contain up to 4 percent vitamin C, whereas a lemon may contain up to 0.5 percent vitamin C. Some researchers estimate that camu camu berries have thirty times as much vitamin C as oranges.

Indigenous Amazonian people have historically picked the camu camu berries in season, dried them, and used them medicinally for the rest of the year. This purplish-red berry becomes light beige in color when dried and powdered.

The camu camu berry is also an excellent source of calcium, phosphorus, potassium, and iron; the amino acids serine, valine, and leucine; as well as small amounts of the vitamins thiamine, riboflavin, and niacin. Camu camu berries especially support the functions of the brain, eyes, heart, liver, and skin. Traditionally, camu camu has been known to:

- support the immune system
- maintain excellent eyesight
- create beautiful skin
- prevent viral infections
- support strong collagen, tendons, and ligaments
- decrease inflammation
- improve respiratory (lung) health
- eliminate heavy-metal toxicity
- help maintain optimal clarity of mind in times of stress and anxiety

Dr. James Duke, author of *The Green Pharmacy,* did a comparative study of botanicals, in order of effectiveness, for various health conditions. Camu camu was ranked among hundreds of herbs as follows:

antimutagenic	#4	gingivitis	#1
antiviral	#6	glaucoma	#1
antioxidant	#4	hepatitis	#1
asthma	#1	infertility	#1
atherosclerosis	#1	migraine headaches	#1
cataracts	#1	osteoarthritis	#1
colds	#1	painkiller	#1
depression	#2	Parkinson's disease	#1
edema	#1		

Note: This comparative study's results are not FDA approved.

Recommended Use: Add one level tablespoon (3 grams) or more to juices, smoothies, raw ice creams, raw desserts, or simply to your drinking water. Camu camu berry powder tastes delicious and tangy. As a natural vitamin C source, this product may be used in conjunction with MSM powder to rejuvenate collagen. Diarrhea symptoms indicate excessive intake.

🌿 Step 3. Krill and Algae Oil, Marine Phytoplankton, Additional Cell-Rejuvenating Supplements, Stone-Breaking Herbs, and Wulzen Factor Foods

Krill and Algae Oil

Figuratively speaking, krill are the "little ants" of the sea, as they are the most common major animal organism in the world. Their biomass spreads across thousands of miles of our planet's oceans. During peak times of reproduction, the seas are literally teeming with these "microscopic shrimp."

Along with phytoplankton, krill are the primary food source of whales. For example, a 200-ton blue whale eats around a ton and a half of krill a day. The whale has the largest nervous system, the largest brain, the largest spinal cord, and the largest nerve fiber network of any organism in the world. All of that nervous-system material is coming from somewhere: krill and phytoplankton.

As humans, we need to get the right nutrition inside our bodies, especially to our brain and nerves. One of the best ways to do this is by ingesting krill oil and/or phytoplankton algae oil. Krill oil or a properly formulated algae oil are the most useable and bio-available sources of EPA and DHA (also known as essential omega-3 fatty acids). Krill and a properly formulated algae oil contain high amounts of phospholipids, which help the EPA and DHA work better. Krill and phytoplankton algae reproduce so rapidly and are so abundant that they can never be fished out of the oceans. In comparison to cod liver oil, krill oil and plant-derived algae oil are a much cleaner and less toxic choice, with krill containing forty times the antioxidants (an exceptionally high content).

Warning: If you have a seafood allergy it is important to know that you cannot consume krill oil. A good substitute in this case, or if you are vegetarian/vegan, is algae oil and/or marine phytoplankton.

Recommended Use: Krill oil usually comes packaged in a gel cap. Soon there will be vegetarian gel caps of krill oil available. David Wolfe Omega 3+ Algae Oil already comes in vegan gel capsules. Currently krill oil is sold in animal factory-byproduct gelatin, which is unfortunate. I recommend biting into the capsules, squeezing the oil out, and then spitting out the gelatin or the soft gel.

> **TIP** Whenever possible, if you purchase encapsulated supplements of any type, make sure that they are vegetarian capsules. Normal capsules used for most pharmaceuticals and supplements are made out of gelatin, which is a byproduct of factory-farmed animals. This is not a product that we recommend putting into your body. Always make sure to select vegetarian capsules versus gelatin. It is a critical distinction with a profound effect on both our health and our environment.

Marine Phytoplankton

The nutritional uses of marine phytoplankton constitute an incredible discovery. This is a category of superfoods containing all known minerals, all known amino acids, and almost everything else that could potentially be missing from our nutrition. Phytoplankton also contains omega-3 fatty acids and phospholipids, which enable the krill oil as well as other superfoods, medicinal mushrooms, and fat-soluble nutrients (such as tocotrienols) to work more effectively.

Certain types of marine phytoplankton help us produce cellular energy without burning calories. This is accomplished by bypassing the mitochondria (the energy powerhouses of the cells) and supplying nucleotides (ATP, ADP, GTP, etc.) directly to the cells. Normally our bodies have to break down everything we eat into little packets of protein, sugar, and oil, which are then put into one end of the mitochondria factory and spit out the other side as nucleotides. These are tiny energy units of ATP, ADP, GTP, etc., that comprise the energy currency of the cell—this is what the cell uses as energy. The phytoplankton actually feed the cells directly with this energy currency, so the cell can produce energy quickly and effectively without having to use energy for digestion. This means energy without stimulation—a high with no crash or hangover.

A team of European doctors, microbiologists, and botanists spent many years and millions of dollars researching forty thousand species of marine phytoplankton to identify the best species to use for biofuel, aquaculture, exotic fish food, and ultimately human consumption. Approximately two hundred species of marine phytoplankton have been isolated and determined to be beneficial for human consumption. As a result of this extensive research, technologically advanced commercial facilities have now been developed and constructed to produce marine phytoplankton in large volume using sophisticated photo-bio-reactors. The bio-reactors consist of extensive clear tubing interconnected in a horizontal grid the size of a football field. A "spring bloom" environment is created that allows natural photosynthesis to occur, using sunlight to grow the marine phytoplankton biomass. The purified seawater solution in which the marine phytoplankton grows ensures that there are no other species contaminating the biomass. This method produces a pure, super-concentrated superfood.

People who consume marine phytoplankton are known to enjoy enhanced brain function, better eyesight, improved immune function, antiviral/antifungal/antibacterial effects, improved cellular repair, radiation protection, detoxification support, anti-inflammatory support, antioxidant support, improved circulation, improved heart function, allergy/asthma relief, suppression of symptoms stemming from degenerative disease, and a residual "grounding energy" overall. There are hundreds of references in peer-reviewed medical journals detailing the vast array of human health benefits from consuming marine phytoplankton and other microalgae.

The high chlorophyll content in marine phytoplankton increases oxygen uptake; higher oxygen uptake means more fuel to muscles, which translates to improved performance and endurance. With the smallest nano-particulate size of all microalgae, marine phytoplankton deliver vital life energy at the DNA level and also penetrate the blood/brain barrier, feeding the higher master glands located deep in the brain and increasing mental clarity.

This unique superfood from the ocean provides the body with an increase in residual energy that builds up significantly when it is ingested on a daily basis. With its abundance of naturally produced vitamins, minerals, nucleotides, antioxidants, polysaccharides, and original life force (absorbed directly from the sun), marine phytoplankton helps to develop a "whole-body" inner strength.

If you are a strict vegan or vegetarian and choose not to consume any animal products whatsoever, I recommend marine phytoplankton. This will supply you with an essential form of omega-3 (EPA) and phospholipids that are different from those found in flax, chia, and hemp seed oil.

For more information on marine phytoplankton, please see my book *Superfoods: The Food and Medicine of the Future.*

Recommended Use: Marine phytoplankton may be taken more frequently and in greater amounts, based upon your personal needs. For a gentler, time-released effect, multiple servings of marine phytoplankton may be mixed into any elixir, hot chocolate, smoothie, beverage, or raw-food dish.

Additional Cell-Rejuvenating Supplements

Lysine

Amino acids were discovered in the last 150 years, and each amino acid is critical to a certain piece of our metabolism. For example, the amino acid tryptophan has been found to help us produce more serotonin, more melatonin, and more of the chemicals we secrete when we dream. Overall, this improves our state of well-being and makes us feel more relaxed. Each of the amino acids has its own unique power, and each works in its own specific way.

In atherosclerosis, lysine can help stop the spread and growth of deposits (atherosclerotic plaques) in the arteries of the heart and brain.... In infectious diseases caused by viruses (such as flu, herpes, and AIDS) or caused by bacteria (such as lung, inner ear, and bladder infections), lysine can stop or slow down an aggressive spread of infection. A combination of high dosages of vitamin C and other dietary supplements can bring additional benefits.... Even in the case of chronic inflammation of the stomach, intestines, joints, and bones, the use of lysine can help keep the inflammation in check.... Even very common allergic problems (such as hay fever, neurodermatitis, or nettle rash) can benefit from the use of lysine, which can relieve the illness or prevent it.

—Mathias Rath, MD, *Cancer*

The therapeutic use of the essential amino acid lysine in the natural treatment of illness is extremely effective, yet largely unknown to healing practitioners and, as a result, vastly underrated. Lysine is critical to building healthy collagen. Decay and disease organisms secrete toxic enzymes that dissolve healthy collagen in order to spread infections. Lysine blocks toxic enzymes from destroying collagen. In addition, it appears that lysine interferes with the reproductive mechanism of viruses and some (or perhaps all) calcium-forming organisms such as nanobacteria. This is supercritical because we want to stop these organisms in their tracks. Lysine is the key amino acid that is able to accomplish this.

Lysine generally exists in a balance with arginine, another amino acid. These two are like opposite ends of the coin: lysine is tails and arginine is heads. They are both important; however, it appears that too much arginine and too little lysine in the body can throw off the balance and contribute to the proliferation of viral and calcium infections. On the other hand, it has been found that if your lysine level is slightly higher than your arginine level, then your health is generally better and your viral count and inflammation levels are much lower.

We naturally absorb amino acids from our food. In our world today, lysine is generally a little harder to come by than arginine. Arginine is common—it predominates in most nuts and seeds. Contrary to online opinions, cacao (raw chocolate) actually has a perfectly balanced arginine to lysine ratio (see the chapter called "Chocolate Science" in my book *Naked Chocolate*). Lysine is a little trickier to get. There are significant quantities present in bee pollen, royal jelly, deer antler velvet, and raw dairy products.

Recommended Use: It is recommended that one experiment with supplemental lysine. If there is a need for lysine, I recommend the powdered form, by itself, and not compounded with a bunch of other nutrients or flow agents (e.g., magnesium stearate). You can take it by mixing directly into water to really experience how powerful an isolated amino acid can be, especially when it comes from a reputable, high-quality source. You can also get encapsulated lysine.

Zinc

Zinc is an essential mineral for increasing health and vitality. Zinc supports our liver, skin, and every single powerhouse (mitochondria) within each cell. These energy-producing mitochondria have a critical component of zinc in them, and if that zinc is missing we cannot produce the right kind of energy in our body. In almost every case, when someone has chronic viral problems they are deficient in zinc.

Zinc acts primarily through the role of enzymes. Zinc is required for the activity of the powerful anti-inflammatory, antioxidant enzyme super-oxide dismutase (SOD). Zinc plays a major role in twenty-five different enzymatic systems involved in digestion and metabolism, and it is part of the molecular structure of eighty or more known enzymes that work with red blood cells to move carbon dioxide from tissues to lungs. Overall, zinc is a vital component of more than two hundred enzymes.

Zinc is required for skin beauty, cell and body growth, sexual development, fertility, night vision, anti-inflammation, and for improving one's sense of taste and smell. It promotes cell division, cell repair, cell growth, and the production of T-lymphocyte white blood cells. It helps the lymphatic organs and the liver eliminate wastes properly. It works through the lymphatic system to assist tissue repair and oxygenation. Zinc is present in insulin and works to balance blood sugar challenges.

Zinc works synergistically with vitamins. For example, zinc in combination with vitamin A and sulfur builds strong hair. Zinc and vitamin E (abundant in tocotrienols, olives, and olive oil) are necessary for the health of the reproductive system in both sexes. Zinc increases female fertility as well as male potency and sex drive. Zinc is present in male sexual fluids. It is an especially important mineral for the prostate, which concentrates zinc up to 2,000 percent above what is found in the blood.

Zinc is essential for a great complexion because it is a key member of a group of enzymes that help the body maintain its collagen supply. Without zinc, the enzymes that digest damaged collagen and rebuild new collagen do not function properly. In this way zinc also helps heal burns. It can even play a role in repairing DNA damage due to viruses, exposure to X-rays, and radiation.

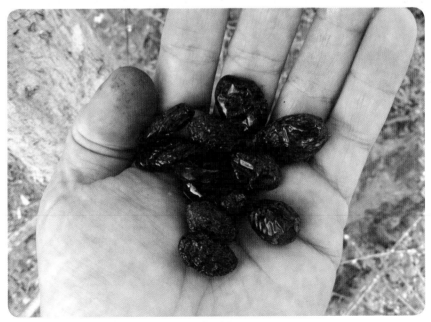

Wildcrafted, ground-ripened black olives offer zinc, vitamin E, and anti-aging oleuropein.

Zinc prevents wrinkling, stretch marks, and the outward signs of aging. Topical zinc (zinc oxide) preparations have long been observed to have an anti-inflammatory effect. Warts, acne, and skin conditions are improved significantly when one consumes more zinc-rich foods and bio-available zinc supplements.

Zinc is one of the most essential trace minerals, yet it has become one of the most common mineral deficiencies in the Western world (along with magnesium, sulfur, calcium, and silicon). One way that deficiency arises is when zinc is displaced from our system by heavy-metal toxicity. When we use the Longevity Now approach, we start breaking down calcification and unloading heavy metals. To resolve difficult zinc-deficiency syndromes, it is critical that we get zinc back into the receptor sites where the heavy metals were previously resting.

As part of the cell rejuvenation process, after we have removed the debris we need to remineralize the "inner soil" and start "growing inner gardens" within our body. This is where zinc continues to be of service. Zinc helps the liver to cleanse and assists the immune system in removing unwanted toxins—especially viral toxins. Zinc is required for the adrenals to function properly, and long-term zinc deficiencies are associated with adrenal exhaustion.

The best natural source of zinc is edible black ants. High zinc content is a trait of all longevity-enhancing black foods. In Taoist tonic herbalism, the polyrachis ant (black Changbai mountain ant) that lives with wild ginseng is utilized as a superherb. It is low on the food chain yet provides essential nutrients often deficient in vegans and vegetarians and thus makes itself useful to folks interested in ethical dietary concerns.

Another extraordinary natural source of zinc is wild chaga mushroom. To get the zinc, one would have to consume wild, cleaned, concentrated whole chaga products.

In a water-soluble form, zinc's bio-availability for absorption by the body is dramatically increased. Water-soluble zinc (zinc in a liquid that does not precipitate) is typically thousands of times smaller than zinc in colloidal form. Unlike colloidal minerals or mineral compounds (e.g., calcium citrate, calcium carbonate, copper glutinate, chromium picolinate, zinc picolinate, potassium sorbate, etc.—all of which are of uncertain origin and variable effect), water-soluble, nonprecipitating minerals are small enough to be actively assimilated by the human body.

Recommended Use: Discover and use a good source of zinc for yourself and your family. Taoist tonic herbalists consider black-colored foods to be rich in zinc and scientific evidence supports this. Consider herbal zinc products (such as the black ant or wild, cleaned, concentrated whole, chaga). Also, look into using liquid zinc (water-soluble) products. Zinc from nuts and seeds is poorly bio-available.

> TIP Store your vitamin B12 supplements away from strong light, as light can degrade vitamin B12.

Vitamin B12

Vitamin B12, like all B vitamins, is water-soluble; therefore, our bodies can store it for a while but not forever. That is why we must replenish B vitamins, especially B12, regularly. Most people in our culture, not just vegans and vegetarians, are chronically deficient in this animal-based vitamin known as vitamin B12, because most people cook their food, and cooking destroys the vitamin B12 that is naturally present. Therefore if you eat cooked meat as a source of vitamin B12, you are probably not going to be able to meet your B12 requirements.

The B12 in plant products (e.g., AFA blue-green algae, spirulina) has not been proven useful for the human body, at least according to current scientific research. Therefore we must sometimes turn to supplementation, raw dairy products, krill oil, the polyrachis black ant, or some other animal-based nourishment that is low on the food chain and less exposed to the toxic environment.

Even though raw animal and raw dairy products can be a source of vitamin B12, the natural soil microbes, bacteria, and insects (aphids, ants, etc.) found on wild food, on unwashed garden plants, in mineral-rich soil, and in plant fermentation (e.g., cultured foods) are also a considerable source and may meet at least minimum vitamin B12 needs. Nutritional yeasts and Brewer's yeasts do not contain vitamin B12 unless they are fortified with it.

I recommend methylcobalamin as the best supplemental form of B12. It is a methylated, more absorbable, more bio-available form of vitamin B12 than what is normally on a store shelf (cyanocobalamin). You can simply put methylcobalamin under your tongue and it absorbs right in. In this way you get a high dosage of vitamin B12. A big problem over the years has been that people cannot get vitamin B12 from traditional cyanocobalamin supplements. Therefore people have had to get more potent vitamin B12 injections. Taking a superior form of methylated B12 helps solve this problem and is less invasive.

To ensure an excellent quality and quantity of vitamin B12 in your diet, take B12 supplements, eat some raw dairy products (if they agree with your digestion), and/or consume some other source of B12 mentioned above.

What does vitamin B12 do in our bodies and why do we require it in effective dosages? Vitamin B12 deactivates homocysteine, a methyl-deficient amino acid byproduct of metabolic aging and/or infections. As the homocysteine level goes up in our bloodstream, inflammation ensues. For example, the number-one marker of a potential heart attack is an elevated level of homocysteine. Testing for elevated levels of homocysteine is more accurate than a cholesterol test in determining the potential of heart disease.*

Once the homocysteine reaches a certain level, a heart attack (bad-calcium occlusion) is inevitable. If this is the case, it is imperative to get homocysteine levels down. We know that homocysteine is related to infections; we know that homocysteine causes all kinds of metabolic disorders; and we know that it will eventually trigger a heart attack or stroke. If one is fifty, sixty, or older and has been following a standard lifestyle, there is no question that homocysteine is beginning to become

---

*Generally, the lower one's cholesterol levels, the more likely one is to die of a heart attack or stroke—exactly the opposite of what we're told. For more on this, see *The Great Cholesterol Con*, by Malcolm Kendricks, MD.

a problem. Because we know that homocysteine can be deactivated by vitamin B12, we must take action.

Vitamin B12 helps maintain the myelin sheaths that insulate nerve fibers. Problems with vitamin B12 absorption and assimilation can result in not only elevated homocysteine levels but also nerve degeneration and anemia. A B12 deficiency in conjunction with a folate (vitamin B9) deficiency can cause pernicious anemia.

Recommended Use: With vitamin B12, it is better to be safe (by having more) than sorry (by not considering it and suffering the consequences). Select a source to meet your requirements.

More on Homocysteine

In a normal metabolism, homocysteine should be recycled into methionine. This process utilizes vitamin B12-related enzymes. Therefore, a B12 deficiency can cause elevated homocysteine. Homocysteine is a marker of a liver methylation problem, as well as an indicator of a high level of calcification, inflammation, and cardiovascular disease. Scientific evidence indicates that homocysteine potentiates calcification. Two important components of Longevity Now, betaine (a methyl donor) and betaine hydrochloride, help deactivate dangerous homocysteine.

Betaine Hydrochloride

Doctors, nutritionists, and health experts have long held the opinion that low stomach acid or hydrochloric acid, the condition known as hypochlorhydria, is a widespread challenge within the general population. My colleague Dr. Marshall believes that folks who have had damage to their center-line (broken nose, broken jaw, breast plate injury, etc.) typically suffer from hypochlorhydria. Damage to the center-line meridian affects the stomach and digestive juices.

Stomach acid (HCl) is a "firewall" that protects our inner terrain from opportunistic infectious organisms that could be in and on our food. Hydrochloric acid is our digestive system's first defense against infection, stopping the growth of bad bacteria and yeast. In individuals who produce sufficient hydrochloric acid, a noted improvement in the cleanliness of the blood chemistry has been observed. In addition to this, stomach acid is essential in assisting the overall cascade of digestion.

A growing body of research suggests that individuals with a wide variety of chronic disorders, such as allergies, asthma, and calcification conditions, benefit from supplementing their meals with betaine hydrochloride, which aids digestion and often reduces food sensitivities. Betaine hydrochloride is a supplement designed to help increase the production of hydrochloric acid in the stomach. It assists the body's natural stomach acids in the digestion and absorption of nutrients, especially protein, good calcium, magnesium, phosphorus, iron, and vitamin B12. Betaine hydrochloride also assists in the detoxification of metabolic protein wastes and toxins.

Betaine hydrochloride is a lipotropic weight-loss supplement that prevents fats from accumulating in the liver. This may prevent gallstone formation and assist the blood in lowering plaque (calcification) deposits.

Betaine hydrochloride is also used to treat spasmodic pain of the facial nerves, cystinuria (a hereditary defect that results in recurrent kidney stone formation), and vitiligo (a condition that is characterized by a lack of skin-color pigments usually around the joints of otherwise normal skin).

Betaine by itself is a wonderful liver-cleansing supplement. Betaine is also known as trimethylglycine or TMG. It was first discovered in sugar beets *(Beta vulgaris)* and is also prevalent in goji berries.

Warning: Individuals with a history of gastrointestinal disorders such as ulcers, heartburn, or hiatal hernias should not take betaine hydrochloride. Excessive amounts can burn the lining of the stomach. If a burning sensation is experienced, betaine hydrochloride should be immediately discontinued.

Those taking nonsteroidal anti-inflammatory drugs (NSAIDs), cortisone-like drugs, or other medications that could cause peptic ulcers should avoid betaine hydrochloride.

Betaine hydrochloride has not been through rigorous safety studies. Its safety in young children, pregnant women or nursing mothers, or those with severe disease is unknown.

Recommended Use: Take one capsule of betaine hydrochloride with each raw-food or cooked-food meal. One may use betaine hydrochloride in between meals also.

Look for betaine hydrochloride brands that are actually made from beets. Betaine hydrochloride is a form of betaine with a chloride ion. It is usually the first crystallized form obtained after extraction from beets. Avoid products containing magnesium stearate, corn, milk, soy, salt, sugar, wheat, yeast, artificial colors, flavors, or preservatives.

Stone-Breaking Herbs

Certain herbs are very highly regarded for their ability to break up and eliminate bad calcium and calcium-forming organisms. Chanca piedra, gravel root, and neem are among this group. Herbs that are known to remove bad calcium, like chanca piedra and gravel root, are called clathrators. Based on my research, clathrators are automatically elevated in the whole spectrum of all herbs. That means they are as powerful as many superherbs (adaptogens) because they're going after a basic type of decay organism—the organisms that are most destructive to us in the long term, the calcium-forming microorganisms.

Chanca Piedra

Chanca piedra *(Phyllanthus niruri)* is one of the most important superherbs because of its ability to fight calcium-forming organisms directly and to remove bad calcium from the urinary tract. Chanca piedra literally means "stone breaker." The name itself indicates its powerful ability to break down calcification. In my opinion, chanca piedra is one of the more important superherbs discovered in the entire history of herbalism.

Chanca piedra has a long history of research and traditional use for breaking up calcification and ridding the body of "stone" formations.

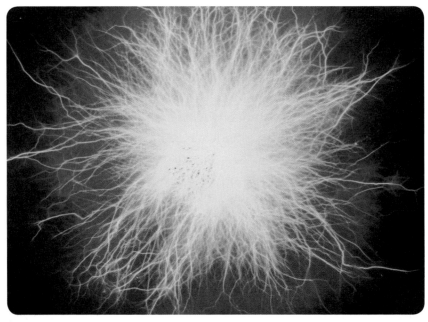

A Kirlian image of chanca piedra

As we have seen, bad calcium or microscopic "stones" are toxic to the body and constitute a primary cause of aging. Chanca piedra has been traditionally recommended for kidney stones and gallstones. Chanca piedra is anecdotally known to dilate the urinary tract and urethral canal during the passing of a kidney stone in order to lessen the pain.

In South America chanca piedra is known for many other healing properties, including easing malaria symptoms, fever and flu, alleviating liver stagnation, aiding digestion, and even working as a mild laxative and pain reliever.

Warning: People with heart conditions or taking prescription heart medications should consult their healthcare practitioner before taking this superherb.

Recommended Use: Chanca piedra may be powdered and consumed whole or taken regularly as a tea.

Gravel Root

Gravel root *(Eupatorium purpureum)* is sometimes known as Joe Pye weed. Joe Pye was a Native American who used this tremendous plant as a cure-all. He gained such a reputation as a healer that his primary herb now bears his name.

Gravel root grows wild throughout the marshy, wetland areas of the temperate regions of North America. It is often found growing on or near beaver dams.

Gravel root earns its name by assisting in the removal of stone formations (gravel) in the gallbladder, kidneys, and perhaps other organs and soft tissue.

About twenty-seven percent of the dry-matter weight of gravel root is mineral matter; this is one of the highest of any land plant (other than tobacco or cannabis). This makes gravel root an excellent source of minerals, in addition to the properties it possesses for dissolving bad calcium. Gravel root also makes for an excellent natural soil fertilizer due to its seaweed-like mineral content.

Recommended Use: Gravel root chunks may be added to teas. Gravel root tinctures may also be tried.

Neem

Neem *(Azadirachta indica)* is a tropical tree from India and Southeast Asia. Neem products (bark, leaf, seed) are aggressive destroyers of many different types of decay organisms, widely used in agriculture. Generally, diluted forms of the seed oil are recommended for topical use or oral hygiene. Neem seed oil is also traditionally used in India and Southeast Asia for body-piercing hygiene and safety because it prevents infections.

Recommended Use: Neem leaf or bark tea may be drunk to support healing. It is very potent and may cause nausea. Neem seed oil can be diluted with other oils, such as olive oil, and encapsulated to become more ingestible.

Neem leaf alcohol tinctures may be used in combination with DMSO, topically, against viral and/or fungal infections that are rooted in one or more joints (i.e., toenail or fingernail fungus).

When eaten, neem supercritical (carbon dioxide) extracts are powerful tools to help assist in a fight against internal dysbiosis and infections.

Neem is primarily recommended in this part of the Longevity Now tools for decalcification because neem seed oil diluted with hemp seed oil or olive oil and then added to small amounts of certain essential oils (cinnamon, peppermint, etc.) makes for a very good toothbrush serum. The neem tooth "truth" serum should not be so strong as to overwhelm a healthy oral environment of friendly bacteria. This is what I personally use to brush my teeth. In the teachings of the great yogis, neem is known to kill all harmful microorganisms like the ones that form plaque on the teeth.

Wulzen Factor Foods

Dutch researcher Rosalind Wulzen discovered a unique property of certain foods to protect against calcification of the joints, hardening of the arteries, cataracts, and the calcification of the pineal gland, and labeled it the Wulzen Factor or "antistiffness" factor—a factor that was never officially recognized in mainstream science.

Sugarcane

Whole sugarcane as an intact and peeled giant grass, or fresh-pressed sugarcane juice, are extraordinary in their ability to dissolve electron-deficient calcium and to build strength. The Wulzen Factor has been linked to the eight (or more) different classes of enzymes found in whole sugarcane. The extraordinary array of enzymes in whole sugarcane is unique among fresh plant foods. Only superfood algae varieties (spirulina, blue-green, chlorella, marine phytoplankton, etc.), grasses, and honey compare.

Raw Butter and Cream

The Wulzen Factor or "antistiffness" factor has been identified in only a few foods: raw butter/cream, raw sugarcane, honeycomb, molasses. This factor is destroyed during pasteurization; therefore we recommend using only raw, organic dairy products.

Oxidation, Oxygen Therapies, MMS, and Ozone

Oxidation is the loss of electrons by a molecule, atom, or ion. One familiar example of this is the process of rust formation on iron exposed to oxygen. Oxidation occurs within the body as a result of physical and mental stress; harmful EMF exposure; consuming overly processed, chemical-laden, and pesticide-sprayed food; drinking tap water; breathing in polluted air; and overall exposure to heavy metals. When this happens, oxygen electrons become wild and unruly "free radicals" that react in a physical way to the electrons of other objects they come in contact with. When the free-radical electrons "bump" into our cells, they cause the cells to decay and mutate. Therefore, oxidation is a causative factor for all things that oppose longevity, including malignant growths and neurodegenerative and cardiovascular diseases.

Generally oxygen therapies, Miracle Mineral Solution (MMS), and ozone therapies are very effective in lowering viral loads, killing de-shelled calcium-forming microorganisms, destroying candida, and destroying cancerous cells. However, the excessive use of oxygen therapies can lead to oxidation and aging. Additionally, oxygen therapies, MMS, and ozone therapies are not capable of correcting the poor-quality terrain of the tissues that have allowed the viral, nanobacteria, candida, and mutated cell growth. Oxygen therapies are like targeted smart bombs, they drop in and kill the harmful organisms and damaged cells, but they cannot replace the consistent patterns of excellent nutrition combined with a solid fitness program that shapes the quality of our internal biological terrain.

Part 4: Longevity Technologies

🔋 Step 1: Zappers

The ark was built by amateurs; the Titanic, by experts.
— ANONYMOUS

In the twentieth century it was discovered that certain types of electromagnetic wave forms (producing EMF fields) are very harmful to the human body. It was also discovered that certain other electromagnetic wave forms (also producing EMF fields) are helpful to the human body—so helpful, in fact, that they have the power to boost our immune system and give us the ability to overcome certain types of chronic conditions. The zapper is the product of one of the friendly electromagnetic wave-form discoveries, and it is a critical part of the Longevity Now approach. Its technology represents one of the great breakthroughs in science, especially because it is so easy to use.

Zappers are simple electronic devices that send "positive offset square wave" electromagnetic waveforms as signals throughout the body that over time fatally damage the circadian rhythms of all viruses, harmful bacteria, fungi, and parasites—and appear to knock out calcium-forming microorganisms as well.

Zappers are small portable electronic devices that need to touch the skin to be effective. Zappers may cause a slight tingling sensation on the skin, or even burn (be careful!). They can be used while resting, working, sitting, driving, or doing daily tasks.

Because they work along pathways of electromagnetic activity, zappers are particularly effective at relieving the emotional trauma caused by tenacious nervous system disorders, such as herpes and Lyme disease. By following the Longevity Now approach and using a zapper, one can stop herpes outbreaks within the first six months in nearly all cases as long as the zapper is close to the area of the outbreaks. The herpes infection may even begin to deactivate and disassemble at its root in the nerve ganglia of the spine (either neck or sacrum).

Zappers with 4, 8, or 12 volts and/or lower (more natural) frequencies (i.e., 0–36 Hz) may be the most effective types of zappers, although it appears all zappers will work at any frequency, as long as they have "positive offset square wave" waveform characteristics. Higher-voltage zappers (I have used up to 16-volt zappers) seem to work more effectively on hard-to-treat cases and deep infections.

Some zappers may have "negative offset square wave" (or both positive and negative) waveform characteristics. Negative offset speeds healing. Positive offset assists the immune system.

Recommended Use: Although sixty-minute sessions of "zapping" are recommended, zappers may be worn all day and all night continuously with only beneficial effects. In general, it is recommended that you zap for one hour before noon, for one hour after noon, and for one hour in the late evening. Any amount of zapping is better than none—even just one minute!

Acidic conditions in the body will give rise to a concentration of toxins on the negatively charged electrode of a zapper. This may cause a slight stinging or even burning reaction on the skin. If this persists, continually move the zapper to avoid stinging and burning. Eventually these reactions will dissipate over weeks, months, and years of zapping with the return of a pure, alkaline state to the body.

Step 2: Grounding Technologies

It is a well-established scientific fact (though not a widely known one) that the Earth's surface is charged with mobile health-giving free electrons. The Earth's surface charge is commonly referred to as "ground" or "the Earth's electrical potential." When grounded or "Earthed," any conductive object, including the human or animal body, gradually becomes negatively charged under the influence of the Earth's healthy free electrons.

Essentially the atmosphere is positively charged and opposes the Earth's negative charge. The positive ions in the atmosphere (e.g., oxygen, ozone) are considered essential, yet corrosive to health over time.

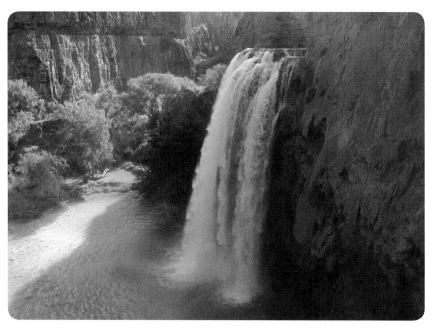

Healthy negative ions are released into the atmosphere by waterfalls.

Excessive positive charge in the atmosphere is linked to not only health problems but also a poor mental attitude. Sometimes, near waterfalls, breaking ocean waves, small campfires, or even a lit beeswax candle, more negative ions (electrons) are released into the atmosphere, causing an improvement in human health and attitude.

From the beginning, all life on Earth has been nurtured within the electromagnetic negatively charged womb of the planet. The original humans lived and slept in direct and virtually constant contact with the Earth. Until recently, the human body has been continually charged with the Earth's free negatively charged electricity.

The concept of grounding to the Earth is based on scientific evidence confirming the long-suspected necessity for barefoot contact with the Earth. A large and growing body of scientific discoveries has determined that standing barefoot on the Earth (or otherwise connecting to the natural frequencies of the Earth, including swimming in the ocean or any natural body of water upon the Earth) has a variety of effects on the human body as it connects with an unlimited supply of free electrons resident in and upon the surface of the Earth.

Being grounded instantly connects the human body with rhythmic cycles of the Earth's energy field. These are essential for synchronizing biological clocks, hormonal cycles, and physiological rhythms. All the years of our life, every ninety seconds, whether we have known about it or not, our bodies have checked for reference frequencies from the Earth in order to synchronize our own circadian rhythms with them.

Today, most people live for extended periods of time completely disconnected from the Earth. For example, we work and often live in high-rise buildings. The use of rubber-soled and synthetic-soled shoes insulates us to an even greater degree so that the human body is no longer in its natural state—connected to the Earth. As a result, the human body is no longer able to receive a constant supply of free electrons.

The immediate result of being disconnected from the Earth's EMF field is that biological challenges in mineralization occur. The further away we are from the Earth's EMF field, the faster and more severe the mineralization problems. A case in point is the extreme osteoporosis seen in astronauts floating in low Earth orbit. To be clear, disconnection from the Earth's natural EMF field will cause bone and teeth mineralization problems.

In addition to this, the lack of negative electrons supplied to us by the Earth appears to cause immune system disorders. An excessive positive charge in the body causes calcification and any number of disorders. When we are grounded, or whenever we are zapping, we are getting a subtle current into our body of negatively charged electrons that help ward off calcification and immune system disorders. Even pipes under the ground will not calcify as long as the predominant current they are carrying is negatively charged. If a pipe's electrical charge is slightly positive, calcification will occur.

Based on scientific evidence, the primary cause of bone-density loss and autoimmune conditions appears to be disconnection from the Earth's EMF field through wearing shoes, living in buildings with insulated floors (dead wood is not a conductor), driving in insulated cars (rubber tires), and flying in airplanes. Mimicking the Earth's EMF field is what any technology that allows us to healthfully leave and live above the surface of the Earth requires—this type of technology is known as magnetic resonance technology.

As a result of having elevated our dwellings, workplaces, and bedding, and having incorporated synthetic materials into our modern lifestyle, we have seen an increase in chronic health problems and sleep disorders that were rare or even unheard of fifty to sixty years ago. Research has revealed that most of our modern diseases are linked with calcification, inflammation, and free-radical damage caused, in part, by a disconnection from the Earth.

Negative electrons are powerful antioxidants. The Earth is the best source of these electrons. Not having enough negative electrons leads to free-radical damage and autoimmune conditions such as osteoporosis, rheumatoid arthritis, and fibromyalgia. The body cannot reach a true state of homeostasis without a direct skin connection to the Earth.

When we stand on the Earth barefoot, we automatically draw these negative electrons into our body. The more inflamed the body is, the more negative electrons it will pull from the Earth. Inflammation is always a precursor to illness. Connecting to the Earth will decrease inflammation within forty-five minutes.

Becoming aware of the importance of our connection to the Earth motivates us to reconnect our bodies with the Earth. This means spending time outdoors as often as possible—without shoes—standing or walking barefoot on the Earth in forests and on beaches; swimming in lakes, rivers, and oceans (all of which are grounded); and getting our bare hands into the Earth while gardening (which instantly grounds us).

Touching our Mother Earth directly has taught me the importance of touching my own mother's skin wherever and whenever I see her. Touching your mother's skin, holding her hand, creates emotional healing and support.

Unfortunately, in today's world, daily barefoot outdoor activities, gardening, and swimming in natural bodies of water are often impractical for

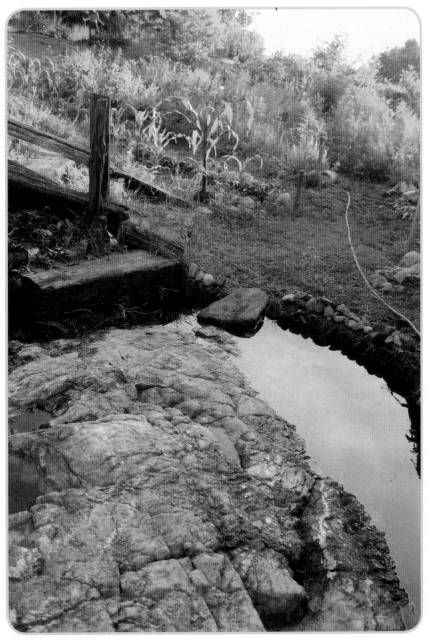

The seepage spring in my garden keeps the Earth wet and the grounding electrons flowing.

many people. When we cannot spend time outside, we can use grounding technologies that will allow us to experience the same effect.

One can imagine how important it is, based on all the information provided thus far, for a pregnant woman to be grounded as much as possible in order to advance the development of a healthy infant. This may be the reason why we have the cultural phrase "barefoot and pregnant." Once born, infants rely on a direct skin connection to their mother, who must be grounded to the Earth in order for both to access the healing and balancing electrons and frequencies that are being emitted from the Earth.

Grounding technologies are based on the fact that metals such as silver, copper, and iron can conduct the electrons, impulses, and frequencies emitted by the Earth. Interestingly, nearly every building in the western world has been installed with a grounding wire as part of the electrical system. This grounding wire is actually conducting Earth electrons and frequencies to the third prong of nearly every electrical plug. Plugging a copper and silver wire of a grounding-technology sleeping sheet, foot pad, or cushion to the grounding wire of nearly any plug allows us access to the electrons and frequencies of the Earth in almost any location. Even if we lack a grounding wire via the plugs in our home or office, we can still use grounding technologies through a metal rod that one sticks into the Earth and connects to a grounding sheet, pad, or cushion.

Plugging in and grounding to the Earth with grounding technologies provides virtually the same effects as standing barefoot on the Earth. People everywhere are reconnecting with the Earth via grounding technologies while sleeping, working, and even during play and exercise.

Here's how it works: The grounding technologies have sheeting fabric containing a grid of conductive, inherently antimicrobial, silver yarn. The fabric snaps to a copper wire system that is connected to the Earth Tap. When the Earth Tap is plugged into a grounded three-prong outlet or directly into the ground, it cancels out the two electrical plugs and uses the current from the ground plug to connect the user into the Earth's natural EMF field. The body is immediately brought to the same electrical potential as the Earth and connected with the Earth's vital electrons and other natural rhythms and frequencies. When a person is in bed—resting or sleeping on grounding technologies—the body is electrically connected to the Earth. All of this occurs at the speed of light and without effort.

Whenever you connect to the Earth, you get in sync with its natural EMF field and immediately discharge any "dirty" EMFs that your body has absorbed from nearby electrical wires, televisions, computers, WiFi, cell phones, etc. The Earth can ground any amount of EMF pollution present in our bodies. Automobiles (especially hybrid vehicles) and airplanes can saturate us with EMF pollution as well. Whenever we step out of a car or airplane it is important to ground ourselves immediately to discharge this EMF pollution by the electron surplus we gather from the Earth.

Connecting to the Earth is known to promote the following benefits:

- heals wounds three times faster
- normalizes cortisol levels
- quiets the brain's left hemisphere and synchronizes brain waves
- allows the natural influences emanating out of the Earth, which have been an integral part of life's process, to flow through our bodies as Nature intended
- discharges the buildup of bioelectrical stress
- neutralizes free radicals that cause pain, chronic inflammation, and autoimmune conditions
- overcomes jet lag (caused by our body not knowing where it is on the planet; standing barefoot on the ground for at least fifteen minutes brings us back in sync)
- supports the synchronization of biological rhythms
- influences the hormones that regulate sleep and many other functions
- re-establishes a negative charge in and around the body (a negative charge automatically begins to break down calcification, caused by an excessive positive charge)

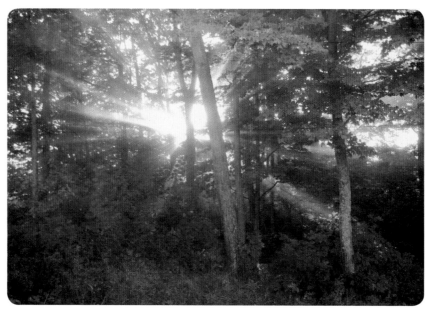

Sungazing: capture with your eyes those first five minutes or last five minutes of sunlight each day.

Is Grounding Always Healthy?

Rudolf Steiner and various dowsers have held the opinion that places above where underwater streams flow are less than excellent for grounding. These places create distorting Telluric forces that rise into homes and especially disturb sleeping environments. Steiner recommended blocking these forces by sleeping on peat bricks, as peat bricks are known to shield from these forces. He also recommended peat-wool fiber clothing, to shield from damaging high-frequency radiation in the atmosphere such as mobile phone signals, WiFi, high-altitude radiation, etc. Peat-wool garments take high frequency radiation and reduce it to low frequency radiation (which the Earth can easily act to protect us from). Therefore, wearing peat-wool garments while being grounded is a wonderful combination (I personally enjoy and recommend this combination).

Qigong and Grounding

When I'm doing my sungazing, during the last five minutes of the day (just before the sun sets), I practice qigong, a soft martial art that emphasizes flowing movement and working with the natural energies of the Earth, the atmosphere, and one's body. As I practice qigong at the twilight hour, I'm looking at the sun (with no eyewear), standing barefoot on stone, and doing gentle exercises. This is connecting me to the natural EMF fields of the Earth (e.g., electrons, telluric forces) and resetting all my circadian rhythms. That, to me, is what qigong is all about. If you are adept at qigong, you can start drawing that energy from the Earth into your body.

For those who practice or are interested in qigong, the potential inherent in grounding more often and for more hours of the day via grounding technologies helps to advance one's qigong practice.

Meditation and Grounding

Meditation reduces and eliminates stress and tension within the body and mind. It's the most effective way to create and cultivate inner peace, time-tested by the Earth's greatest masters. A healthy body requires a healthy, happy heart and mind. If you feel that you're emotionally upset or mentally confused, just go into a beautiful area in Nature and sit down on the bare Earth. While being quiet, close your eyes and relax. Breathe deeply. This is the best thing you can do for both your physical and mental health. If you cannot get to a place where you have a direct skin-to-skin connection with the Earth, use grounding technologies in your home to make the connection. If you are already a meditator, over time you'll notice a significant difference meditating while grounded.

The benefits of meditation are both physical and mental. Mental benefits include the following:

- reducing stress and tension
- increasing concentration
- calming the mind
- creating inner peace and harmony
- improving problem-solving abilities

Physical benefits include:

- relaxing the body
- lowering blood pressure
- helping open the energy meridians
- quick recovery from stress
- reduced LDL or "bad" cholesterol levels
- reduced chronic and acute pain

Researchers have published hundreds of studies, the results of which indicate that people who meditate regularly have better health than people who don't. Meditation has become an enormous part of our current culture because it is simple, effective, and practical. Anybody can meditate! Now we can amplify our results by being grounded and connected directly to all the telluric forces that arise from the Earth.

Sleeping and Grounding

Over the years, raw-food pioneer Dr. Gabriel Cousens has taught me about the enormous value of sleep. When you get enough sleep, your immune system is able to rejuvenate, you're able to release a lot of internal stress, and your body gains much-needed rest and relaxation.

The environment surrounding your bed greatly enhances the benefits of sleep. First of all, it is important to get some fresh air while you are sleeping. Many people suffer from all kinds of health disorders because they're breathing mold spores and dust inside their own homes. If you can keep your window open just a little bit, even in the middle of winter, the fresh air circulating around your house can be very beneficial.

Use only natural bedding—organic sheets, pillow, and blankets and/or the grounding technology bedding. This latter type of bedding helps you connect to the EMF field of the Earth. I have already talked extensively about the benefits of using this incredible technology (see above). Remember that by connecting barefoot to the Earth, and by picking up healthy electrons and the EMF signals of the Earth, we remove physical and mental stress from our body and support our immune system. We can do this while we sleep using grounding technology. It will help us

Meditation in Five Simple Steps

1. Find a quiet place and sit down in a comfortable position with a straight spine.
2. Close your eyes, take a few deep breaths in and out of your nostrils, and try to relax your body.
3. Focus your awareness on a specific object. This could be any of the following: a word or a phrase that has a special meaning to you (a.k.a. a mantra), a specific chakra on your body, an image of strength or beauty (internal or external), or even the simple sensation of air as it enters and exits the nostrils.
4. Repeat the word, phrase, or mantra silently to yourself (not out loud). If you get distracted, don't worry; gently bring your attention back to the object and focus once again (like training an unruly puppy to sit).
5. Try to stay focused in your meditation for at least two to five minutes. Then gently relax your concentration and open your eyes.

Now check in with your body and mind. Do you feel more calm and peaceful? Is your body more relaxed? As you become more familiar with the practice of meditation, your experience of inner peace, calmness, and happiness will deepen. Now try to maintain this experience of peacefulness for as long as you can throughout the day!

get the best sleep ever! Nearly 100 percent of users of grounded bedding report better sleep.

Also, be sure that when you sleep the environment around your bed is free from EMF fields. For example, if you have an alarm clock, especially a digital plug-in alarm clock, it can be creating a huge EMF field right next to your head. Keep all those things at least two meters away from you, and make sure that all plugs, even if there's nothing plugged into them (and they appear to be off) are far away from your bed because they can be producing EMF fields even if you don't know it.

Part 5: Yoga and Deep-Tissue Bodywork

Massage, bodywork, and physical self-activated squeezing and twisting are part of any holistic healing system and critical to the overall decalcification strategy. It is youthening and rejuvenating to squeeze those often-neglected areas of the body, to move energy around, and to break up stagnation. Through various modalities we can release toxins and dislodge them permanently from their hiding places.

Modalities for physically breaking up stagnation include yoga, rebounding, bongers, and various kinds of deep-tissue massage.

Yoga

The fundamental three yogic ingredients are pranayama (breathing), basti, and inversions.

Pranayama

The average person breathes between fifteen and twenty times per minute, taking in more than 22,000 breaths per day. What are we breathing in? Because of all the toxicity we are dumping into our environment, we are now assaulted with air pollutants, both indoors and outdoors. Dr. Howard Fisher's book *Extreme Toxic Times* lists in comprehensive detail the challenges we face every day:

> *Aside from the particulate matter such as dust, pollen, smoke, we are also exposed to: ammonia from household cleaners, acetone from nail polish remover and solvents, benzene from carpets, furniture, and paint, carbon tetrachloride vapors from your dry cleaning, carpets, drapes, and paint, formaldehyde vapors from your pressed-wood furniture, plywood, plastic, carpets, drapes, or tobacco smoke. But wait, that's not all. The list continues. Mildew, molds, dust, dust mites, dust mite feces, viruses, bacteria, fungi, and more all challenge your health.*

Please keep in mind that we inhale these substances regularly.

Clean air and deep breathing are an essential part of optimal detoxification and health. A good friend, longevity expert Peter Ragnar, claims that 70 percent of the toxins in our body can be eliminated by proper breathing. That's one of the reasons to get into a yoga class, it's one of the reasons to walk in a forest and take deep breaths, it's one of the reasons to get out of an office building regularly. The deep breathing helps to move and eliminate toxins better than anything else. Breathing is an excellent way to open up the channels of elimination in one's body.

The heart is the regulator that keeps the cardiovascular system going. The lymphatic system doesn't have that kind of regulator; it has a pump—the lungs. Deep breathing functions to move our lymphatic fluid around. So we have to breathe in order to squeeze that lymphatic fluid and move it from one node to the next.

The power of breath is fourfold. First and foremost, the breath controls the energy levels in the body. When people have low energy, they're probably shallow breathers. You can see it in the way they carry themselves, slumping over, humped down a little bit; and you can see that their breathing is shallow. People who are energetic breathe in deeply and have an open chest.

Second is the fact that the lungs play a major role in the immune system. This is a big key. When we breathe in, the lymphatic fluid moves around and allows our immune system, our white blood cells, to do their job properly.

Third, controlling the breath allows us to begin to also control the automatic functions of the body. We were told that we can't control our heart rate or our blood flow or our body temperature, but the yogis of India never believed that. They knew that if they could control their breath, they could control their heart rate. Once you can control your heart rate, then you can control your body temperature. Once you can control your body temperature, then you can control your response to stresses caused by the environment.

Fourth, when we are touching the ground barefoot or are connected to the Earth via grounding technology, simply breathing in oxygen eliminates pain. If we have pain in our body, deep breathing can help us. Deep breathing is the single easiest technique to improve health and decrease pain.

I'm like you—I forget a lot of the time. I'll be in the middle of so many millions of things that I will literally forget to take a deep breath. But I'm telling you, this is something that is a great little trigger to have in the back of your mind. If you feel the stress increasing moment to moment, day by day, go outside barefoot and take ten deep breaths; that will do more for you than practically anything else, and the effects are immediate.

Through deep breathing you'll find that you immediately calm down. This is because your mental state is related to how you're breathing. What you want to do is breathe in slowly and hold three or four times the length of the in-breath. Then breathe out. You'll notice a difference if you do it right now: breathe in, through the nose, hold, breathe out through the mouth. What I have just described is a ratio of breathing that we call the 1:3:2 ratio. If you breathe in for five seconds, you hold for fifteen seconds (or three times the in-breath), then you breathe out for ten seconds (or twice the in-breath).

To reiterate, anxiety is related to shallow breathing and can be relieved by standing barefoot on the Earth or via grounding technologies in your home or office and taking ten long, deep, meditative breaths.

Another breathing ratio that is very simple and easy to do is the 1:1:1:1 ratio. You breathe in for one, hold for one, breathe out for one, and then hold again for one. Then you breathe back in for one, hold for one, breathe out for one, and hold for one.

I've been extremely fortunate to study with some of the most wonderful advanced yogis throughout my travels all over the world. Their instruction enabled me to heal myself from a crippling back injury that I suffered from for a long time. One of the things I've learned is you don't need to be an expert on five hundred different breathing techniques. All you need is one that you actually use—that's the key.

Basti

Basti, the ancient yogic practices of enemas and colonics, has now become more common in our society. Colon hydrotherapy is a very effective method for speeding up detoxification. It allows a great amount of toxicity to be flushed out quickly, so we can continue with our daily lives without enduring extreme detoxification symptoms. Colon hydrotherapy is simple and relatively painless.

By regularly visiting a colon hydrotherapist you will extend your life and increase your health. The raw-foodist Dr. Norman Walker had two series of six colon cleanses done every year in the second half of his life—he lived to be at least 109 (some say older). I've found that one colonic every four to six months has been effective for me—although I am sure that more would do me good. I always recommend starting with a series of four to six sessions even if you think you do not need it.

The primary goal of colon hydrotherapy is to empty the bowels completely in order for the lymph system to drain. The secondary goal is to remove encrusted mucus (which feeds unwanted parasites and poisons the system) from the inner intestinal lining. The third goal is to allow the liver to flush and release.

Colon hydrotherapy is a mechanical way to keep our colon operating properly; it is not a crutch to help us eliminate. Good elimination comes from eating a healthy diet and exercising regularly.

You can also speed up the detoxification process by doing enemas coupled with fasting on Superhero beverages (see pages 105, 115, and 262) and celery-based vegetable juices.

Even after fifteen years of clean living and raw foodism, I get colonics whenever I have a chance. This is because it is important to invest in your health not just when you are sick but also when you are healthy. With the colonics and the cleansing, you'll be younger, you'll be healthier, you'll be happier, and you will feel good, even in spite of all the catastrophes and stresses of our world.

Inversions

Before our eyes, every day, is the force of levity that allows everything to grow, evolve, and move from the Earth toward the heavens.

In the yogic sense, an inversion means inverting the forces of gravity and levity, which also means inverting the forces of death and life. Yoga teaches us that inversions activate glandular secretions that make us younger. Due to the forces of gravity, most of the toxic sediment in our body ends up below our knees in our calves, ankles, and feet. Whenever we practice the sacred science of yoga and the inversions that are part of it, we allow gravity to work for us. (An inversion is typically defined as a bodily position in which the hips are above the heart or the feet and legs are above the torso). During inversions, especially on a yoga swing that allows us to get upside down, we can practice deep-tissue massage, have Bongers used on us (springy sticks with rubber balls at the tip for thumping muscles), extend our spine, and experience the magic of gravity as it helps to push sediment out of our lower extremities, all while we elongate the spine.

Bad-calcium sediments that accumulate in the lower legs are assisted in being churned up for detoxification by the gravity-levity flip. While one is inverted, the added blood flow to the head and neck activates the brain and the hypothalamus, pituitary, pineal, and thyroid glands. More blood flow occurs in the upper portion of the body, including the heart and lungs.

The elongation of the spine, while inverted, removes chronic gravitational pressure from the vertebrae and creates space for expansion.

Again, yogic inversions help to reverse the forces of levity and gravity, stimulating the energies that make us younger. You'll notice that the great poses in yoga—such as backbends, shoulder stand, headstand, handstand, downward dog, waterfall, etc.—are all inverted postures, which flip the levity and the gravitational forces around.

Whenever we stand upright we significantly activate noradrenaline and adrenaline. Symptoms ranging from anxiety to lack of energy to unclear thinking are immediately improved by becoming inverted. Such positions immediately take the metabolic pressure off one's system and encourage the adrenals to relax. The yogis say that we only need eleven minutes of sleep each night. This sounds impossible until one begins to invert and purify. I have had dozens of moments in my life where inverting has immediately restored strength, energy, and clarity before important public performances.

Sometimes we're functioning on such high levels of adrenaline for such extended periods of time that we never de-adrenalize. Getting horizontal or inverted during rest or sleep actually de-adrenalizes our bodies and calms our adrenals down. Again, this is really important because adrenaline is one of the main neurotransmitters/hormones needed to keep us walking upright. When we walk upright, we use adrenaline all day, especially if we have to stand on our feet all day long. When we lie horizontal or invert, our adrenals have that time to shut off.

When our hips are above our heart in any inverted position, we can actually rejuvenate very quickly. I generally sleep that way (in an inversion with my hips above my heart) so that I can rejuvenate and get less sleep without having any immune system compromise.

Rebounding

Rebounding, or jumping on a trampoline or a mini-tramp, is absolutely one of the most extraordinary things you can do to keep every one of your buoyant cells free of debris. When you jump on a trampoline, you are actually moving the g-forces up and down throughout every cell in your body. Literally every little water bag in your body, namely every cell, is getting squeezed and then is suddenly having zero gravity, then getting squeezed, then suddenly having zero gravity again. This repeated squeezing activates all the cells and tissues, eliminates stagnation, and displaces calcification. The squeeze happens at the bottom of the trampoline, when you hit with your feet; the zero gravity happens when you're at the peak of the jump.

Jumping around on a trampoline creates lean, powerful muscle. It moves the lymphatic fluid around. It has been shown to increase oxygenation. There's no question that rebounding can deliver to you the best exercise, in the shortest period of time.

Efficiency in exercise is critical if you're a busy person like I am. I need to be able to jump on that thing for twenty minutes and get a workout in; that way I feel like I really got something done. Some days I literally don't have more than twenty minutes to do an exercise program.

🎵 Bongers

Bongers are a brand-name pair of handheld devices. They are the length of a percussionist's drumstick or slightly longer and have a hardened rubber ball at one end and a handgrip on the other. They are used to soften hardened body tissue and to break up calcification conditions such as cellulite. They flex when swung, thus allowing more momentum to be generated when they hit the skin. A good thirty-minute session of using Bongers on yourself or another can do wonders to bring healthy bloodflow into stagnant, hardened areas.

Other products and brands similar to Bongers that are longer and have spiked, hardened plastic balls at each end are available. These are slightly more aggressive. All products of this kind are recommended.

🎵 Deep-Tissue Bodywork

Massage has always been the number-one modality of healing—and it's hands-on healing. Give yourself the gift of more bodywork and massage in your life. Being grounded during bodywork sessions for more hours of the day via grounding technologies helps to advance and increase energy levels for both the practitioner and the receiver.

Deep-tissue bodywork is an absolutely essential part of the Longevity Now approach because of its ability to squeeze and break up toxic organisms and debris. Deep-tissue work stirs up the dirt and breaks up the bad calcium deposits, in the system and on the bones, in order for the immune system and cleansing organs of the body to remove them. With the other parts of the decalcification system, we have the power to cleanse, detoxify, and decalcify; however, only with the deep-tissue bodywork can we directly manipulate and break up the calcification and eliminate it.

The pain one feels from deep-tissue bodywork—whether it is Rolfing, Body Electronics (pointholding), Chinese *gua sha,* or Romi Romi—is not real pain in most cases. It is actually the dislodging of toxicity, the breakup of toxic calcium crystals, and the breakup of calcium-forming organisms and other organisms that are attached to the nervous system (e.g., nanobacteria, fungi, unwanted guests), along with the dissolving of stuck emotional energy.

The nervous system can be compared to the monetary system of the body politic. Parasites on the nervous system eventually manifest outwardly, as do parasites in the monetary system of our world. Why are there governments and usury banking and corporations who, like parasites, destroy their hosts? Because these classes of microorganisms rule the bodies of people in every strata of civilization and they are hooked directly into the nervous system of each individual. Because they attach directly to the nerves, they cause pain when they are broken off the bones and tissues.

The pain of deep-tissue work will eventually be transformed into pleasure as one breaks up the calcification, removes toxins, eliminates unwanted debris, and uplifts emotional-spiritual stagnation from the body.

Rolfing

In 1920, Ida Rolf received a PhD in biochemistry from the College of Physicians and Surgeons at Columbia University. She subsequently furthered her education through research in organic chemistry at the Rockefeller Institute. Dr. Rolf was driven by the desire to heal her own and her family's health problems. She spent many years studying and experimenting with different systems of alternative healing including homeopathy, osteopathy, chiropractic, and yoga. Eventually Dr. Rolf became a leader and pioneer in the fields of soft-tissue manipulation and movement, as well as movement and bone structure education.

Based on her research, Dr. Rolf found that imbalances in bone structure are exacerbated by gravity, putting pressure on the soft-tissue network of the body including muscles, fascia, tendons, and ligaments.

This creates compensations throughout the bone structure. Dr. Rolf concluded that when the bone structure is in proper alignment, an overall sense of well-being can be experienced.

Dr. Rolf posed the following question: "What conditions must be fulfilled in order for the human body-structure to be organized and integrated in gravity so that the whole person can function in the most optimal and economical way?" The answer to this question became Rolfing—a system of soft-tissue manipulation and movement, as well as bone structure education. In order to make her process accessible, she developed a ten-session series of treatments known as the Ten Series.

Rolfing Structural Integration is a form of deep-tissue bodywork that reorganizes the connective tissues through release and realignment. This improves our range of motion, flexibility, posture, and bone structure. Rolfing helps break down calcification in the connective tissue and fascia, thereby assisting the resolution of physical discomfort, chronic tension, and pain. People from all walks of life have benefited from Rolfing, including dancers, athletes, yogis, mothers, business professionals, and children. Rolfing assists in easing pain and chronic stress and has been shown to improve performance in professional and daily activities. Since its inception, Rolfing has touched the lives of more than one million people.

Dr. Rolf passed from the Earth in 1979 at the age of eighty-three. Since that time the Rolf Institute of Structural Integration has continued to share her inspirational work by certifying Rolfers and Rolf Movement Practitioners. At the moment of this writing, there are more than 1,550 Rolfers and Rolf Movement Practitioners worldwide.

Body Electronics

Body Electronics is one of the most interesting natural healing systems to come out of America in the last century. Body Electronics was founded by the late John W. Ray, ND, who developed it during the 1950s, 1960s, and 1970s in Oregon, California, Utah, and Wisconsin. Ray was an innovator and a powerful intuitive who managed to rediscover several highly important and powerful principles of healing, on which Body Electronics is based. As you'll see, these principles are in alignment with the Longevity Now approach.

Dr. Ray taught a combination raw vegetarian and raw animal food diet, with the fervent belief that it is impossible to ignore a raw-food diet due to its healing power. In addition to raw food, he recommended various vitamin and mineral supplements, including digestive enzymes and "chelated" colloidal prehistoric minerals rich in humic and fulvic acids from a mineral deposit in Utah.

Ray understood the calcium crystals that were embedded in people's bodies in an emotional sense; he believed that each crystallization was associated with a suppressed emotion. To break up these crystals, he recommended holding specific points on the body, nonstop, for periods ranging from thirty minutes to over a dozen hours, where the point-holder presses down on a specific point on a person's body with a finger, thumb, or elbow. The person receiving the treatment lies on a massage table perfectly still for the duration of the pointholding.

According to Body Electronics, suppressed patterns of negative thoughts, words, emotions, toxins, imbalances, memories, reactive karmic patterns, and traumas are stored in the body in crystals. We now more clearly understand these crystals in a physical sense as calcium deposits, a.k.a. calcification. Energetically, they are concentrates of low-energy karmic information. Healing takes place as this information is unlocked and transformed with the intent of unconditional love and unconditional forgiveness. Ray taught that as long as this karmic information remains locked in the crystals, it will exist within us at an unconscious level and manifest emotionally. The process of true healing begins by dissolving these crystals. During this process, the karmic information in them is released, along with negativity, traumatic memories, debilitating emotions, etc. Ray's unique method of sustained acupressure and pointholding accelerates the speed of dissolving the crystals.

The ultimate goal of Body Electronics is to remove resistance patterns that develop into outer physical symptoms. Once these resistance patterns are removed, one's consciousness may be transformed. When a change of consciousness occurs, the associated crystals that have been dissolved are removed permanently. If crystals simply dissolve or are broken up without any change of consciousness, they will eventually reform somewhere else in the body.

According to internet research and anecdotal reports, John Ray was a wonderful healer, teacher, and developer of self-healing methods who occasionally flew off the deep end with bizarre, controversial, and exaggerated claims. Nevertheless, the nutrition and pointholding system he offered is valuable.

David Wolfe Neckwork Protocol

Most of the immune system's activity occurs in the area surrounding the mouth and in the front of the neck. Approximately thirty lymph nodes are present in the neck. Any stagnation in this area can have catastrophic effects on the body over the long term. The chronic jaw tension created by stress, the grinding of teeth, the presence of mercury amalgam fillings in the mouth, emotional holding patterns in the front of the neck due to issues with one's father or mother, and immune-response burdens on the lymphatic system in this area all add up to create astonishing acute subconscious pain and tenderness in the neck and jaw that is just below daily awareness, until someone presses into the area.

As you might guess from the name, the Neckwork Protocol is my own contribution to longevity bodywork technologies. Over the last twenty years I have rediscovered a system of reflexology in the front of the neck and underneath the jaw. This system is similar to classic reflexology and Rolfing. It is extremely effective at relieving TMJ (temporomandibular joint) syndrome, headaches, jaw troubles, and a host of emotional holding patterns. This Neckwork Protocol is a very powerful adjunct to any bodywork system. I teach it to groups at some of my events and retreats. The Neckwork Protocol consists of massaging the front of the vertebrae behind the esophagus as well as the jaw joint, jaw bone, and face. This area can build up an enormous amount of tension, and requires at least some attention. Fortunately, this area releases tension very quickly, and relief soon follows.

Chinese *Gua Sha*

Gua sha bodywork techniques from China utilize a hardened natural tool (such as a fossilized rib or turtle shell spoon), instead of a finger or knuckle, to drive into the tissues and bones to break off barnacles, dig up stuck energy, and activate tender body parts.

Coconut oil may be used to lubricate the skin in order to assist the *gua sha* tool in sliding over its surface and digging into the muscle tissue. Please see a trained *gua sha* practitioner to learn how to perform these techniques on yourself and others. *Gua sha* can be used on all areas of the body in order to break up stagnant energy, activate tender areas with blood flow, and remove unwanted guests and calcification under the skin or muscles, or on the bones.

My friend Dr. Robert Cassar, an expert in *gua sha* techniques, recommends scrubbing the skin with the following formula before engaging in *gua sha:*

- 1.5 liters organic vodka
- 200 drops liquid fulvic acid (200,000–350,000 parts per million)
- 50 drops liquid silica (Bio-Sil or Orgono)
- 1 tbsp MSM
- 1 tsp cayenne pepper

A clean, organic, slightly abrasive towelette is wetted with this formula and then the skin is scrubbed as if you were scrubbing with soap in the shower. The entire 1.5 liter (in the recipe above) would not be used in one scrubbing, one would use as needed.

Maori Romi Romi Bodywork

The Maori are the indigenous peoples of Aotearoa (New Zealand), whom I believe are descended from the Egyptians, and later the Polynesians. The Maoris are the greatest indigenous force in Polynesia today. In past ages they sailed the entire Pacific and maybe even further into other seas with their handcarved kauri-wood ships. They landed in Hawaii and were particularly fond of Kauai. The Maori word for heaven is *Wairua*, probably referencing the Wailua River Valley of Kauai. Over their history, they have developed an extraordinary system of deep-tissue bodywork that breaks up scar tissue and calcification and reactivates stagnant necrotic tissue.

Romi Romi practitioners use hands, elbows, forearms, and their body weight to dig into muscles and other tissues in order to move stuck energies and calcified debris. Coconut oil is used on the skin, and ocean water is used to clear negative energies.

Romi Romi focuses on spiritual healing through bodywork. On the physical level, the primary focus is the legs and especially the calves. The pain created by deep-tissue work in this area can be more intense than in any other part of the body. Due to gravity, all the detritus, debris, heavy metals, bad calcium residues, and uric acid crystals typically settle in the areas from the knees down. Generally, from a simple glance at one's ankles, it is possible to estimate how much calcification is present, and how many years one has left—through determining the level of inflammation visible there.

Romi Romi bodywork can be very intense. One should approach Romi Romi with a spiritual commitment to receive deep healing.

AFTERWORD

In spite of all the propaganda and health claims, calcium and calcium supplements have never been scientifically proven to be a safe and effective method for increasing bone density. With the identification of the danger of calcium supplements and making the distinction between good and bad calcium, a new awareness is brought forth. In the same way, in spite of all the estrogen replacement therapies and claims, estrogen dominance has been implicated in being fundamental to numerous degenerative conditions. Nurturing an androgenic metabolism stacks the odds in your favor, to activate rejuvenation and youthening. Let us move forward with ease and grace, and let us make clear, informed decisions about our future.

> *A long habit of not thinking a thing wrong gives it a superficial appearance of being right.*
> —THOMAS PAINE (INTRODUCTION TO *COMMON SENSE*, 1776)

Add silicon-rich herbs, superfoods, and supplements as well as alkaline magnesium (from raw chocolate and chlorophyll) in order to detoxify and remineralize. Activate the Longevity Now approach as best you can, in any way you can, with everything you've got. Take careful notes of your results.

Notice that as your inner energies increase, your fears decrease. The dissipation of common fears (including the fear of death, the fear of failure, and the fear of rejection) will have a remarkable positive influence on your will to live. Finding the joy and love in living is an essential component of the longevity experience.

Absorb all the information provided in these pages with an inner realization that through continual study of the material you will master it swiftly. Remember the difference between good calcium (from plants, pure raw dairy, and some superherbs) and bad calcium (from naturally contaminated water or from strata in the Earth). Good calcium is essential for detoxification, muscle relaxation, lowering tension, and creating alkalinity. Bad calcium gets deposited as sediment and allows for the creation of "golems in the gears."

Remember, you are what you eat. The technology behind the nutrition section of Longevity Now is designed to bring you to superhero levels of performance. Build a body out of the best foods ever so that the body can eliminate estrogen dominance, lower calcification, and maintain flexibility. We have the potential to live free from arthritis, inflammation, joint problems, heart problems, wrinkles, cancer, cellulite, cysts, etc.

Incorporating raw and living foods into our diet, at whatever level we can right now, is the best investment we can make in our health. The more we rely on Mother Nature's abundance and her living waters, the better the results we will achieve with the Longevity Now approach.

Learning is growing. Being a lifelong learner is also a key aspect of longevity—it's a key aspect of inspiration, which instantly empowers us. Now all the tools are available for anyone to become a longevity specialist. As we become inspired, we activate genius and our imagination and we feel the wonder of a big four letter word coming toward us: H-O-P-E.

Only passions, great passions, can elevate the soul to great things.
    —DIDEROT

Discovering and/or activating a mission that you are passionate about appears to be a key aspect of why we are all here on Earth. Making a contribution to our planet and its residents gives life meaning, creates magical synchronicities, and allows us to unfold into true happiness. Inside your mission is the essence of your longevity.

To hell with circumstances; I create opportunities.
    —BRUCE LEE

The spiritual concept of free will indicates that we can alter our fate. It is possible, even probable, that our fate is not predetermined. The power of our thoughts, words, and deeds appears to exert strong influences upon our destiny. When backed by noble intentions, our thoughts, words, and deeds may escalate beyond ourselves to even influence the fate of our world.

It is interesting to notice the way the substances we ingest become interwoven with our thoughts, words, and deeds. For example: How often do we think of food? How often do we talk about food? How often do we eat?

Have we backed our food and supplement choices with noble intentions and goals? Do they align with our mission? Are they in accordance with longevity?

Most of the foods and supplements we have eaten in our lifetime have been completely random. There was no rhyme or reason to our choices beyond simply "needing protein," "filling up on fuel," "being hungry," or "needing vitamins and minerals."

With our commitment to Longevity Now we are invited to put every choice under the light of overarching noble intentions such as increasing longevity, increasing flexibility, building up core life-force energy, regaining the vigor of our youth, activating our mission, fostering androgenic metabolism, and eliminating calcification. Making appropriate choices from a perspective of noble ideals inevitably delivers us into a transformed destiny.

What is possible for each one of us is miraculous. By the power of free will, you can regain your youth.

Have The Best Life Ever!!!

—David "Avocado" Wolfe

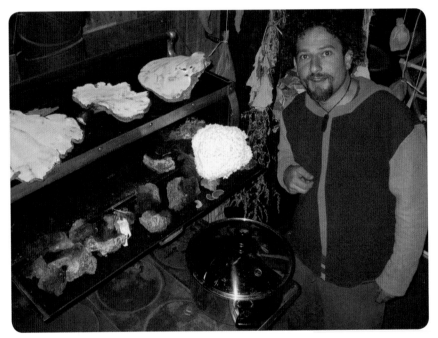

My wood-burning stove with wild mushrooms and Saladmaster teapot

Jing Master Tea

½ tsp cordyceps

½ tsp *ho shou wu*

½ tsp eucommia bark

½ tsp cistanche

2 droppers deer antler (optional)

Sweetener of choice (stevia, lo han guo, xylitol, inulin, jerusalem artichoke syrup, yacon syrup, maple syrup, birch syrup, and/or raw honey)

Immune Mushroom Master Tea

½ tsp reishi

½ tsp chaga

½ tsp cordyceps

½ tsp agaricus

½ tsp astragalus

Sweetener of choice (stevia, lo han guo, xylitol, inulin, jerusalem artichoke syrup, yacon syrup, maple syrup, birch syrup, and/or raw honey)

The Metabolizer Tea

2 tbsp goji berries

1 tbsp coconut oil

2 caps rhodiola

½ tsp vanilla bean *or* 1 dropper vanilla stevia

Sweetener of choice (stevia, lo han guo, xylitol, inulin, jerusalem artichoke syrup, yacon syrup, maple syrup, birch syrup, and/or raw honey)

Reishi Cappuccino Tea

½ tsp reishi

½ tsp *ho shou wu*

1 tbsp cacao powder

1 tbsp coconut oil

A dash Cinnamon

Sweetener of choice (stevia, lo han guo, xylitol, inulin, jerusalem artichoke syrup, yacon syrup, maple syrup, birch syrup, and/or raw honey)

Kefir Margarita

⅔ cup iced coconut water kefir (coconut water with probiotics added that's been allowed to culture/ferment for twenty-four hours)

2–3 oz. spring water

2–3 oz. lemon juice

1 tbsp tocotrienols

½ tbsp coconut oil

2 droppers ocean minerals

1 dropper ginger extract

1 pinch Himalayan salt

½ tsp vanilla bean *or* 1 dropper vanilla stevia

Sweetener of choice (stevia, lo han guo, xylitol, inulin, jerusalem artichoke syrup, yacon syrup, maple syrup, birch syrup, and/or raw honey)

The $18,000 Jing Master Smoothie

2 tbsp cacao powder

1 tbsp maca

1 tbsp mesquite

2 tbsp hemp seeds

2 tbsp tocotrienols

1 tbsp coconut oil

1 tsp vanilla bean

2 droppers ocean minerals

½ tsp cordyceps

½ tsp *ho shou wu*

½ tsp eucommia bark

½ tsp cistanche

½ tsp chaga

Sweetener of choice (stevia, lo han guo, xylitol, inulin, jerusalem artichoke syrup, yacon syrup, maple syrup, birch syrup, and/or raw honey)

Neem Clean Green Drink

12 oz. water

4–8 leaves neem (depending on size)

¼ tsp sea salt

Juice from one lemon

Blend on high until mildly warm from blender, then drink.

Seaweed Soup

1 cup kelp strips, cut up

2 tbsp coconut oil

½–1 tbsp lemon juice

½–1 tbsp *nama shoyu*

½ tbsp *hacho miso*

1 tsp kuzu root

1 tsp umeboshi plum puree

½–1 tbsp organic curry powder

½–1 tbsp organic Mexican spice blend

1 dropper daily ginger extract

1 cup twig tea with gynostemma base

To prepare the kelp: Soak kelp strips in hot water or tea for a few minutes, then strain. Once the kelp strips are prepared, blend all ingredients.

Unwanted Guest Removal Tonic

    3 tbsp raw pumpkin seeds (dry)

    4 oz. beet juice

    4 oz. apple juice

    4 oz. coconut water kefir or Rejuvelac

    ½ tsp ginger juice

    1 squirt ocean trace minerals

    2 drops peppermint essential oil

    2 squirts olive leaf tincture

    Juice from one lemon

Preblend raw pumpkin seeds, stir powdered pumpkin seeds into juice, add the rest of the ingredients, and serve.

Agariki Mushroom Soup

Immune Mushroom Broth

    10 oz. hot gynostemma tea

    1 tbsp miso paste

    1 tbsp coconut oil

    6 capsules agaricus mushroom, opened (1 tsp extract powder)

    3 capsules lion's mane mushroom, opened (½ tsp extract powder)

Blend well and serve.

Clove Bud Chai Tea

    12 oz. water

    1 tsp clove buds

    ¼ tsp ginger juice *or* 1 squirt ginger tincture

    ⅛ tsp cardamom powder

    1 tbsp coconut oil

    2 oz. raw nut milk *or* 1 tbsp raw cashews

    A dash cinnamon

Sweetener of choice (stevia, lo han guo, xylitol, inulin, jerusalem artichoke syrup, yacon syrup, maple syrup, birch syrup, and/or raw honey)

Boil the water with the clove buds for 10 minutes, strain tea, add to blender. Add the other ingredients to the blender. Blend on high for 40 seconds and serve!

Vanilla Shilajit Latte

10 oz. hot gynostemma tea *or* other mild tea as base

1–2 tsp shilajit powder

1 tsp vanilla powder

1 tbsp coconut oil

2 oz. raw nut milk *or* 2 tbsp raw cashews

1 squirt ocean trace minerals

Sweetener of choice (stevia, lo han guo, xylitol, inulin, jerusalem artichoke syrup, yacon syrup, maple syrup, birch syrup, and/or raw honey)

Cordyceps Ice Cream

20 oz. ice cubes

1 heaping tbsp raw maca

1 heaping tbsp mesquite meal

1 heaping tbsp lucuma powder

3 heaping tbsp tocotrienols

6 capsules cordyceps mushroom, opened (or 1 tbsp extract powder)

1-½ tbsp birch xylitol

½ tsp vanilla powder

1 squirt stevia

1–2 oz. raw nut milk

Use a blender with plunger capability. Put all ingredients in blender. Turn blender on high and plunge vigorously until you have an ice cream texture. Scoop out and serve as ice cream!

Reishi Chagaccino

Immune Mushroom Drink

10 oz. hot gynostemma tea

6–9 capsules chaga, opened (1 to 1-½ tsp extract powder)

2–4 capsules reishi, opened (⅓ to ⅔ tsp extract powder)

1 heaping tbsp raw cacao powder

1 tbsp cacao nibs

1 squirt ocean trace minerals

1-½ tbsp coconut oil

2–3 oz. raw nut milk *or* 2–3 tbsp raw cashews

Dash of cinnamon

Sweetener of choice (stevia, lo han guo, xylitol, inulin, jerusalem artichoke syrup, yacon syrup, maple syrup, birch syrup, and/or raw honey)

Blend on high 40 seconds and serve.

Immune Balance Tea

10 oz. hot gynostemma tea

3 capsules coriolus versicolor mushroom, opened (½ tsp extract powder)

4 capsules maitake mushroom, opened (⅔ tsp extract powder)

4 capsules shiitake mushroom, opened (⅔ tsp extract powder)

1–2 tsp camu

1 squirt ocean trace minerals

Sweetener of choice (stevia, lo han guo, xylitol, inulin, jerusalem artichoke syrup, yacon syrup, maple syrup, birch syrup, and/or raw honey)

Blend and serve.

Super Vitamin C Berry Anti-Inflammatory Smoothie

1–2 tbsp goji berries

2 tsp non-GMO lecithin powder (or granules)

2 tbsp coconut oil

2 tbsp unheated raw honey

4 oz. hot gynostemma tea *or* other mild tea *or* water

1 piece fresh ginger (1-½ by ½ inches)

1 piece fresh turmeric (1-½ by ½ inches)

1 apple, peeled and chopped

2 kiwis, peeled and chopped

1 lime, peeled and chopped

12 oz. orange juice

8 oz. coconut water kefir

12 oz. ice

4 squirts ocean trace minerals

3 tbsp flax oil

3 tsp camu

To a clean blender, add the goji berries, lecithin, coconut oil, honey, and hot gynostemma tea. Blend on high for 40 seconds. Add the rest of the ingredients and blend on high for 40 seconds more. Serve.

Noni Colada

1 tsp noni powder

4 oz. pineapple, chopped

⅛ tsp cinnamon

⅛ tsp nutmeg

1 tbsp raw unheated honey

Coconut water kefir

Ice cubes

This tart, effervescent drink tastes great! Fill a 12 oz. cup with ice cubes, then cover the ice with the coconut water kefir until the cup is ¾ full. Pour the ice and kefir into a blender and add the other ingredients. Blend and serve.

Berry AO Immune Boost

AO = Anti-Oxidant

½ cup ice

8 oz. coconut water kefir *or* Rejuvalac

1 tbsp freeze-dried açaí powder

1 oz. black elderberry syrup

1 capsule rhodiola, opened

1 tbsp colloidal silver

1 squirt ocean trace minerals

Sweetener of choice (stevia, lo han guo, xylitol, inulin, jerusalem artichoke syrup, yacon syrup, maple syrup, birch syrup, and/or raw honey)

"AO" means "antioxidant." This rejuvenating and refreshing drink tastes excellent! Just blend all ingredients and serve.

Fulvic Diet Soda Detox

4 oz. fulvic *or* humic/fulvic liquid minerals

6 oz. coconut water kefir

1 squirt ocean trace minerals (optional)

½ to 1 squirt stevia

Give the combined ingredients a quick stir, and serve.

Probiotic Margarita

½ cup ice

8 oz. coconut water kefir

1 tbsp lemon juice

¼ tsp ginger juice *or* 1 squirt ginger tincture

1 tbsp acidophilus powder (dairy-free)

1 tbsp bifidus powder (dairy-free)

2 tbsp tocotrienols

1 squirt ocean trace minerals

Sweetener of choice (stevia, raw honey, clear agave)

Blend and serve.

Macro Digestive Tea

12 oz. water, plus ½ tsp water

1 kukicha twig tea bag

1 tsp wild kuzu root starch

½ tsp umeboshi plum paste

½ tsp *nama shoyu*

¼ tsp ginger juice

Boil the 12 oz. water and pour over tea bag in a mug. In a second mug, add the rest of the ingredients (including the ½ tsp of water) and stir into a smooth paste—the back end of a chopstick works well for this. Pour the tea over the paste, stir, and serve.

Antistress Adaptogenic Tonic

- 12 oz. hot gynostemma tea
- 2 softgels Supercritical Holy Basil
- 1 capsule rhodiola, opened
- 3 squirts Siberian ginseng *or* ½ tsp powder
- 3 squirts American ginseng *or* ½ tsp powder
- 3 capsules reishi (½ tsp powder)
- 3 squirts Chinese asparagus root *(tain mein dong)* or ½ tsp powder
- 6 capsules *ho shou wu,* opened (½ tbsp powder)
- 1 tsp mucuna powder
- 1 squirt ocean trace minerals
- Sweetener of choice (stevia, lo han guo, xylitol, inulin, jerusalem artichoke syrup, yacon syrup, maple syrup, birch syrup, and/or raw honey)

Blend and serve.

Brazil Nuts for Strawberry Gelato

- 1 bag organic frozen strawberries
- 4 oz. ice cubes
- 1 heaping tbsp mesquite meal
- 1 heaping tbsp lucuma powder
- 3 heaping tbsp tocotrienols
- 1 tbsp raw unheated honey
- 4 Brazil nuts
- ½ tsp camu
- 1 oz. nut milk (optional)

Using a blender with plunging capacity, blend all ingredients on high, pounding with plunger vigorously until smooth like gelato (the optional nut milk can make this easier). Scoop out of the blender and serve!

Note: Recipes courtesy of Los Angeles–based herbalist Truth Calkins

LONGEVITY NOW SHOPPING LIST

This is your shopping list! Please be "underwhelmed" by it. Remember: Just add. Add a little bit at a time (or a lot!). This list represents the best superfoods, superherbs, super supplements, and healing longevity products on the planet!

- acerola
- agaricus blazei
- aged garlic extracts
- amla
- angelica root
- ashwagandha
- asparagus root
- astragalus
- betaine hydrochloride
- black walnut
- Bongers
- brahmi (bacopa)
- camu camu
- cat's claw (extract, powder and/or tea)
- chaga
- chanca piedra
- citric acid (citrate)
- cloves
- cordyceps
- crystal energy
- deer antler
- DMSO
- EDTA (optional)
- enzymes
- eucommia bark
- fulvic acid
- ginseng
- gravel root
- grounding technologies
- gua sha tool
- gynostemma
- ho shou wu
- jujube
- krill oil *or* algae oil
- licorice
- lion's mane
- Longevity Zapper
- lysine
- maitake
- mangosteen
- marine phytoplankton
- megahydrate
- MSM
- neem
- noni fruit-seed powder
- probiotics (friendly bacteria)
- raw butter and cream

- rebounder
- reishi
- rhodiola (arctic root)
- Schizandra berry
- shiitake
- shilajit (optional)
- sugarcane
- trametes versicolor (PSP and PSK)
- tulsi
- vitamin B12
- wormwood
- zeolites
- zinc

I believe strongly that I am presenting a leading edge in nutrition information—information that has literally been gifted forward to me by the world's experts. An entire history of discoveries has been stacked together to allow for the creation of Longevity Now. The valuable resources listed in this section will help you continue with your studies.

Other Books by David Wolfe

- *Amazing Grace,* by David Wolfe and Nick Good
- *Chaga: King of the Medicinal Mushrooms,* by David Wolfe
- *Eating for Beauty,* by David Wolfe
- *Naked Chocolate,* by David Wolfe and Shazzie
- *The Sunfood Diet Success System,* by David Wolfe
- *Superfoods: The Food and Medicine of the Future,* by David Wolfe

Nutrition and Health

- *The Ancient Wisdom of the Chinese Tonic Herbs,* by Ron Teeguarden
- *The Body Ecology Diet,* by Donna Gates
- *The Calcium Bomb,* by Douglas Mulhall and Katja Hansen
- *Cancer,* by Dr. Matthias Rath
- *Chew on This,* by Eric Schlosser and Charles Wilson
- *The Coconut Oil Miracle,* by Bruce Fife
- *Conscious Eating,* by Dr. Gabriel Cousens
- *Control for Life Extension,* by Valery Mamanov
- *The Cure for All Diseases,* by Dr. Hulda Clark
- *The DMSO Handbook,* by Dr. Bruce Halstead
- *DMSO: Nature's Healer,* by Dr. Morton Walker
- *Doctor Yourself,* by Andrew Saul

- *Dr. Spock's Baby and Child Care,* by Benjamin Spock, MD, and Stephen J. Parker, MD
- *Enzyme Nutrition,* by Dr. Edward Howell
- *Extreme Toxicity,* by Howard Fisher
- *Flood Your Body with Oxygen,* by Ed McCabe
- *Food Combining and Digestion,* by Steve Meyerowitz
- *Food Combining Made Easy,* by Dr. Herbert Shelton
- *Food Enzymes for Health and Longevity,* by Dr. Edward Howell
- *The Garlic Cure,* by James F. Scheer, Lynn Allison, and Charlie Fox
- *Honey in Nutrition,* by William Miller
- *The LifeFood Recipe Book,* by Dr. David Jubb
- *Minerals for the Genetic Code,* by Charles Walters
- *Mycelium Running,* by Paul Stamets
- *MycoMedicinals,* by Paul Stamets
- *New Foods Encyclopedia,* by Rebecca Wood
- *Parasites: The Enemy Within,* by Hanna Kroeger
- *The Rainbow Green Live-Food Cuisine,* by Dr. Gabriel Cousens
- *Sea Energy Agriculture,* by Dr. Maynard Murray
- *Spiritual Nutrition,* by Dr. Gabriel Cousens
- *Trace Minerals and Man,* by Henry Schroeder
- *Wild Fermentation,* by Sandor Katz

Betaine Hydrochloride

- http://altmedicine.about.com/cs/homeremedies/a/Betaine.htm

Body Electronics

- www.howweheal.com/be.htm
- http://rawpaleodiet.vpinf.com/healing-body-electronics.html

Deer Antler

- www.LongevityWarehouse.com

Milk

- www.notmilk.com
- *Milk: The Deadly Poison,* by Robert Cohen

Soy

- *Myths and Truths about Soy Foods,* by Sally Fallon, Mary G. Enig, PhD, and Mike Fitzpatrick, PhD
- For references and additional information, send $12 to Soy Alert!, 4200 Wisconsin Avenue #106-336, Washington, DC 20007.

NOTES

Chapter 1. Nutrition and Diet

1. W. Schuphan, "Nutritional Value of Crops as Influenced by Organic and Inorganic Fertilizer Treatments. Results of 12 Years' Experiments with Vegetables (1960–1972)," *Qual. Plant Pl. Fds. Hum. Nutr.* 23, no. 4 (1974): 333–58.
2. Bob L. Smith, "Organic Foods vs Supermarket Foods: Element Levels," *Journal of Applied Nutrition* 45, no. 1 (1993): 35–39.
3. "Body Burden: The Pollution in Newborns," www.ewg.org/research /body-burden-pollution-newborns.
4. E. Fombonne, "The Prevalence of Autism," *JAMA* 289 no. 1 (2003): 87–9; L. Wing and D. Potter, "The Epidemiology of Autistic Spectrum Disorders: Is the Prevalence Rising?" *Ment Retard Dev Disabil Res Rev.* 8, no. 3 (2002): 151–61.
5. Paul Kouchakoff, MD, "The Influence of Food Cooking on the Blood Formula of Man," Proceedings: First International Congress of Microbiology, Paris 1930. Translation by Lee Foundation for Nutritional Research, Milwaukee, Wisconsin. Available in pdf form at www.igien -enaturale.it/Post-Prandial Leucocytosis.pdf.
6. Victor Kulvinskas, "Don't Dine without Enzymes," a booklet available digitally at http://loveinservice.tripod.com/viktoraskulvinskas/id2.html.
7. Maynard Murray, MD, *Sea Energy Agriculture* (Austin, TX: Acres USA, 2003).
8. Bernard Jensen, *Dr. Jensen's Juicing Therapy: Nature's Way to Better Health and a Longer Life* (Lincolnwood, IL: Keats Publishing, 200).

Chapter 2. The Essential Raw Plant Food Groups

1. Dr. William Davis, *Wheat Belly* (Toronto, ON: HarperCollins, 2011), 43–54.
2. I. Tomida et al., "Effect of Sublingual Application of Cannabinoids on Intraocular Pressure: A Pilot Study," *J Glaucoma* 15, no. 5 (Oct 2006): 329–53; Alison Mack and Janet Joy, *Marijuana as Medicine: The Science beyond the Controversy* (Washington, DC: National Academies Press, 2001).

3. J. Thomas Ungerleider, et al., "Delta-9-THC in the Treatment of Spasticity Associated with Multiple Sclerosis," *Advances in Alcohol & Substance Abuse* 7, no. 1 (1998), 39–50; John Zajicek et al., "Cannabinoids for Treatment of Spasticity and Other Symptoms Related to Multiple Sclerosis (Cams Study): Multicenter Randomised Placebo-Controlled Trial," *The Lancet* 362 (Nov. 8, 2003), 1517–26; Derick T. Wade et al., "Do Cannabis-based Medicinal Extracts Have General or Specific Effects on Symptoms in Multiple Sclerosis? A Double-Blind, Randomized, Placebo-controlled Study on 160 Patients," *Multiple Sclerosis* 10, no. 4 (August 2004), 434–41.

4. M. M. el-Sheikh et al., "The Effect of Permixon on Androgen Receptors," *Acta Obstet Gynecol Cand* 67, no. 5 (1988), 397–99.

5. "Believed to Be World's Oldest, Woman in France Dies at 122," *Houston Chronicle,* August 4, 1997.

6. P. Bucheli et al., "Goji Berry Effects on Macular Characteristics and Plasma Antioxidant Levels," *Optom Vis Sci* 88, no. 2 (February 1988): 257–62.

7. Jae-Dong Lee, et al., "An Overview of Bee Venom Acupuncture in the Treatment of Arthritis," *Evidence-Based Complementary and Alternative Medicine* 2, no. 1 (2005) 79–84.

Chapter 3. Foods to Avoid

1. Romina Pedreschi et al., "Andean Yacon Root (*Smallanthus sonchifolius* Poepp. Endl) Fructooligosaccharides as a Potential Novel Source of Prebiotics," *Agric. Food Chem.* 51, no. 18 (2003): 5278–84.

2. For just one example, Gilles-Eric Séralini, "Long Term Toxicity of a Roundup Herbicide and a Roundup-Tolerant Genetically Modified Maize," *Food and Chemical Toxicology* 50, no. 11 (Nov. 2012), 4211–31.

3. Institute for Responsible Technology, "State-of-the-Science on the Health Risks of GM Foods." Excellently referenced paper on current GMO research. Found online at www.saynotogmos.org/paper.pdf.

4. Jean Weiss, "12 Food Additives to Avoid," MSN Health & Fitness, http://healthyliving.msn.com/nutrition/12-food-additives-to-avoid-1.

5. Mary G. Enig, "The Soy Controversy," presented on May 25, 2001 at the 8th International Symposium of the Institute for Preventive Medicine in Vancouver, Canada. Summary available online at www.nutritions-playground.com/soycontroversy.

6. "Greenland Ice Core Reveals History of Pollution in the Arctic," National Science Foundation press release 08-142, August 18, 2008, www.nsf .gov/news/news_summ.jsp?cntn_id=112074.

7. United States Environmental Protection Agency, "Water on Tap: What You Need to Know," December 2009, United States Environmental Protection Agency, available at www.epa.gov/ogwdw/wot/pdfs/book_wate-rontap_full.pdf.

**Chapter 5. Hormones: The Natural Approach
for Women and Men**

1. References for this hormone health section include the following: E. I. Barengolts et al., "Effects of Progesterone on Postovariectomy Bone Loss in Aged Rats," *Journal of Bone and Mineral Research* 5, no. 11 (1990): 1143–47; E. I. Barengolts et al., "Comparison of the Effects of Progesterone and Estrogen on Established Bone Loss in Ovariectomized Rats," *Scanning Microscopy International,* Cell and Materials Supplement 1 (1991), 108; Dr. John Lee and Virginia Hopkins, *What Your Doctor May Not Tell You about Menopause* (New York, NY: Warner Books, 2004); Dr. John Lee and Virginia Hopkins, *What Your Doctor May Not Tell You about Pre-Menopause* (New York, NY: Warner Books, 1991); Dr. John Lee and Virginia Hopkins, *Dr. John Lee's Hormone Balance Made Simple* (New York, NY: Warner Books, 2006).

2. North American Menopause Society, "Estrogen and Progestogen Use in Postmenopausal Women: 2010 Position Statement of the North American Menopause Society, *Menopause* 17, no. 2 (2010): 242–55, www.menopause.org/PSht10.pdf; Million Women Study Collaborators, "Breast Cancer and Hormone-Replacement Therapy in the Million Women Study," *Lancet* 362, no. 9382 (2003): 419–27; Women's Health Initiative Steering Committee, "Effects of Conjugated Equine Estrogen in Postmenopausal Women with Hysterectomy," *JAMA,* 291, no. 14 (2004): 1701–712; L. Speroff et al., "Menopause and the Perimenopausal Transition," in *Clinical Gynecologic Endocrinology and Infertility,* 7th ed. (Philadelphia: Lippincott Williams and Wilkins Philadelphia: Lippincott Williams and Wilkins, 2005), 621–88; G. A. Bachmann et al., "Lowest Effective Transdermal 17beta-Estradiol Dose for Relief of Hot Flashes in Postmenopausal Women," *Obstetrics and Gynecology* 110, no. 4 (2007): 771–79.

3. Olivia A. M. Franks, ND, and Jonathan V. Wright, MD, "Estriol: Its Weakness Is Its Strength," *Life Extension Magazine,* August 2008. www.lef.org /magazine/mag2008/aug2008_Estriol-Its-Weakness-is-its-Strength_01.htm.

4. The source for this information on foods and breast cancer is D. T. Zava et al., "Estrogen and Progestin Bioactivity of Foods, Herbs, and Spices," *Proc Soc Exp Biol Med.* 217, no. 3 (March 1998): 369–78.

5. Research in support of cannabis use to treat hormonal cancers includes María M. Caffarel et al., "Cannabinoids: A New Hope for Breast Cancer Therapy?" *Cancer Treat Rev.* 38, no. 7 (Nov. 2012): 911–18. Research against using cannabis for hormonal cancers includes S. Takeda et al., "Delta(9)-Tetrahydrocannabinol Enhances MCF-7 Cell Proliferation via Cannabinoid Receptor-Independent Signaling," *Toxicology* 245, no. 1–2 (March 12, 2008): 141–46.

6. Dr. Daniel Cramer, "Coffee May Boost Estrogen Levels on Women," *Fertility and Sterility* 76 (October 2001): 723–29.

7. Ray Peat, "Progesterone Summaries," http://raypeat.com/articles/articles/progesterone-summaries.shtml.

8. International Osteoporosis Foundation, "Facts and Statistics," www.iof bonehealth.org/facts-statistic.

9. H. S. Aiyer, "Dietary Berries and Ellagic Acid Diminish Estrogen-Mediated Mammary Tumorigenesis in ACI Rats," *Nutr Cancer* 60, no. 2 (2008): 227–34.

10. Z. Papoutsi et al., "Evaluation of Estrogenic/Antiestrogenic Activity of Ellagic Acid via the Estrogen Receptor Subtypes ERalpha and ERbeta," *J Agric Food Chem.* 53, no. 20 (October 5, 2005): 7715–20.

11. For more on I3C's antiviral effects, see Terry Dorene Stoner, "Indole-3-Carbinol Inhibition of Herpes Simplex Virus Replication," a December 2008 dissertation submitted to Kent State University, available at http://tinyurl.com/n3doq25.

12. Amy Norton, "Estrogen-like Lignan Diet, Less Breast Cancer Linked," Reuters, June 4, 2010, http://tinyurl.com/mmlnqb3.

13. Here is the controversial Israeli study connecting melatonin to lowering estradiol: R. Luboshitzky et al., "Melatonin Administration Alters Semen Quality in Healthy Men," *J Androl.* 23 no. 4 (July–Aug. 2002): 572–78. See also T. Kiefer et al, "Melatonin Inhibits Estrogen Receptor

Transactivation and Camp Levels in Breast Cancer Cells," *Breast Cancer Res Treat* 71 no. 1 (Jan. 2002): 37–45.

14. BioInitiative 2012 report, available at www.bioinitiative.org.

15. J. Zhao et al. "Antiaromatase Activity of the Constituents from Damiana *(Turnera diffusa),*" *Journal of Ethnopharmacology* 120 (December 2008): 387–93.

16. Rosário Monteiro, "Effect of Hop (*Humulus lupulus* L.) Flavonoids on Aromatase (Estrogen Synthase) Activity," *J. Agric. Food Chem.* 54, no. 8 (2006): 2938–43.

17. J. Strathmann et al., "Xanthohumol from Hops Prevents Hormone-Dependent Tumourigenesis In Vitro and In Vivo," *Acta Hort. (ISHS)* 848 (2009): 179–90.

18. M. M. el-Sheikh et al., "The Effect of Permixon on Androgen Receptors," *Acta Obstet Gynecol Cand* 67, no. 5 (1988), 397–99.

19. D. T. Zava et al., "Estrogen and Progestin Bioactivity of Foods, Herbs, and Spices," *Proc Soc Exp Biol Med.* 217, no. 3 (March 1998): 369–78.

20. G. Zhang et al., "Epimedium-derived Phytoestrogen Flavonoids Exert Beneficial Effect on Preventing Bone Loss in Late Postmenopausal Women: A 24-Month Randomized, Double-Blind and Placebo-controlled Trial," *J Bone Miner Res.* 22, no. 7(2007): 1072–79.

21. M. M. el-Sheikh et al., "The Effect of Permixon on Androgen Receptors," *Acta Obstet Gynecol Cand* 67, no. 5 (1988), 397–99.

Chapter 6. Calcification, the Great Undertaker

1. The research results can be found at http://www.yourncdinfo.com /clinoptilolite-affinity-schedule.pdf. The same report states, "Clinoptilolite zeolite safely removes mercury, lead, tin, cadmium, arsenic, aluminum, antimony, nickel and all other toxic heavy metals."

Hormones and Longevity

Henry A. Feldman, Christopher Longcope, Carol A. Derby, Catherine B. Johannes, Andre B. Araujo, Andrea D. Coviello, William J. Bremner, and John B. McKinlay, "Age Trends in the Level of Serum Testosterone and Other Hormones in Middle-Aged Men: Longitudinal Results from the Massachusetts Male Aging Study," *The Journal of Clinical Endocrinology & Metabolism* 87.2 (2002): 589–98.

Stephanie J. Fonda, Rosanna Bertrand, Amy O'Donnell, Christopher Longcope, and John B. McKinlay, "Age, Hormones, and Cognitive Functioning Among Middle-Aged and Elderly Men: Cross-Sectional Evidence From the Massachusetts Male Aging Study," *Journal of Gerontology: Medical Sciences* 60 (2005): 385–90.

Martin Hermann and Peter Berger, "Hormonal Changes in Aging Men: A Therapeutic Indication?," *Experimental Gerontology* 36.7 (2001): 1075–82.

Martin Hermann and Peter Berger, "Hormone Replacement in the Aging Male?," *Experimental Gerontology* 34.8 (1999): 901–1036.

B. Lapauw, S. Goemaere, H. Zmierczak, I. Van Pottelbergh, A. Mahmoud, Y. Taes, D. De Bacquer, S. Vansteelandt, and J. M. Kaufman, "The Decline of Serum Testosterone Levels in Community-Dwelling Men Over 70 Years of Age: Descriptive Data and Predictors of Longitudinal Changes," *European Journal of Endocrinology* 159.4 (2008): 459–68.

E. Leifke, V. Gorenoi, C. Wichers, A. Von Zur Mühlen, E. Von Büren, G. Brabant, "Age-related Changes of Serum Sex Hormones, Insulin-Like Growth Factor-1 and Sex-Hormone Binding Globulin Levels in Men: Cross-Sectional Data from a Healthy Male Cohort," *Clinical Endocrinology* 53.6 (2008): 689–95.

D. Rudman, A. G. Feller, H. S. Nagraj, G. A. Gergans, P. Y. Lalitha, A. F. Goldberg, R. A. Schlenker, L. Cohn, I. W. Rudman, and D. E. Mattson, "Effects of Human Growth Hormone in Men Over 60 Years Old," *New England Journal of Medicine* 323 (1990): 1–6.

Stefan Schlatt, Clifford R. Pohl, Jens Ehmcke, and Suresh Ramaswamy, "Age-Related Changes in Diurnal Rhythms and Levels of Gonadotropins, Testosterone, and Inhibin B in Male Rhesus Monkeys (Macaca mulatta)," *Biology of Reproduction* 79 (2008): 93–99.

Dominique Simon, Paul Preziosi, Elizabeth Barrett-Connor, Marc Roger, Michel Saint-Paul, Khalil Nahoul, and Laure Papoz, "The Influence of Aging on Plasma Sex Hormones in Men: The Telecom Study," *American Journal of Epidemiology* 135.7 (1992): 783–79.

Johannes D. Veldhuis, Ali Iranmanesh, and Thomas Mulligan, "Age and Testosterone Feedback Jointly Control the Dose-Dependent Actions of Gonadotropin-Releasing Hormone in Healthy Men," *Journal of Clinical Endocrinology & Metabolism* 90.1 (2005): 302–309.

Xanthohumol (Hops Extract)

B. B. Aggarwal, H. Ichikawa, P. Garodia, et al. "From Traditional Ayurvedic Medicine to Modern Medicine: Identification of Therapeutic Targets for Suppression of Inflammation and Cancer." *Expert Opinion Therapeutic Targets* 10. (2006): 87–118.

A. Albini, R. Dell'Eva, Vene R, et al. "Mechanisms of the Antiangiogenic Activity by the Hop Flavonoid Xanthohumol: Nf-Kappa B and Akt As Targets." *Faseb J.* 20 (2006): 527–529.

W. J. Chen, J. K. Lin. "Mechanisms of Cancer Chemoprevention by Hop Bitter Acids (Beer Aroma) Through Induction of Apoptosis Mediated by Fas and Caspase Cascades." *J Agric Food Chem.* 52 (2004): 55–64.

E. C. Colgate, C. L. Miranda, J. F. Stevens, et al. "Xanthohumol, a Prenylflavonoid Derived from Hops Induces Apoptosis and Inhibits NF-Kappa B Activation in Prostate Epithelial Cells." *Cancer Lett.* 246 (2007): 201–9.

E. C. Colgate, C. L. Miranda, J. F. Stevens, T. M. Bray, E. Ho. "Xanthohumol, a Prenylflavonoid Derived from Hops Induces Apoptosis And Inhibits NF-Kappab Activation in Prostate Epithelial Cells." *Cancer Lett.* 246 (2007): 201–209.

L. Delmulle, T. V. Berghe, D. D. Keukeleire, P. Vandenabeele. "Treatment of PC-3 and DU145 Prostate Cancer Cells by Prenylflavonoids from Hop (Humulus Lupulus L.) Induces a Caspase Independent Form of Cell Death." *Phytother Res.* 22 (2008): 197–203.

B. M. Dietz, Y. H. Kang, G. Liu G, et al. "Xanthohumol Isolated From Humulus Lupulus Inhibits Menadione-Induced DNA Damage Through Induction Of Quinone Reductase." *Chem Res Toxicol.* 18 (2005): 1296–1305.

C. Gerhauser, A. Alt, E. Heiss, et al. "Cancer Chemopreventive Activity of Xanthohumol, a Natural Product Derived From Hop." *Mot Cancer Thor.* 1 (2002): 959–969.

K. Goto, T. Asai, S. Hara, et al. "Enhanced Antitumor Activity of Xanthohumol, a Diacylglycerol Acyltransferase Inhibitor, Under Hypoxia." *Cancer Lett.* 219 (2005): 215–222.

M. C. Henderson, C. L. Miranda, J. F. Stevens, M. L. Deinzer, D. R. Buhler. "In Vitro Inhibition of Human P450 Enzymes by Prenylated Flavonoids from Hops, Humulus Lupulus." *Xenobiotica.* 30 (2000): 235–251.

S. H. Lee, H. J. Kim, J. S. Lee, I. S. Lee, B. Y. Kang. "Inhibition of Topoisomerase I Activity and Efflux Drug Transporters' Expression by Xanthohumol from Hops." *Arch Pharm Res.* 30 (2007): 1435–1439.

S. Lust, B. Vanhoecke, A. Janssens, J. Philippe, M. Bracke, F. Offner. "Xanthohumol Kills Bchronic Lymphocytic Leukemia Cells by an Apoptotic Mechanism." *Mol Nutr Food Res.* 49 (2005): 844–850.

C. L. Miranda, J. F. Stevens, A. Helmrich, et al. "Antiproliferative and Cytotoxic Effects of Prenylated Flavonoids From Hops (Humulus Lupulus) in Human Cancer Cell Lines." *Food Chem Toxicol.* 37 (1999): 271–285.

R. Monteiro, A. Faria, I. Azevedo, C. Calhau. "Modulation of Breast Cancer Cell Survival by Aromatase Inhibiting Hop 4 (Humulus Lupulus L.) Flavonoids." *1 Steroid Biochem Mal Biol.* 105 (2007): 124–130.

L. Pan, H. Becker, C. Gerhauser. "Xanthohumol Induces Apoptosis in Cultured 40-16 Human Colon Cancer Cells by Activation of the Death Receptor and Mitochondria Pathway." *Mol Nut Food Res.* 49 (2005): 837–843.

J. F. Stevens, A. W. Taylor, M. L. Deinzer. "Quantitative Analysis of Xanthohumol and Related Prenylflavonoids in Hops and Beer by Liquid Chromatography-Tandem Mass Spectrometry." *J Chromatogr A.* 832 (1999): 97–107.

N. Tabata, M. Ito, H. Tomoda, S. Omura. "Xanthohumols, Diacylglyceral Acyltransferase Inhibitors, from Humulus Lupulus." *Phytochemistry.* 46 (1997): 683–687.

H. Tobe, Y. Muraki, K. Kitamura, et al. "Bone Resorption Inhibitors from Hop Extract." *Biosci Biotechnol Biochem.* 61 (1997): 158–459.

B. Vanhoecke, L. Derycke, V. Van Marck, H. Depypere, D. De Keukeleire, M. Bracke. "Anti-invasive Effect of Xanthohumol, a Prenylated Chalcone Present in Hops (Humulus Lupulus L.) and Beer." *Int J Cancer.* 117 (2005): 889–895.

J. Y. Yang, M. A. Della-Fera, S. Rayalam, C. A. Baile. "Effect of Xanthohumol and isoXanthohumol on 3T3-L1 Cell Apoptosis and Adipogenesis." *Apoptosis.* 12 (2007): 1953–1963.

F. Zhao, H. Nozawa, A. Daikomiya, K. Kondo, S. Kitanaka. "Inhibitors of Nitric Oxide Production from Hops (Humulus lupulus L.)." *Biol Pharm Bull.* 26 (2003): 61–65.

Nanobacteria (Calcium-Forming Micro-Organisms)

Amit Asaravala, "Are Nanobacteria Making Us Ill?" *Wired,* March 14, 2005.

J. Kelly Beatty, "Life at the Limit," *Sky & Telescope,* September 1999.

Mikael Bjorklund, Neva Ciftcioglu, and E. Olavi Kajander, "Extraordinary Survival of Nanobacteria under Extreme Conditions," *Society of Photographic Instrumentation Engineers Journal* (SPIE) 3441 (1998): 123–29.

Neva Ciftcioglu, Mikael Bjorklund, and E. Olavi Kajander, "Stone Formation and Calcification by Nanobacteria in Human Body," SPIE 3441 (1998): 105–11.

David S. Goldfarb, "Microorganisms and Calcium Oxalate Stone Disease," *Nephron Physiol* 98 (2004): 48–54.

Professor Allan Hamilton, "Nanobacteria: Gold Mine Or Minefield of Intellectual Enquiry?," *Microbiology Today* (November 2000): 182–184.

Jenny Hogan, "Are Nanobacteria Alive Or Just Strange Crystals?" *New Scientist* 182, 2448 (2004): 6–7.

G. Hudelist, C. F. Singer, E. Kubista, M. Manavi, R. Mueller, K. Pischinger, K. Czerwenka, "Presence of Nanobacteria in Psammoma Bodies of Ovarian Cancer: Evidence for Pathogenetic Role in Intratumoral Biomineralization," *Histopathology* 45 (2004): 633–37.

Tomislav Jelic, Amer Malas, Samuel Groves, Bo Jin, Paul Mellen, Garry Osborne, Rod Roque, James Rosencrance, Ho-Huang Chang, Case Report: "Nanobacteria-caused Mitral Valve Calciphylaxis in a Man with

Diabetic Renal Failure," *Southern Medical Journal* 97.2 (February 2004): 194–98.

Fred Jueneman, "Life Size," *R&D Magazine* (February 2000), www.rdmag.com.

E. Olavi Kajander and Neva Ciftcioglu, "Nanobacteria as Extremophiles," *SPIE* 3755 (1999): 106.

Benedict S. Maniscalco, Karen A. Taylor, "Calcification in Coronary Artery Disease Can Be Reversed by EDTA-Tetracycline Long-Term Chemotherapy," *Pathophysiology* 11.2 (October 2004): 95–101.

Virginia M. Miller, George Rodgers, Jon A. Charlesworth, Brenda Kirkland, Sandra R. Severson, Todd E. Rasmussen, Marineh Yagubyan, Jeri C. Rodgers, Franklin R. Cockerill, III, Robert L. Folk, Ewa Rzewuska-Lech, Vivek Kumar, Gerard Farell-Baril, and John C. Lieske, "Evidence of Nanobacterial-Like Structures in Calcified Human Arteries and Cardiac Valves," *Am J Physiol Heart Circ Physiol* 287 (2004): H1115–H1124.

Michael Morgan, "Nanobacteria and Calcinosis Cutis," *Journal of Cutaneous Pathology* 29 (2002): 173–75.

Douglass Mulhall, "The Nanobacteria Link to Heart Disease and Cancer," *Nexus Magazine* 12.5 (August–September 2005).

A. M. Pretorius, A. P. Sommer, K. M. Aho, E. O. Kajander, "HIV and Nanobacteria," *HIV Medicine* 5 (2004): 391–93.

Reuters, "Calcium Pills May Boost Heart Attack Risk," (January 16, 2008) www.canada.com.

Zoltan Rona, "The Nanobacteria Revolution: The Real Cause of Calcium Deposits?," *Alive: Canadian Journal of Health & Nutrition* (May 2005): 34–36.

Eric Taylor, Gary Curhan, "Role of Nutrition in the Formation of Calcium-Containing Kidney Stones," *Nephron Physiol* 98 (2004): 55–63.

Wulzen Factor

"A Study of the Assay Method for the Guinea Pig Anti-Stiffness Factor," by Bert E. Christensen, M.B. Naff, Vernon H. Cheldelin, Rosalind Wulzen (from the Departments of Chemistry and Zoology, Oregon State College) (Received for publication, April 16, 1948).

"The Wulzen Calcium Dystrophy Syndrome in Guinea Pigs," by Hugo Krueger, PhD.

Other Sources

Aspartame (Nutrasweet): Is It Safe?, by H. J. Roberts, MD (The Charles Press, Publishers, Inc. 1990).

The Calcium Bomb, by Douglas Mulhall and Katja Hansen (The Writer's Collection, 2005).

The Desktop Guide to Herbal Medicine, by Brigitte Mars, A.H.G. (Basic Health Publications Inc., 2007).

Don't Eat This Book: Fast Food and the Supersizing of America, by Morgan Spurlock (G.P. Putnam's Sons 2005).

The Essential Kombucha: The Manchurian Mushroom, by Andra Anastazia Malczewski (The Kombucha Network, 1995).

Excitotoxins: The Taste That Kills, by Russell L. Blaylock, MD (Health Press, 1997).

Extreme Toxic Times: How to Escape on Your Own Two Feet, by Dr. Howard W. Fisher (Wood Publishing, 2004).

Kombucha: Healthy Beverage and Natural Remedy from the Far East, by Gunther W. Frank (Publishing House W. Ennsthaler, 1995).

Silica: The Amazing Gel, by Klaus Kaufmann (Alive Books, 1993).

Silica: The Forgotten Nutrient, by Klaus Kaufmann (Alive Books, 1990).

INDEX

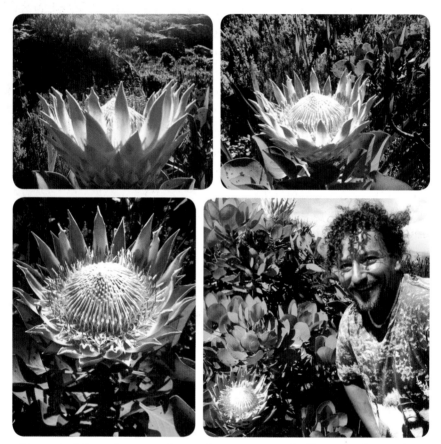

Everything in moderation, especially moderation. Glow like the sun. Live young as long as possible. Immortality is the only cause worth dying for.

ABOUT THE AUTHOR

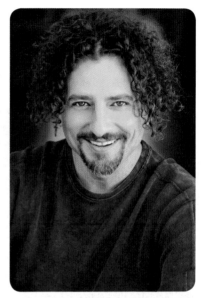

David "Avocado" Wolfe

Source: Michael Roud

You'd think David "Avocado" Wolfe was a rock star, with a fanbase like his: America's top CEOs, global ambassadors, Hollywood celebrities, busy professionals, and even the world's most powerful influencers—moms! But it's not rock 'n' roll that they flock to him for... it's his nutrition mission, and the natural health and beauty eco-revolution that he champions.

With a master's degree in nutrition and a background in science and mechanical engineering, David is considered one of the world's top authorities on natural health, beauty nutrition, herbalism, chocolate, organic superfoods, superherbs, and living spring water. Leading the field with his vision, education, and business, David has more than twenty years of dedicated professional experience in the health field.

With a lifelong passion for inspiring people to "Have The Best Day Ever," David has touched the hearts and minds of millions of people across the world. Through his down-to-earth and simple approach, David shows us that no problem is created without a solution, and that we have the opportunity, right at our fingertips, to make new choices about our lifestyle and take our health back into the power of our own hands.

David is the author of the following best-selling books:

- *Eating for Beauty*
- *The Sunfood Diet Success System*
- *Superfoods: The Food and Medicine of the Future*
- *Naked Chocolate*

379

- *Amazing Grace*
- *Chaga: King of the Medicinal Mushrooms*

He has also appeared in the following breakthrough films:

- *Food Matters*
- *Hungry for Change*
- *Discover the Gift*
- *The Frequency of Genius*
- *The Raw Natural*
- *Simply Raw: Reversing Diabetes in 30 Days*
- *The Serpent & the Sun*
- *Semisweet: Life in Chocolate*

David Wolfe empowers and inspires people to take charge of their health, even up against all the modern-day demands of bills, technology, environmental pollution, commuting, and inflation. David shows us that by making simple, informed decisions, we can all enjoy quality time for ourselves and with our family, because, after all, Health Is Wealth!

David currently represents his favorite blender kitchen appliance, the NutriBullet, on television and on the internet. David has founded several all-green and ecofriendly businesses that continue to lead the world with the most innovative, highest-quality organic superfoods and healthy lifestyle-related products and information. David Wolfe's leadership has been inspired by principles of sustainable agriculture, living in harmony with Nature, and ethical global cooperation.

Taking the world by storm with a trendsetting sense of ecochic style, David, groundbreaking businessman, entrepreneur, and lecturer, is like many other successful forty-somethings who are turning conventional living on its head and bringing awareness of green living and natural health into mainstream consciousness. By championing an environmentally friendly business, he is a living example of the next frontier of success technology. He is a sound believer in the power of the dollar to bring ecofriendly living into the mainstream, and he teaches, through his work, that by practicing just a few key principles, anyone can improve his or her health, fashion, physical appearance, and sense of well-being.

As an innovative environmentalist, David Wolfe is also the president and founder of The Fruit Tree Planting Foundation (www.ftpf.org), a nonprofit organization with a mission to plant eighteen billion fruit trees on planet Earth. David's organization has planted, to date, tens of thousands of fruit trees in locations spanning from Africa to Canada, from India to Hawaii.

In addition to running one of the busiest schedules anyone has ever seen, and setting the standard and precedent for the highest-quality level of clean, organic, and fair-trade superfoods and superherbs, David Wolfe privately consults and inspires the ordinary into the extraordinary, and the extraordinary into peak states of experience. A highly sought-after health and personal-success speaker, David has given more than 2,700 live lecture events in the past twenty years.

David is also a gourmet chocolatier. He is a passionate proponent of the healing and beautifying power of raw chocolate (cacao beans). By bringing cacao beans and nibs into mainstream distribution throughout North America, David has continued to promote the economies of indigenous cultures through ethical business. Just ask him—he won't be shy to tell you why chocolate is the greatest, most prosperous, nutritious, energizing, and top weight-loss aphrodisiac food on the planet! To try some of David's exotic chocolate, visit: www.sacredchocolate.com.

David Wolfe:

- Cofounder: TheBestDayEver.com online health magazine, Sacred Chocolate
- President: The Fruit Tree Planting Foundation, a nonprofit, www.ftpf.org
- Star: *The NutriBullet Show,* www.nutribullet.com
- Educator: Raw Nutrition Certification course, www.rawnutritioncertification.com
- Product Innovator: www.SacredChocolate.com, www.LongevityWarehouse.com

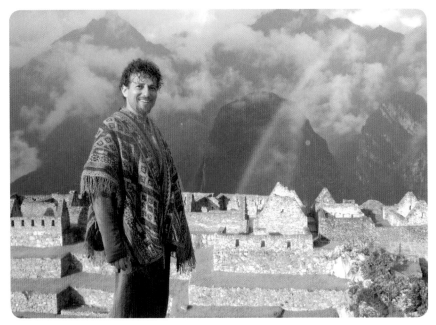

David "Avocado" Wolfe (Machu Picchu, Peru)

- Adventurer: Explore Exotic Locations with David, www.David WolfeAdventures.com
- Website: www.DavidWolfe.com
- Twitter: www.twitter.com/DavidWolfe
- Facebook: www.facebook.com/DavidAvocadoWolfe
- YouTube: www.youtube.com/DavidAvocadoWolfe
- Instagram: www.instagram.com/DavidAvocadoWolfe

Sacred Chocolate: The Best Source of Alkaline Magnesium

> Sacred Chocolate is clearly the best chocolate bar ever. Take one bite and you will know that Sacred Chocolate has cracked the cacao code!
>
> —DAVID WOLFE

Sacred Chocolate™ is committed to bringing you the highest-quality chocolate ever. From the cacao bean to each chocolate bar, Sacred Chocolate is infused with love, prayer, and gratitude. We honor, respect, and give thanks to all beings that make possible the amazing superfood known as chocolate. *Theobroma cacao,* which means the "food of God," is the scientific name for the chocolate tree. To our Sacred Chocolate team, this food is a holy sacrament, an offering to the higher power and a superfood for positive life transformation.

Our special chocolate is made over several days, the old-fashioned way: we slowly stone-grind raw cacao beans at a low temperature. Our cacao beans are never roasted, and all processes are kept below 114° F to ensure maximum antioxidant retention and zero trans-fatty acid production.

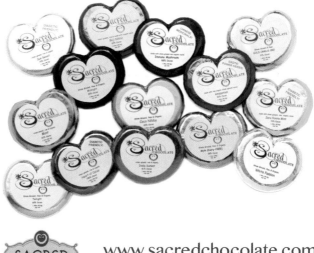

 www.sacredchocolate.com

Sacred Chocolate has an antioxidant rating (ORAC score) three to four times higher than that of a cooked dark chocolate bar of comparable cacao content. Our ingredients are raw (unroasted) wherever possible and always certified organic and/or wildcrafted. Sacred Chocolate is also certified vegan, kosher, and halal.

Our cacao is sold above fair-trade standards. We never use weak cacao "filler" beans to boost the cacao percentages of our bars, and we completely avoid cane sugar in all our products. Sacred Chocolate comes in rectangular bars as well as in the shape of a heart to symbolize that raw chocolate is good for the heart and that great love and care go into the making of this superfood treat.

Sacred Chocolate is extremely low in caffeine and, like all chocolate, contains theobromine, which is greatly superior to caffeine, since theobromine has cardiovascular- and lung-healing properties. Theobromine does not affect the central nervous system or constrict blood vessels. For those who want to reduce their coffee consumption, Sacred Chocolate is the healthiest alternative.

Theobromine dilates blood vessels and relaxes smooth muscle tissue, reducing the risk of cardiovascular challenges. For four decades (1890–1930), theobromine was injected into the bloodstream to revive heart attack victims. Theobromine also relaxes bronchial muscles in the lungs. Studies indicate that theobromine acts on the vagus nerve, which runs from the lungs to the brain. For this reason, chocolate has been found to be effective in reducing asthma symptoms.

Sacred Chocolate is the only chocolate product in the world that includes the microbe-free skin of the cacao bean for flavor and nutritional purposes. The delicate skin adds a fruity complexity to the flavor of Sacred Chocolate and also contains concentrated phytonutrients, analogous to the nutrition found in the skin of most fruits and vegetables. Sacred Chocolate uses certified vegan, organic maple sugar in all sweetened recipes. The maple bouquet adds a rich complexity to the cacao bean. Also, using maple helps old-growth forests thrive—trees are not cut down to produce it. Maple rates low on the glycemic index with a score of fifty-five, and it contains manganese, zinc, and potassium, as well as antioxidants including antiaging epicatechins and quercetin.

Sacred Chocolate's Longevity Bliss chocolate bar is the only chocolate bar currently formulated to have antiaging, longevity qualities, activated by the unique hops extract xanthohumol it contains. This bar is designed to: help the body build healthy hormones, act as a natural aromatase inhibitor, prevent metabolic syndrome, and improve immunity.

A portion of Sacred Chocolate profits is donated to the Fruit Tree Planting Foundation (ftpf.org).

Now is the best time ever to visit www.SacredChocolate.com.

"Open the Heart... Discover the Magic!"

Hops X Factor: Cell Protector

Hops X Factor is the most promising anti-aging, longevity product I know of. It works by itself and also in conjunction with other longevity compounds such as resveratrol and astragaloside IV (TA 65, Superpill 2) as well as high-dose omega-3 fatty acids. I drink a dropper-full every day and use Hops X Factor topically as well.

—David Wolfe

Hops X Factor contains a natural molecule extracted from hops flowers (Humulus lupulus) called Xanthohumol (Xn). Hops flowers are most well-known for their use as a flavoring agent and natural preservative in beer. The Hops X Factor molecule (Xn) is a flavonoid phenol compound that has been the subject of more than seventy-five research papers due to its role as a cell protector, preventative phytochemical, and as a potentially longevity-enhancing compound.

Research into Hops X Factor was initially inspired by discoveries concerning resveratrol. The active ingredient in Hops X Factor is a prenylated chalcone similar in structure and action to resveratrol.

Worldwide, hundreds of scientific studies focusing on resveratrol and its effects on health have been conducted. Many of these studies have been promising, while some are controversial. Discrepancies in the efficacy of resveratrol may be due to the short window of bio-availability upon ingestion, which is only three hours.

Unlike Resveratrol and other extracts of hops (which are typically not bio-available), Hops X Factor's Xanthohumol has twelve hours to reach the cells once ingested.

Hops X Factor Scientific Properties

The active compound in Hops X Factor is a prenylated chalcone phenol antioxidant called Xanthohumol (Xn), which some scientists and researchers believe is two hundred times more powerful than resveratrol. It has been shown to:

- inhibit NF-k B (nuclear factor kappa beta) activation in cells
- lower isoprostanes in humans by 36 percent within three weeks (measured in urine)
- downregulate aromatase (natural aromatase inhibition)
- inhibit nitric oxide and prostaglandin E2 production
- inhibit phase I cytochrome P450 enzyme, which is involved in the metabolic activation of carcinogens

These properties and dozens more have earned Hops X Factor its title as "cell protector."

Hops X Factor FAQ

Question: Do hops flowers or Hops X Factor products contain phytoestrogens?
Answer: Hops flowers are known to contain some phytoestrogens, however, Hops X Factor contains no phytoestrogens due to the proprietary extraction process it undergoes, which isolates xanthohumol. Xanthohumol is not a phytoestrogen.

Question: Can I take Hops X Factor with other products such as resveratrol or TA65?
Answer: Yes. Hops X Factor is compatible with other anti-aging products.

Question: Does Hops X Factor contain alcohol?

Answer: No. Hops X Factor contains no alcohol or artificial preservatives.

Question: Why should I choose Hops X Factor over other hops extracts?

Answer: Other hops extracts may or may not contain the super-antioxidant xanthohumol. If other products contain xanthohumol, they lack the proprietary, highly bio-available delivery mechanism of the xanthohumol found in Hops X Factor. The delivery mechanism of xanthohumol in Hops X Factor is what makes Hops X Factor unique in the world.

Question: Are there any foods that contain the active ingredient in Hops X Factor?

Answer: Yes. Please try Sacred Chocolate's Longevity Bliss chocolate bar. The Longevity Bliss chocolate bar uses the exact highly bio-available form of xanthohumol found in Hops X Factor.

- Hops X Factor ingredients: hops xanthohumol extract, distilled water, castor oil, and citric acid.
- Hops X Factor bottle size: 50 ml Miron glass bottle
- Dosage: 1 dropper-full per day (each dropper-full contains 5 mg of active ingredient)
- May be mixed with water or other beverages.
- Frequency: Use twenty-five days a month (take a day or two off each week)

At this dosage and frequency rate each bottle of Hops X Factor contains an estimated two-month supply.

Note: This product may also be used topically on aged or damaged skin.

Recommended for those over 18 years of age. Do not use if pregnant. Consult with your physician before using this product if you have a medical condition or are taking medication.

Hops X Factor is a dietary supplement that has been developed as a complete wellness solution that supports multiple biochemical functions within the body and helps maintain its natural balance for a healthier life.

Hops X Factor is available from www.sacredchocolate.com and www.longevitywarehouse.com

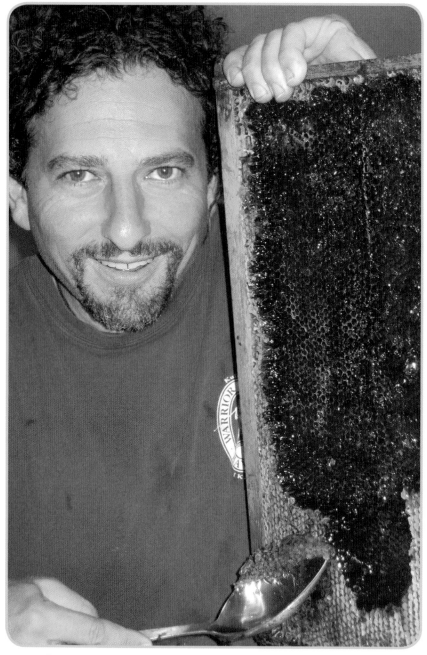

Fresh NoniLand BlackGold Honey

NoniLand Hawaiian Agricultural Research Center and Bee Sanctuary

Our story begins in the midst of an abundant tropical jungle within a paradise setting on the north shore of one of the Hawaiian Islands: this is NoniLand. These trees are some of the happiest, most fruitful trees on the planet. With the tropical sun warmth, and the ocean nearby, the mana is high.

At NoniLand, we are continuously nourishing the trees and garden with rock dust minerals, diluted ocean water, Dead Sea salts, spirulina, Ormus elements, blue volcanic rock silt, compost teas, and love.

You can order NoniLand's certified organic noni powder, noni products, honey, bee products, coconut chips, specialty chocolate superfoods, and other organic superfood items from: www.LongevityWarehouse.com.

The Fruit Tree Planting Foundation

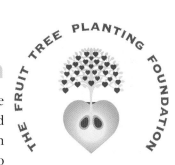

Nothing in the world gives me more satisfaction than planting fruit, nut, and medicinal trees. As I have always chosen to channel my energy and finances into environmentally friendly, sustainable, and healthy directions, I founded the nonprofit Fruit Tree Planting Foundation so that we can all vote with our money for a better, happier, more abundant, forested future on Earth. Please read about our foundation and decide that you want to donate your time, energy and/or finances to this worthy cause.

—DAVID WOLFE

The Fruit Tree Planting Foundation (FTPF) is a unique nonprofit charity dedicated to planting edible, fruitful trees and plants to benefit needy populations and improve the surrounding air, soil, and water. We strategically plant orchards where the harvest will best serve the local community for decades to follow, at places such as Native American reservations, city parks, homeless shelters, drug rehab centers, low-income areas, international hunger relief sites, and animal sanctuaries. FTPF's projects benefit the environment, human health, and animal welfare—all at once!

FTPF's goal is straightforward: to collectively plant eighteen billion fruit, nut, and medicinal trees for a healthy planet (approximately three for every person alive).

Fruit, nut, and medicinal trees heal the environment by cleaning the air, improving soil quality, preventing erosion, creating animal habitats, sustaining valuable water sources, and providing healthy nutrition. We envision a place where one can have a summer picnic under the shade of a fruit, nut, or medicinal tree, breathe the clean air it generates, listen to the songbirds it attracts, and not have to bring anything other than an appetite for the healthy foods growing overhead.

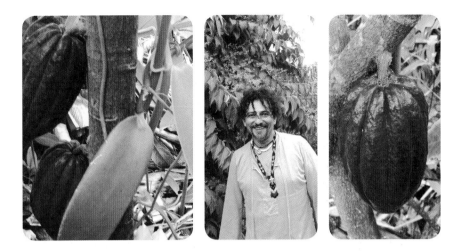

We envision and act to create a world where one can take a walk in the park during a lunch break, pick and eat a variety of delicious fruits, plant the seeds so others can eventually do the same, and provide an alternative to buying environmentally destructive, illness-causing, chemically laden products. FTPF has planted hundreds of thousands of fruit trees all over the world and provided advice and training for others to do the same.

We have launched a series of exciting new programs, and we need your help! Your tax-deductible, charitable investment will help us realize our dream of a sustainable planet for generations to come.

As you find you are interested in donating, please send a check or money order payable to:

- The Fruit Tree Planting Foundation
- P.O. Box 81881
- Pittsburgh, PA 15217

Donations may also be made online at **www.ftpf.org** or by contacting the foundation by phone (831) 621-8096, toll-free (877) 884-7570, fax (831) 621-7978, or email: info@ftpf.org.

We will send a receipt for your tax-deductible donation, but you may also want to make a note of this transaction for tax purposes. Thank you for taking action.

David Wolfe's Peak Performance Archives

www.thebestdayever.com

Warning! The contents of this website may cause you to have The Best Day Ever!

This peak-performance website features a priceless amount of the most valuable information ever assembled in one place on peak performance and longevity, including nutritional seminars, documents, interviews, videos, product reviews, and product discounts for www.LongevityWarehouse.com.

As soon as you join, you'll immediately have access to hundreds of MP3s, videos, PDFs, and much more.

Even more important, inside www.thebestdayever.com is a community of individuals just like you. You can meet hundreds of new friends with the same passions for health, wellness, and success.

You'll learn how to:

- achieve an extraordinary level of energy
- achieve healthy hormone levels
- shed those stubborn, unwanted pounds
- utilize superfoods, superherbs, raw foods, and chocolate
- discover up-to-date information from America's foremost healthy-lifestyle authorities
- leap ahead of the curve in health, longevity, success technology, and peak performance
- radically rejuvenate yourself physically, emotionally, and spiritually
- enjoy every second of life, a second chance at life, and really experience the Best Day Ever
- explode your creativity and imagination
- sleep two to four fewer hours each night, and wake up feeling better than ever
- add years (if not decades) to your life span

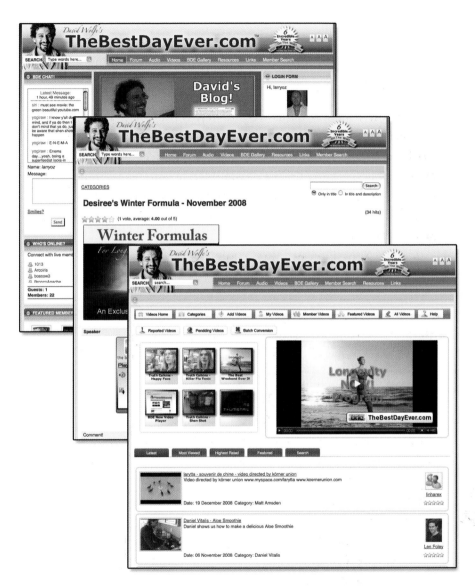

This incredible website gives you complete access to my text, audio, and video library, which contains hundreds of lectures and files on superfoods, superherbs, raw foods, chocolate, health, beauty, minerals, and rejuvenation programs, including information on how to heal some of the most stubborn ailments known to humanity. The website also includes professional nutrition coaching forums where you can get answers to your questions. You will hear live interviews with me on a monthly basis, where I answer your questions and bring you up to date on the latest and greatest news.

Also, if you are interested, you can tap into my monthly blog on the site. I am a strong believer in saturating oneself with positive, empowering information, so www.thebestdayever.com has been designed to bombard you with inspirational text, audio, and video.

All I do, all day, every day, is pursue and live the cutting edge of health, success, beauty, nutrition, longevity science, peak performance, and superfood/superherb diets. This information allows you to create astounding rejuvenation and healing now, without having to make the same mistakes that tens of thousands of others have made.

No more waiting by the mailbox. My website was created to give you immediate access to cutting-edge information that helps you instantly enhance the quality of your life. It is a constantly updated, ever-growing resource for you and your whole family to enjoy. This is the first time in the history of my career as a peak-performance consultant that I've grouped so many compelling, life-changing programs into one jam-packed website. Nothing else like this website is available on the Internet—it is truly a one-of-a-kind phenomenon. If you are inspired to achieve an exceptional state of health, success, beauty, fitness, awareness, joy, sensuality, accomplishment, peak performance, and, most important, fun, then thebestdayever.com is for you!

JOIN TODAY and HAVE THE BEST DAY EVER!

Longevity Products, Superherbs, and Superfoods

Explore your vast library of choices—what's in the cupboard of possibility? Today is the best day ever to experiment with longevity technologies, raw foods, supplements, superfoods, superherbs, and more! The following superfood and superherb products (and other unique products) are organically grown or wildcrafted and available now for your enjoyment at health-food stores and the online shop www.LongevityWarehouse.com.

- ant (Changbai mountain ant)
- ashwagandha
- asparagus root (shatavari)
- astragalus
- baobab
- betaine (TMG)
- cacao beans
- cacao butter
- cacao nibs
- cacao paste
- cacao powder
- camu berry powder
- cashews
- cat's claw
- cayenne
- chaga (unique products including wild Canadian chaga and chaga tinctures)
- chanca piedra
- chia
- chlorella
- chocolate (including Sacred Chocolate™)
- coconut cream (coconut butter)
- coconut oil
- deer/elk antler
- E3 live™ (blue-green algae)
- earthing technology (grounding)
- enzymes
- EstroGuard (indole-3-carbinol/DIM)
- ginseng (world's leading selection of extracts)
- goji berries
- gynostemma (capsules, powders, and tea)
- Hawaiian Superfood Formula (drink mix)
- hemp seeds and their oil
- ho shou wu (fo-ti)

- honey (exclusive, rare NoniLand™ honey)
- Immortal Machine (superfood drink mix)
- Incan berries
- iodine
- kelp (and other seaweeds)
- maca (regular, red, black, etc.)
- mangosteen powder
- moringa
- mucuna
- noni
- marine phytoplankton
- medicinal mushrooms (all types)
- olive oil (ice-pressed)
- pau d'arco
- pine pollen products
- probiotics
- progesterone cream
- reishi (unique products, including wild reishi tincture)
- rhodiola
- schizandra berry
- shilajit
- spirulina
- tulsi
- vanilla

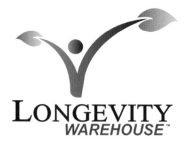

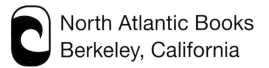 North Atlantic Books
Berkeley, California

Personal, spiritual, and planetary transformation

North Atlantic Books, a nonprofit publisher established in 1974, is dedicated to fostering community, education, and constructive dialogue. NABCommunities.com is a meeting place for an ever-growing membership of readers and authors to engage in the discussion of books and topics from North Atlantic's core publishing categories.

NAB Communities offer interactive social networks in these genres:

NOURISH: Raw Foods, Healthy Eating and Nutrition, All-Natural Recipes

WELLNESS: Holistic Health, Bodywork, Healing Therapies

WISDOM: New Consciousness, Spirituality, Self-Improvement

CULTURE: Literary Arts, Social Sciences, Lifestyle

BLUE SNAKE: Martial Arts History, Fighting Philosophy, Technique

Your free membership gives you access to:

Advance notice about new titles and exclusive giveaways

Podcasts, webinars, and events

Discussion forums

Polls, quizzes, and more!

Go to www.NABCommunities.com and join today.